Collana scientifica

Fondazione Carlo Erba

STANDARDIZATION IN HEMATOLOGY

Editors: G. Astaldi
C. Sirtori
G. Vanzetti

Franco Angeli Editore

Prima edizione: 1970

Contents

6

8

Part I

Proceedings of the Open Session of Hemoglobinometry Expert Panel of ICSH (New York, September 3, 1968). Moderator: R.J. Eilers

Proceedings of the Symposium of the International Committee for Standardization in Hematology (New York, September 2, 1968). Moderator: G. Brecher

Reports of Proceedings of the 7th Board Meeting and 5th General Assembly of ICSH (New York, September 4, 1968)

Editors:

G. Astaldi, Editor in Chief
W. Crosby, President of ICSH
J. Spaander, President Elect of ICSH
K. G. von Boroviczény
J. Coster
R. J. Eilers　　　　　　　　Members of the ICSH Secretariat
G. Izak
S. M. Lewis

Open Session of Hemoglobinometry Expert Panel of ICSH
Moderator: R. J. Eilers

1. *Criteria for the International Cyanmethemoglobin Reference Solution - Challenges to and Verification of*

1.1. *Spectral Characteristics of the International Haemiglobincyanide Reference Solution*
W.G. Zijlstra, O.W. van Assendelft and E.J. van Kampen
Groningen, the Netherlands

The international haemiglobincyanide reference solution is prepared on behalf of ICSH by the Dutch Institute of Public Health (R.I.V., Utrecht, the Netherlands), using the following procedure [1, 4]. Fresh donor blood is collected in 1/5 the volume of 3.2% sodium citrate, centrifuged and the plasma removed. The cells are washed twice with 0.9% NaCl and twice with 1.2% NaCl solution. To the cells is added an equal volume of twice distilled water and 0.4 volume of highly purified toluene. The mixture is thoroughly stirred and stored at 4°C for 12 h. After centrifugation the mixture displays three clearly distinct layers. The upper layer consists of toluene, the middle one is a turbid suspension of erythrocyte stromata and the third a clear haemoglobin solution. The first two layers are removed and the remaining haemoglobin solution filtered through ash-free filter paper. Drabkin's reagent is then added to obtain a HiCN solution of about 60 mg/100 ml. This solution is sterilized by means of Seitz filtration and transferred to 10 ml brown borosilicate glass ampoules.

The absorption spectrum of this HiCN solution is shown in Fig. 1. The $\lambda \varepsilon$ curve is based on data obtained with three different spectrophotometers of which wavelength and optical density scales had been checked using mercury emission lines and a NBS carbon yellow filter respectively. Optical density values have been converted into quarter-millimolar extinction coefficients (i.e. conversion of D-scale into ε-scale) on the basis of $\varepsilon_{HiCN}^{540} = 10.99$ [5].

Although a carefully measured $\lambda \varepsilon$ curve over the 1000-480 nm range

14

Figure 1

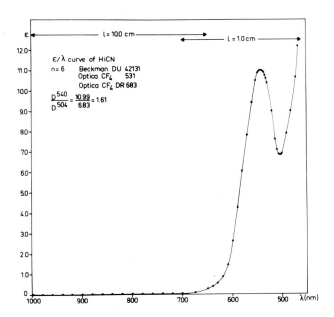

is the best criterion to judge a HiCN solution, reliable characterization of the absorption spectrum by means of but a few measurements is desirable for checking the international reference solution as well as secondary HiCN standard solutions. Inspection of the absorption spectrum immediately suggests the ratio $\varepsilon^{540}/\varepsilon^{504} = D^{540}/D^{504}$ as a quantity of sufficient significance. Its theoretical value is $10.99/6.83 = 1.61$. In the Recommendations put forward by ICSH, it is stated that D^{540}/D^{504} should lie between 1.63 and 1.59 [2]. As HiCN solutions follow Lambert-Beer's law at $\lambda = 540$ nm as well as at $\lambda = 504$ nm, the ratio D^{540}/D^{504} may be expected to be independent of concentration. That this actually is the case is shown in Fig. 2. The slightly too low value at $c_{Hb} = 4.6$ mg/100 ml may be dismissed on the ground of the rapidly decreasing accuracy of optical density measurements when D falls below 0.050 [3].

Turbidity tends to decrease the D^{540}/D^{504} ratio, increasingly so when the HiCN concentration is lowered. Thus when a slightly turbid HiCN solution, which at $c = 60$ mg/100 ml may still have a D^{540}/D^{504} ratio within the tolerated range, is diluted, a decrease of the ratio is observed. Even though the ratio D^{540}/D^{504} is to a certain extent an indicator of

Figure 2

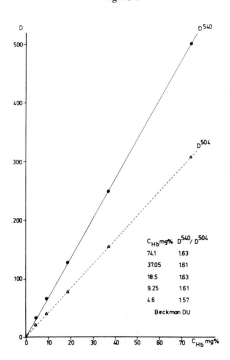

$C_{Hb}mg\%$	D^{540}/D^{504}
74.1	1.63
37.05	1.61
18.5	1.63
9.25	1.61
4.6	1.57

Beckman DU

turbidity, it was felt necessary to have a more specific measure for the presence of light scattering particles in the HiCN solution.

Quantitative turbidimetry being difficult and expensive, measuring the optical density at a wavelength of zero absorption appeared the most suitable approach to the problem. As shown in Fig. 1, optical density is zero when $\lambda > 710$ nm. Dark red light is not particularly suitable for measuring turbidity, because light scattering decreases with increasing wavelength. Moreover, measuring very low optical density values is inaccurate. Nevertheless, the measurement of D^{750}, especially when performed in a cuvette providing a 10 cm lightpath, proved to be of value as a turbidity check. This has been demonstrated by measuring D^{750} of a HiCN solution made by diluting whole blood with Drabkin's reagent, before and after filtration through millipore filters of various pore size and before and after centrifugation. Of these solutions the ratio D^{540}/D^{504} has also been measured. The results are shown in Table 1. The recommendation by ICSH that the optical density of the international reference solution in the near infrared region should be < 0.002 per cm pathlength thus may be considered appropriate. The exact wording of the recommendation, however, should be changed to: « Measurement in near infrared (1000 > λ > 710 nm) to check turbidity, e.g. at $\lambda = 750$ nm ».

Table 1 – D^{750} and D^{540}/D^{504} values of 2 blood samples diluted 200 fold with Drabkin's solution before and after filtering through millipore filters or centrifuging for 15 min. Beckman DU spectrophotometer, layer thickness 1.000 cm for D^{540} and D^{504} measurement, 2.0 cm for D^{750} measurement. Martin Christ UJ15 centrifuge, 15000 rpm.

	sample 1		sample 2	
Filter	D^{750}	D^{540}/D^{504}	D^{750}	D^{540}/D^{504}
none	0.010	1.54	0.0095	1.54
pore size 3.0 μ	0.0035	1.59	0.0025	1.59
pore size 0.8 μ	0.002	1.60	0.0015	1.60
pore size 0.45 μ	0.0005	1.61	0.0005	1.61
centrifuged	0.002	1.60	0.001	1.60

Table 2 – Mean $D^{750}/D^{540}/D^{504}$ values of International HiCN Reference Solutions, as measured by different laboratories.

solution		n	D^{750}	s	D^{540}/D^{504}	s
40400	(April 1964 – Jan. 1967)	20	0.001	0.001	1.61	0.009
60400	(April 1966 – Jan. 1968)	38	0.001	0.0008	1.61	0.006
70400	(April 1967 –	28	0.0005	0.0006	1.61	0.008
80400	(April 1968 –	6	0.000	–	1.61	0.004

n = number of results, each result being based on at least one operator measuring at least 3 ampoules on at least one spectrophotometer

$$s = \sqrt{\frac{\Sigma (x - \bar{x})^2}{n - 1}}$$

Table 2 shows the results of measuring D^{750} and the ratio D^{540}/D^{504} by the ICSH nominated laboratories for international HiCN reference solution 40400, 60400, 70400 and 80400. These data are in close agreement with the theoretical values (Fig. 1) and well within the limits put forward by ICSH [2].

References

[1] Holtz, A.H., « Some Experience with a Cyanhaemiglobin Solution », *Bibl. Haemat.,* *21,* 75, 1965

[2] International Committee for Standardization in Haematology, « Recommendations for Haemoglobinometry in Human Blood », *Brit J. Haemat., 13* (Suppl.), 71, 1967

[3] Van Kampen, E.J., Zijlstra, W.G., Van Assendelft, O.W. and Reinkingh, W.A., « Determination of Hemoglobin and its Derivatives », *Advanc. clin. Chem., 8,* 141, 1965

[4] Zijlstra, W.G. and Van Kampen, E.J., « Standardization of Hemoglobinometry. III. Preparation and Use of a Stable Hemiglobincyanide Standard », *Clin. chim. Acta, 7.* 96, 1962

[5] Zijlstra, W.G., Van Kampen, E.J. and Van Assendelft, O.W., *Standardization of Haemoglobinometry: Establishing the Reference Point,* Symposium on the Haematology of Normal Man. Haemoglobin concentration, XII Congress of the International Society of Haematology, New York City 1968

1.2. *Challenge to the Criteria*

John J. Moran, President, Hycel, Inc., USA

In the definition of a cyanmethemoglobin standard we must be concerned with the nature of the standard and with its measurement.

Many unanswered questions still remain with respect to the nature of cyanmethemoglobin. Among these are the differences in stability in cyanmethemoglobin solutions prepared from crystallized hemoglobin and fresh erythrocytes. Similarly, small but persistent spectral differences are encountered in cyanmethemoglobin solutions prepared from sickle cell patients. Additionally, the long range effects of various solubilizers or detergents require further study . However, the major factors of the cyanmethemoglobin complex are sufficiently well established that my challenge is not addressed to them.

It can be assumed that everyone present strongly endorses the use of the cyanmethemoglobin method for hemoglobinometry. The challenge in point, then, concerns itself with the feasibility of the techniques of measurement.

The content definition for the ICSH standard is given by the formula,

$$c = \frac{A \times 64{,}500}{44.0 \times d \times 10} = 146.5 \; A \qquad [1]$$

The formula and its derivation are well known to the participants in this meeting. c refers to the concentration in mg/100 ml, d refers to the thickness of the sample in cm, and A is the measured absorbance

18

at 540 nm. Any fluctuation in A or d will proportionately change the value of c. The ICSH proposal under *Evaluation and Control* permits d to be 1.000 cm ± 0.5 %. This automatically introduces a possible variation of ± 0.5 % in c. In then follows that allowable cuvette differences alone could result in two laboratories differing by as much as 1 % in determining the content of a cyanmethemoglobin standard for evaluation or control.

However, as serious as are the differences occasioned through varying cuvettes, more serious differences arise from the measurement of absorbance. These errors come from instrumental fluctuation, from human differences in technique and from the spectral characteristics of cyanmethemoglobin itself. Evidently, the cumulative erratic nature of these errors has already been encountered in the preparation and evaluation of the ICSH standard since the criteria state, « ... erratic results are discarded in accordance with current statistical practice ».

I must definitely challenge this statement. Acceptable statistical practice most assuredly does not permit discarding erratic results if the purpose of the statistical evaluation is to establish correlation between different sets of data. If this is not the case, then the entire program is subject to human judgment and bias, which is inadmissable in any scientific program of standardization.

I believe it is the practice, in some laboratories, of discarding supposed erratic data rather than recording all data that has resulted in certain technical parameters not within the experience of our laboratories. For example, on the ICSH standard 60400, A at 540 nm on a Beckman DU varied from .385 to .391 for the Cleveland laboratory and from .385 to .390 for the Freiburg laboratory. The Utrecht laboratory reported absolutely no deviation from .385, despite the fact the Utrecht measurements were made by two different operators. Our experience is in line with that of the Cleveland and Freiburg laboratories. We are unable to make any series of absorbance measurements without some fluctation.

I am indebted to Dr. Klein-Wisenberg [2] for pointing out that common experience of a relatively broad uncertainty factor in measuring absorbance was supported by the careful work of W.O. Coaster [3]. Dr. Coaster settled upon a figure of ± 2 % encompassing the average uncertainty factor of the Beckman DU. Since his work appeared in 1951, undoubted improvements in instrumentation have probably reduced the uncertainty factor to the order of ± 1.5 %.

The uncertainty factor certainly must be taken in consideration with respect to measurements of a single instrument, and in correlating results between two instruments. On a single instrument absorbance data held within ± 1.5% of a mean figure at 540 nm and 504 nm may be assumed to be reproducible. In establishing any ratios between A at 540 nm and 504 nm, the ± 1.5% uncertainty factor for each parameter must, through simple mathematics, become an uncertainty factor of ± 3.0%.

With respect to the intrinsic value of the ratio of A at 540 nm and 504 nm, serious reservations exist in my mind.

The value of the ratio in our laboratories fluctuates according to the mode of preparing the standard. Eliminating toluene washing of the erythrocytes results in a lowering of the ratio. The addition of non-ionic detergents to the standard results in an increase in the ratio. The ratio is depressed in a higher concentration of cyanmethemoglobin. Although I do not believe the absolute value of the ratio has been fully explored, I agree that changes in an observed initial value indicate changes in the standard. The ratio may thus be important in evaluation and control work, particularly with determining the stability of the standard. However much more work is required to establish the permissible range of the ratio. Certainly, based upon present work, the variation should be at least ± 3% of the most common ratio, 1.60, i.e., 1.55 to 1.65.

It is interesting to note that ICSH standard 60400 exhibited ratios from 1.58 to 1.63 in the reference laboratories. If this much variation is obtained upon a single ICSH standard, is it not reasonable to expect greater variation in different batches of standards, prepared in differing fashions and by different laboratories or manufacturers?

I seriously question the value of measurements at 750 nm. With a red tube, the absorbance of the reagent is less than that of distilled water and measurements must be made against reagent. Thus any turbidity in the reagent is automatically compensated. Changing from a blue tube to a red tube introduces needless source of error and variation. Certainly, changing cuvettes or otherwise introducing other changes into the measuring system should be avoided if at all possible. There is no proof that any absorbance value at 750 nm, whether employing a blue tube or a red tube, is solely a measurement of turbidity. This is an assumption not yet borne out by laboratory proof.

Dr. Matsubara and Dr. Shibata [4] have recently concluded an evaluation of the ICSH standard 70400. Their turbidity measurements at 750 nm, employing a red tube, definitely indicate the absorbance value to be a function of hemoglobin concentration.

Without introducing any changes in the measurement system, except for wavelength setting, the A at 685 nm may be employed as a check upon less than visual turbidity. Absorbance at this wavelength is still a factor of cyanmethemoglobin concentration, being approximately equivalent to 3% of the absorbance at 540 nm. Turbidity sufficient to affect the 540 nm or 504 nm values would have a greatly enhanced effect at 685 nm since the turbidity value is an absolute. Our experience indicates that 685 nm values fluctuate between 2.5% to 3.5% of the 540 nm value.

In summation, I challenge the required reproducibility and correlation factors as being outside the realm of our experience. My challenge is supported by a critical evaluation of the factors which indicates the technical parameters. I am certain all of us are most desirous that these parameters be within the realm of sound laboratory practice.

References

[1] Standardization Committee, ICSH, August, 1966
[2] Communication to Dr. A.H. Holtz, June 3, 1966
[3] W.O. Coaster, *Anal. Chem.*, 23, 1229, 1951
[4] Matsubara T. and Shibata S., unpublished paper on evaluation of ICSH standard

1.3. *The How? Why? The Intercalibration of Spectrophotometers*

Charles E. Willis, Assistant Director, Standards Laboratory, College of American Pathologists, USA

The standardization of spectral performance involves measurement of a multitude of parameters. In practical laboratory everyday usage it becomes a tremendous task to daily check each factor such as stray light, spectral band width, effective sample path length due to beam convergence or divergence. These and many other factors lead to photometric error. Furthermore, if we did check each parameter, we would have no assurance that two spectrophotometers from the same manufacturing source would give the same absorbance value for a non-variable standard glass.

Herein lies our dilemma. How can absorbance values obtained from one laboratory be related to values obtained in another laboratory even when similar instruments are employed in this measurement? It is impossible to build two instruments exactly alike. Hence, it will be impossible to have values exactly alike. Furthermore, human factors in setting the wavelength scale, slit width, and voltage fluctuations all add to our dilemma. We must then accept a reasonable probable error between laboratories.

How can we best calibrate our instruments within our own laboratory on a day to day basis and further, how to calibrate instruments on an interlaboratory basis? Photometric standards have been evaluated by various groups of spectroscopists. In 1934, Gibson [1] and later, Vandenbelt [2] and Haupt [3] at NBS, investigated chromate solutions. Glass filters were investigated by Keegan and Schleter [4] at NBS, and Slavin [5] and ASTM committee A-13 [6].

It has now become obvious that a completely reproducible standard glass or solution does not exist. However, even if it did exist, the final absorbance values would exceed the accuracy or precision of the instrument as stated by the manufacturer. In the conclusion of the paper by Keegan and Schleter [4] it states that three of the reference standards of spectral transmittance (selenium red, carbon yellow, copper green) are subject to slight impermanence. It is suggested that exposure to high energy particles, ultraviolet radiation, temperature variations, and chemical fumes cause these phenomena. The date for following this variation goes back to 1946 for the carbon yellow, the copper green and the cobalt blue.

We (the CAP) as physicians are not spectroscopists; however, our daily life in the chemistry laboratory depends upon this instrument as does the chemical quantitation of the values we send out to the practicing physician. With this obvious deficiency in our knowledge, we consulted the National Bureau of Standards for their expert opinion. They have recommended for our consideration the use of a glass photometric standard. This could be the Chance or carbon yellow filter with which they have had considerable experience over the last 22 years. This glass is to be used *only* as an absorbance (or transmittance) check of the photometric scale of the Beckman DU and similar spectrophotometers. The wave length scale *must* be checked *prior* to making the absorbance reading for obvious reasons. This can be performed in a few minutes using the mercury arc quartz lamp. There is a single peak at 546.07 nm and a doublet in the ultra violet at 253.48 nm. These emissions are quite intense and small slit openings can be used. Emission sources such as the mercury quartz, helium, neon, aluminum spark, hydrogen arc, sodium arc, or cesium arc can be used depending upon the desired range to be calibrated. In the Standards Laboratory we use the mercury arc because of its peak at 546 nm is close to the 540 nm hemoglobin standard peak. These emission sources can be used for both recording and non-recording instruments. The use of the Holmium oxide glass is for gross checks on wavelength in recording instruments only and is not considered to be as accurate as the narrow emission lines of mercury. The calibration of wavelength is performed according to the recommendations of the NBS [7]. Following wavelength calibration, the photometric absorbance is checked with a clean carbon yellow glass fitted in an aluminum holder. The variation with temperature is negligible however thermospacers at 25 °C are used. This is recorded daily. One must realize that at 540 nm one is reading on the slope of the carbon yellow glass. This may lead to wider variations than the Chance ON-10 glass which has a broad peak at this wavelength. The day-to-day variations in reading both of these glasses has been reported by Copeland [8], and they report a seven year experience with these standard glasses.

Obviously, a neutral glass which had a constant absorbance value over the desired wavelength range would be less subject to wavelength changes and hence could reflect photometric errors more precisely. However, no such filters are presently available. Until such a set of glasses becomes available, it is our recommendation, backed by the NBS, that the carbon yellow or Chance glass be used for calibration of the photometric scale for both recording and non-recording spectrophotometers.

Other glasses could undoubtedly be used; however, because of the experience of NBS over a two decade period and the relative stability and availability of this glass, we have felt that this conservative approach to a difficult and controversial subject is the best available route to take at the present time.

We have recently taken our standard filters, the carbon yellow, Chance ON-10, and Holmium oxide, back to the NBS for a complete recalibration on their Cary 14. It has been gratifying to note the close correlation of these glasses on their instrument and our Cary 14. We are attempting to keep our spectrophotometer as close as possible to their instrument. These transmittance values are run in triplicate and averaged in their computer and kept on file in the CAP laboratory.

We have been sending an NBS calibrated glass to anyone interested in checking his photometric scale, but as stated previously, he must have accurately calibrated his wavelength scale prior to running the photometric scale. These curves from our Cary 14 will shortly be made available to manufacturers and any interested laboratory at no cost and will cover the visible range from 400-700 mu. It will include the carbon yellow, Chance ON-10 and Holmium oxide glasses.

23

We are hoping that this will provide a method for interlaboratory calibration and an attempt to have these instruments as close to the NBS instrument as possible. Any suggestions as to how this inter laboratory monitoring can be expedited will certainly be appreciated.

References

[1] Gibson, K. S., Walker, G. K., and Brown, M. E., « Filters for Testing the Reliability of Spectrophotometers », *J. Opt. Soc. Am.*, 24, 58, 1934
[2] Vandenbelt, J. M., *J. Opt. Soc. Am.*. 50, 24-27, 1, 1960
[3] Haupt, G. W., *J. Res. Nat. Bur. Stand.*, 48, 414, 1952 & *J. Opt. Soc. Am.*, 42, 441, 1952
[4] Keegan, H. J., Schleter, J. C., Belknap, M. A., *J. Res. Nat. Bur. Stand.*, 67 A, 577-584, 6, 1963
[5] Slavin, W., *J. Opt. Soc. Am.*, 52, 1399-1401, 12, 1962.
[6] ASTM Committee E-13, *Proposed Methods for Evaluation of Spectrophotometers*, ASTM, 1916 Race Street, Phila. Pa., 1958
[7] U. S. Dept. of Commerce, Nat. Bur. Stand., Washington, D.C., Jan. 1955 (reissued 1967), Letter LC-1017, « Standards for checking the calibration of Spectrophotometers (200-1000 nm) »
[8] Copeland, B. E., King, J. W., and Willis, C. E., *Am. J. Clin. Path.*, 49, 459-466, 4, 1967

1.4. The Measurement of International Haemiglobincyanide Reference Solutions by Various Operators Using Various Spectrophotometers

E.J. van Kampen, O.W. van Assendelft and W.G. Zijlstra, Groningen, the Netherlands

Although rather extensive experience has been acquired in the measurement of international haemiglobincyanide (HiCN) reference solutions [2, 3], it was thought interesting to look into the measurement results of one operator using a variety of different spectrophotometers and of a large number of operators using one and the same instrument. These data could be useful to judge the significance of differences in measurement results obtained in different laboratories for the international reference solution, as well as for secondary standard solutions.

In all measurements the spectrophotometric procedure adhered to by the ICSH nominated control laboratories, was followed. This procedure is as follows. After adjusting zero and sensitivity controls, the instrument is balanced with the sample in the lightpath. The sensitivity and zero are then checked and only if no shift has occurred the absorption scale is read. If a shift has occurred, the entire procedure is repeated.

Table 1 – D^{540} measurement of International HiCN Reference Solution 70400. Beckman DU spectrophotometer. 14 Operators, slit width and wavelength setting fixed.

operator	D^{540}		
1	0.404	0.404	0.404
2	0.402	0.401	0.401
3	0.402	0.402	0.402
4	0.400	0.400	0.402
5	0.402	0.403	0.402
6	0.402	0.402	0.403
7	0.404	0.404	0.403
8	0.403	0.402	0.402
9	0.401	0.401	0.401
10	0.402	0.401^5	0.401^5
11	0.404	0.404	0.404
12	0.403	0.403	0.403^5
13	0.403	0.403	0.402
14	0.402	0.404	0.404

Table 2 – D^{540} and D^{504} measurements of International HiCN Reference Solution 60400. Beckman DU spectrophotometer. 20 Operators, slit width fixed.

operator	D^{540}	D^{504}	D^{540}/D^{504}
1	0.385	0.240	1.60
2	0.385	0.240	1.60
3	0.385	0.240	1.60
4	0.385	0.240	1.60
5	0.385	0.240	1.60
6	0.384	0.239	1.61
7	0.385	0.240	1.60
8	0.385	0.239	1.61
9	0.385	0.239	1.61
10	0.385	0.240	1.60
11	0.384	0.239	1.61
12	0.385	0.240	1.60
13	0.385	0.239	1.61
14	0.384	0.239	1.61
15	0.386	0.241	1.60
16	0.384	0.239	1.61
17	0.385	0.240	1.60
18	0.385	0.239	1.61
19	0.385	0.240	1.60
20	0.384	0.240	1.60

Table 3 – D^{540} and D^{504} measurements of International HiCN Reference Solution 70400. Beckman DU spectrophometer. 21 Operators, slit width fixed.

operator	D^{540}	D^{504}	D^{540}/D^{504}
1	0.404	0.251	1.61
2	0.404	0.251	1.61
3	0.404	0.252	1.60
4	0.404	0.252	1.60
5	0.404	0.253	1.60
6	0.405	0.252	1.61
7	0.404	0.252	1.60
8	0.402	0.250	1.61
9	0.405	0.252	1.61
10	0.402	0.250	1.61
11	0.404	0.250	1.62
12	0.405	0.252	1.61
13	0.404	0.251	1.61
14	0.403	0.251	1.61
15	0.402	0.250	1.61
16	0.404	0.252	1.60
17	0.404	0.252	1.60
18	0.402	0.251	1.60
19	0.404	0.251	1.61
20	0.402	0.251	1.60
21	0.402	0.251	1.60

Table 4 – Mean D^{540} and D^{504} measurement of International HiCN Reference Solutions. Beckman DU spectrophotometer, slit width fixed. Different operators.

HiCN solution	n	D^{540}	s	$s/\sqrt{n}$	D^{504}	s	$s/\sqrt{n}$	D^{540}/D^{504}	s	$s/\sqrt{n}$
60400	20	0.385	0.0005	0.0001	0.240	0.0006	0.0001	1.60	0.006	0.001
70400	21	0.4035	0.001	0.0003	0.251	0.0008	0.0002	1.61	0.007	0.002

$$s = \sqrt{\frac{\Sigma(x-\bar{x})^2}{n-1}}$$

Table 1 shows the results of the first measurement series, using the international HiCN reference solution 70400 and a Beckman DU spectrophotometer, wavelength fixed at 540 nm, slit width 0.02 mm. 14 Different operators took 3 consecutive readings each. The highest and lowest value found differ only 0.004.

In the next two measurement series, using a second Beckman DU spectrophotometer, the optical density at both $\lambda = 540$ and $\lambda = 504$ nm was read (Tables 2 and 3, solutions 60400 and 70400). Each operator thus also performed the wavelength setting. The results, including the mean value and scatter of D^{540}/D^{504}, have been summarized in Table 4. It is clear from these 3 measurement series that any laboratory technician, properly using a good instrument, can obtain quite accurate results.

Finally, one operator measured D^{540} and D^{504} of solution 70400 on 12 different spectrophotometers, of which three were of the recording type (Table 5, instruments 1, 2 and 3). To insure measuring on a

Table 5 D^{540} and D^{504} measurements of International HiCN Reference Solution 70400. One operator, different spectrophotometers.

spectrophotometer	D^{540}	D^{504}	D^{540}/D^{504}
1. Cary 15 nr. 225	0.405	0.251	1.61
2. Cary 14	0.405	0.250	1.62
3. Optica Cl 4 DR nr. 683	0.404	0.251	1.61
4. Beckman DU nr. 42151	0.402	0.248	1.62
5. Beckman DU nr. 42183	0.403	0.248	1.63
6. Beckman DU nr. 20694	0.403	0.250	1.61
7. Unicam SP600	0.403	0.249	1.62
8. Optica Cl 4 nr. 531	0.403	0.249	1.62
9. Zeiss PMQ II nr. 29010	0.402	0.248	1.62
10. Zeiss PMQ II nr. 48449	0.402	0.248	1.62
11. Zeiss PMQ II nr. 18169	0.402	0.248	1.62
12. Zeiss PMQ II nr. 29380	0.400	0.249	1.61

reliable instrument in good condition, both the wavelength and the optical density scale should have been calibrated first, using mercury emission lines and a reference filter, e.g. NBS carbon yellow [1], respectively. However, since this proved to be too laborious, only a carbon yellow filter, the λ D curve of which is shown in Fig. 1, certified by the National Bureau of Standards, was used to check the optical density reading at $\lambda = 540$ nm. Spectrophotometers giving D^{540} values

Figure 1

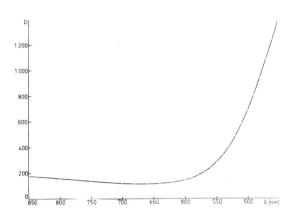

within 0.005 of the certified value were accepted for use, as it was thought improbable that in such cases a possible wavelength error would be compensated for by a coincidental optical density error. The results obtained on the 12 instruments used (Table V) show good agreement.

It may be concluded from the results presented, that accurate values as regards the measurement of HiCN reference solutions, can be obtained by any laboratory technician when reliable spectrophotometers, regularly calibrated as to wavelength and optical density, are used. Quality control of HiCN reference solutions on the basis of spectro-photometric measurements thus is justified and claims that wide scatter of spectrophotometric measurement results may discredit a good HiCN reference solution must be rejected.

References

[1] Copeland, B.E., King, J. and Willis, C., « The National Bureau of Standards' Carbon Yellow Filter as a Monitor for Spectrophotometric Performance », *Amer. J. clin. Path.*, *49*, 459, 1968

[2] Van Assendelft, O.W., Holtz, A.H., Van Kampen, E.J. and Zijlstra, W.G., « Control Data of International Haemiglobincyanide Reference Solutions », *Clin. chim. Acta, 18,* 78, 1967

[3] Zijlstra, W.G., Van Assendelft, O.W. and Van Kampen, E.J., *Spectral Characteristics of the International Haemiglobincyanide Reference Solution*, Proceedings Open Session of the ICSH Expert Panel on Haemoglobinometry, New York City, 1968

28

1.5. *Nomographic and Numeric Corrections for Background Absorption of Turbid Haemiglobincyanide Solutions*

A. von Klein-Wisenberg, Medizinische Universitaetsklinik Freiburg im Breisgau, Germany

Determination of haemoglobin is done through spectrophotometric measurement after conversion of all haemoglobin derivatives into haemoglobincyanide. This is the standard procedure as adopted by the International Committee for Standardization in Haematology (ICSH). Agreement has been achieved in defining the absorptivity

at 540 nm (peak absorbance in the visible spectrum)	to be	11,0	per milliatom of iron in haemiglobincyanide
at 504 nm (minimum in absorption spectrum in the visible)	to be	6,9	»
at 750 nm	to be less than	0,05	»

[1]

The characteristic absorption spectrum of pure HiCN solutions as resulting from a multitude of measurements in the visible and near infrared (NIR) region with an uncertainty of less than ± 2 % in absorbance is illustrated in fig. 1.

Storage capability of solutions more concentrated than approximately 70 mg HiCN/100 ml is still a point in discussion, although it would be highly desirable — after the introduction of auto-analysers in clinical laboratories — to have available a haemoglobin quality control standard of about the concentration of blood. However, shelf-life of such preparation, even when stored cool, is still unsatisfactory and a tendency towards increasing apparent haemiglobin concentration could be observed in the author's laboratory. Simultaneous with this apparent increase in absorbance in the visible an increase of NIR absorption took place. So this apparent increase in concentration resulted from increasing background. In absence of other coloured matter and excluding the possibility of its formation by a slight decomposition it is justified as well as customary to attribute NIR background absorption to turbidity. This absorbance will show a dependence inverse to some power of the wave-length. Assuming the particle diameter causing the light scattering to be small in comparison with the incident wavelength ($< \lambda/20$, Rayleigh scattering [2]) absorbance increases inverse to the fourth power

29

Figure 1

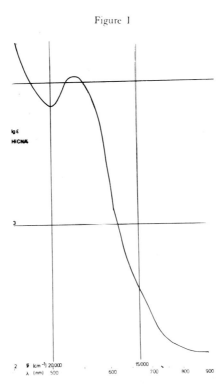

lg E
HiCN

3

2   ν̃ (cm⁻¹) 20000   15000
     λ (nm) 500   600   700   800   900

of the wavelength. In ultramicrospectrophotometry of cells use has
been made of corrections after Rayleigh [3]. With particle diameter
approaching the magnitude of the wavelength ($> \lambda/15$, Mie scattering [4]) the mathematical expression is more complicated [5].

The absorbance increases inverse with the wavelength to a power
less than four which can be evaluated empirically [6 a-d].

In clinical chemistry this correction has found application in elimination of plasma turbidity effect in Evans blue plasma volume determination through measurement at different wavelengths [7].

The change of absorption spectrum of a pure HiCN solution assumed to contain 58,6 mg HiCN/100 ml with A_{750} amounting to 10 %
of A_{540} and exponents rising from 0 (constant background absorption)
to 4 (Rayleigh scattering) is schematically illustrated in fig. 2. Attributing
the NIR background absorbance of turbid although otherwise unchanged HiCN solutions solely to turbidity, and expressing c, the concentration of HiCN in mg/100 ml for ease of subsequent calculations, the
apparent absorbance per cm cell path length of turbid HiCN solutions

are:

$$A_{750} < 0,034 \cdot 10^{-3}\,c + A_\infty\,750^{-p} \qquad (I)$$
$$A_{540} = 6,826 \cdot 10^{-3}\,c + A_\infty\,540^{-p} \qquad (II)$$
$$A_{504} = 4,266 \cdot 10^{-3}\,c + A_\infty\,504^{-p} \qquad (II)$$

which practically reduces to

$$A_\infty \backsim A_{750} \cdot 750^{p} \qquad (I\,a)$$
$$A_{540} = 6,826 \cdot 10^{-3}\,c + A_{750}\,(750/540)^{p} \qquad (II\,a)$$
$$A_{504} = 4,266 \cdot 10^{-3}\,c + A_{750}\,(750/504)^{p} \qquad (III\,a)$$

By elimination of c from equations (II a) and (III a) we obtain

$$A_{540} = 1,60\,A_{504} - A_{750}\,(1,60 \cdot 1,4881^{p} - 1,3889^{p}) \qquad (IV)$$

Figure 2

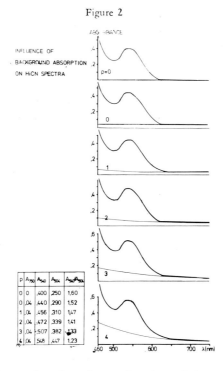

INFLUENCE OF BACKGROUND ABSORPTION ON HiCN SPECTRA

p	A_{750}	A_{540}	A_{504}	A_{540}/A_{504}
0	0	,400	,250	1,60
0	,04	,440	,290	1,52
1	,04	,456	,310	1,47
2	,04	,472	,339	1,41
3	,04	,507	,382	1,33
4	,04	548	,447	1,23

Hence, 1,60 A_{504} — A_{540} is a linear function of A_{750} with the slope depending on p. This deduction is confirmed by observation: fig. 3 is showing for Hb and HiCN preparations of different origin and several concentrations:

— overall regression line is 1,6 A_{504} — A_{540} = 3,12 A_{750} + 0,0045 with a coefficient of correlation r = 0,7 and a slope corresponding to

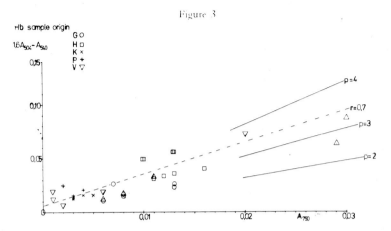

Figure 3

$3 < p < 4$. The intersection with the ordinate is not significantly different from 0.

— For any single connecting line of an observed point with the origin a slope corresponding to $p = 4$ is never significantly exceeded.
— Experimental points of series of samples of equal origin are co-linear with the same slope.

Therefore, the initial assumptions are justified and the problem of getting the real HiCN concentration in turbid solutions from data A_{504}, A_{540}, and A_{750} is reduced to the elimination of p from equations (II a) and (IV). This is not possible by straightforward operation; however, both equation (II a) and (IV) can be shaped into a nomograph, using the simple geometric relations illustrated in fig. 4. The parameter p obtained from a nomograph according to key equation (IV) is used to link by pivotal lines a compound nomograph according to key equa-

Figure 4

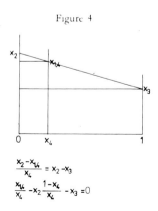

$$\frac{x_2 - x_4}{x_4} = x_2 - x_3$$

$$\frac{x_4}{x_4} - x_2 \frac{1 - x_4}{x_4} - x_3 = 0$$

tion (II a) to the former, the sought-for concentration can be read from. Fig. 5 shows the nomograph constructed on the outlined principles. For details of application of this nomograph the reader is referred to the legend, for those on construction of nomographs to the appropriate chapters in textbooks on practical mathematics [8, 9].

Figure 5

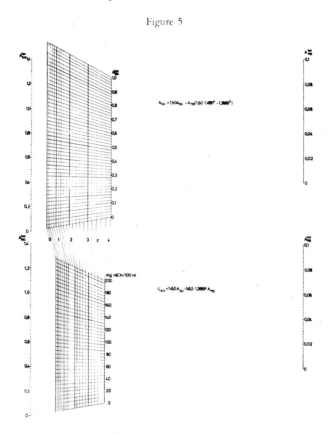

For numeric correction of background absorbance three procedures are proposed: the first being an iterative procedure useful for eventual computer operation; the second is an approximation with one correction term in exponential form, adequate for slide rule operation; the third is a different approximation having only linear terms.

Procedure 1 eliminates p from equation (II a) and (III a) by rearranging and converting into logarithms, to give

$$c = 146{,}5 \cdot A_{540} - 1{,}6114 \cdot A_{750}^{0{,}1736} \; (234{,}4 \cdot A_{504} - c)^{0{,}8264} \qquad (V)$$

Although this expression is not explicitly solvable for c it is useful for an iterative numerical treatment by successively refining preliminary values of c by insertion into the right side of equation (V):

$$c_0 = 146{,}5 \, A_{540} \tag{V a}$$

$$c_1 = 146{,}5 \, A_{540} - 99{,}341 \, A_{750}^{0,1736} \, (1{,}60 \, A_{504} - A_{540})^{0,8264} \tag{V b}$$

$$c_2 = 146{,}5 \, A_{540} - 1{,}6114 \, A_{750}^{0,1736} \, (234{,}4 A_{504} - c_1)^{0,8264} \tag{V c}$$

In procedure 2 iteration (V b) is transformed for ease of slide rule calculation as follows:

Absorbancies A are multiplied with a factor of 1000

$$A \cdot 10^3 = A' \quad \text{(dimension: } - \text{millibel)}$$

to get positive logarithms throughout. The correction term is written in exponential form, expanded in power series, which is disrupted after the first term. It is assumed that

$$A'_{750} \geqslant 10 \quad \text{and} \quad A'_{540}/A_{504} \geqslant 1{,}50$$

Thus finally results:

$$c'_1 \sim 0{,}1465 \, A'_{540} - 10^{-1,468} + 0{,}174 \lg A'_{750} + 0{,}826 \lg A'_{504} \tag{VI}$$

Procedure 3: From observation of the spacing of lines corresponding to parameter p in both half nomographs in fig. 5 one might infer a near to linear relationship between the factors of A_{750} in equations (IV) and (II a). Fig. 6 shows this actually to be the case: plotting $(750/540)^p$ as

Figure 6

p	x	y	$y_{approx.}$	difference %
0	0,6000	1,0000	1,0897	+ 9,0
1	0,9921	1,3889	1,3955	+ 0,5
2	1,6141	1,9290	1,8807	− 2,5
3	2,5933	2,6792	2,6444	−1,3
4	4,1248	3,7211	3,8390	+ 3,2

34

function of $[1,6\,(750/504)^p - 750/540)^p]$ in the range $0 < p < 4$, yields a slightly convex curve with respect to the abscissa. The mathematical technique for finding the best linear approximation function is described in the legend to fig. 6. Denoting the exponential function of p which is the factor of A_{750}

in equation (II a) with y and in equation (IV) with x, the aforementioned calculation yields

$$y = 0,780\,x + 0,622 \qquad (VII)$$

transforming equation (IV) into

$$(1,60 \cdot 1,4881^p - 1,3889^p) = x = \frac{1,60 \cdot A_{504} - A_{540}}{A_{750}} \qquad (IV\,a)$$

and inserting (IV a) and (VII) into equation (II) and rearranging we obtain

$$c = 260,8\,A_{540} - 182,8\,A_{504} - 91,1\,A_{750}\ (mg\ HiCN/100\ ml) \qquad (VIII)$$

This probably is the most expedite and illustrative technique for numerically calculating the true HiCN content with an error less than ± 1 mg/100 ml as long as NIR background absorption does not exceed $\sim 0{,}01$.

It may be mentioned that the procedures now outlined for nomographic and numerical corrections for background absorption due to turbidity are by no means restricted to HiCN solutions; they are quite universally applicable as long as spectral characteristics of pure substances are known on three different wavelengths.

References

[1]   Expert Panel on Haemoglobinometry, *Bibl. Haemat.* 21, 213, Basel 1965
[2]   Lord Rayleigh, *Philos. Mag.* 41, 107, 274, 447 and subsequent volumes, 1871
[3]   Thorell B. in Merker H. Ed., *Zyto- und Histochemie in der Hämatologie*, p. 22, 1963, Berlin-Göttingen-Heidelberg
[4]   Mie G., *Ann. Physik*, 25, 377, 1908
[5]   Jaenicke W., *Z. Elektrochem.*, 60, 163, 1956
[6 a] Schramm G., Dannenberg H., *Ber. d. chem. Ges.*, 77, 53, 1944
[6 b] Treiber E., Schauenstein E., *Z. Naturforsch.*, 4 b, 252, 1949
[6 c] Schauenstein E., Bayzer H., *J. Polym. Sc.*, 16, 45, 1955
[6 d] Treiber E., Berndt W., Toplak H., *Angew. Ch.*, 67, 69, 1955
[7]   Nielsen M.H., Nielsen N.C., *Scand. J. clin. & lab. Invest.*, 14, 605, 1962
[8]   Mauser H., p. 911 *Ullmanns Encyclopädie der technischen Chemie*, Vol. 2/1, München-Berlin, 1961
[9]   von Klein-Wisenberg., *Z.f. Ernährungswissenschaft*, 8, 66, 1967

1.6. *Evaluation of the International Method for Hemoglobinometry*
Takakata Matsubara, The Second Department of Internal
Medicine, Kumamoto University Medical School,
Kumamoto, Japan
and Susumu Shibata, Department of Medicine (The Third
Division), Yamaguchi University School of Medicine,
Ube, Japan

The recommendations of ICSH for a standard method in hemoglobinometry are very carefully laid down, but we believe that they can be improved if a few minor faults mentioned below are eliminated.

1. *Standard solution*

The ICSH specifies that the optical density of a standard HiCN solution should be less than 0.002 per cm path length in the near infrared between 670 to 800 nm (Tab. 1). In our opinion this statement should be corrected, because the standard solutions of about 60 mg/dl prepared by us as well as those prepared by the ICSH gave an optical density

Figure 1

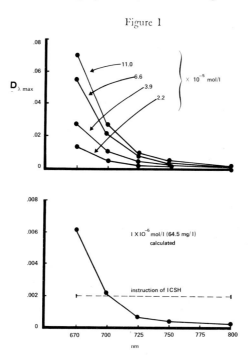

larger than 0.002 between 670 and 700 nm, and smaller than 0.002 only in the range between 750 and 800 nm.

Moreover, we calculated the optical density of a 64.5 mg/dl HiCN solution from that of more concentrated solutions and we obtained the same values (Fig. 1). According to these data the recommendations of ICSH should be modified as follows: « optical density should not be larger than 0.002 in the range between 750 and 800 nm ».

The ICSH specifies that the standard solution should be prepared by dissolving the hemolysate in Drabkin's reagent. We examined the stability of standard solutions dissolved at a pH of 8.6 in Drabkin's reagent and at a pH of 7.2 in van Kampen's reagent in which the detergent was omitted. Kept at 5 °C both standards showed no sign of deterioration for more than a year. At 37 °C, however, both standards showed deterioration within a year, as evidenced by a decrease in optical density at 541 nm and by a decrease in the ratio $D_{\lambda max}/D_{\lambda min}$: the deterioration appeared earlier with Drabkin's reagent. Fig. 2 shows an example of such an experiment. Accordingly, 7.2 rather than 8.6 is recommended as pH for the standard solution.

Figure 2

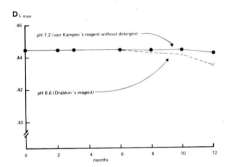

2. Diluting reagents

The ICSH recommends three reagents, i.e. van Kampen's, Drabkin's and modified Drabkin's. The latter two reagents, however, have some shortcomings.

Allowing for 1 % error, the time required for the conversion of Hb to HiCN at 25 °C was 1.5 minutes with van Kampen's reagent, 10 minutes with Drabkin's, and 30 minutes with modified Drabkin's reagent respectively; at 15 °C the corresponding times were 4, 40 and 120 minutes.

Table 1 — *Optical density of standard HiCN solutions of about 60 mg/dl in the infra-red region*

	prepared by	670 nm	700 nm	725 nm	750 nm	800 nm
determined	the authors	.0050 S .0080	.0023 S .0040	.0004 S .0025	.0 S .0015	.0 S .0015
	ICSH	.0059	.0028	.0011	.0010	.0010
	instructions of ICSH			$< .002$		

Table 2 — *Conversion time of HbO$_2$ → HiCN*

	allowed	reagent		
^oC	error %	van Kampen's	Drabkin's	modified Drabkin's
25	2.0	1.25	7	20
	1.0	1.5	10	30
	0.5	2	15	60
15	2.0	3	25	60
	1.0	4	40	120
	0.5	5	60	$>$120

(minutes)

Table 3 — *Error of Hb value caused by turbidity*

blood samples	reagent		
	van Kampen's	Drabkin's	modified Drabkin's
previous hemolysis	0.44%	6.48%	1.53%
direct addition	0.36%	1.16%	0.70%

(%)

Addition of a blood sample to the reagents caused some turbidity: the degree of turbidity was different according to the procedure (Table 2). When a blood sample was added to the reagents after hemolysis with water, van Kampen's reagent gave an optical density 0.44 % higher than the centrifuged sample, Drabkin's 6.48 %, modified Drabkin's 1.53 %. When a blood sample was dissolved directly in the reagents, van Kampen's reagent gave an optical density 0.36 % higher, Drabkin's 1.16 % higher and modified Drabkin's 0.70 % higher (Tab. 3).

Accordingly, we suggest that van Kampen's reagent be recommended as the most suitable for pratical use.

3. Other improvements of the ICSH's instructions (Tab. 4)

In the ICSH recommendation it is stated that the optical densities should be measured at 540 and 504 nm. We believe, however, that the correct designation should be: at the wavelengths of maximum and minimum light absorption. We have found the maximum to be at 540 to 542 nm, the minimum at 503 to 504 nm.

Table 4 – Other changes recommended for the ICSH's instruction.

	item	ICSH	the authors
standard solution	wavelength nm	measure at 540 504	measure at λmax, λmin max 540 – 542 min 503 – 504
standard solution	quotient D λmax D λmin	1.59 – 1.63	1.60 – 1.62
van Kampen's reagent	pH and amount of KH_2PO_4	KH_2PO_4 140mg/l pH 7.0 – 7.4	pH 7.0 – 7.4 (20°C) with an adequate amount of KH_2PO_4 (usually 140 – 160 mg/l)

The ratio $D_{\lambda max}/D_{\lambda min}$ gave a value of 1.60 to 1.62. Values of 1.59 or 1.63 were only found when standards were impure or deteriorating. We thus believe that the range of 1.59 to 1.63 recommended by the ICSH should be restricted to 1.60 to 1.62.

Finally, we have found that the amount of 140 mg of KH_2PO_4 in the reagent according to van Kampen is not always sufficient to bring the solution to a pH 7.0 to 7.4, e.g. in those cases where KCN had attracted excess moisture. We would thus recommend to change the ICSH recommendations as follows: « the pH pf the reagent should be brought to a value between 7.0 and 7.4 at 20 °C with an adequate amount of KH_2PO_4 (140 to 160 mg)».

1.7. Discussion

First Dr. Shibata presented Dr. Matsubara's and his results with the haemiglobincyanide method in Japan. This was followed by Dr. Spaander who noted an invitation by W.H.O. to make a physical device for the calibration of instruments used for the determination of haemoglobin. Dr. Zettner showed a photomicrograph of red cell ghosts encountered when diluting blood with Drabkin's reagent; Dr. von Klein Wisenberg presented a possible method of correcting the D_{HiCN}^{540} reading for turbidity, using D_{HiCN}^{750} and D_{HiCN}^{504} reading of the same samples.

W.G. Zijlstra. « As regards to Dr. von Klein Wisenberg's correction method of D_{HiCN}^{540} readings for turbidity, I should like to say that this does indeed offer us new possibilities as regards corrections when determining the haemoglobin content of whole blood samples. I would like to emphasize, however, the necessity of our having clear, i.e. non-turbid, reference solutions as a standard at all times.

I agree with Dr. Matsubara that the range given by the requirements for $D_{HiCN}^{540} / D_{HiCN}^{504}$ is too wide. Our measurements always fall well within this required range. The wide range was a concession for the benefit of the manufacturers of haemoglobin standards. As regards Mr. Moran's paper I can only say that we are not working on what Mr. Moran would like to call an esoteric plane but on a scientific plane. If Mr. Moran does not wish to work on a scientific plane he had better keep out of this field. I believe that sufficient solid evidence has been presented here today proving that it is well possible to perform spectrophotometric measurements quite accurately».

Dr. Klein (Hoffman La Roche) questioned the haemoglobin measurement in the many laboratories not equipped with precise spectrophotometers but with simple filter photometers and using commercial reagents not containing detergents. He called for a return to the measurement of haemoglobin iron and stated that his company offers a simple and reliable method.

Mr. Moran returned to the stand and stated he is not used to being first invited to meeting, then being asked to leave. He stated that he knows of no laboratory in the U.S. which is able to repeat the measurement series as presented by Dr. van Kampen. He wished to know how the HG reference laboratories are getting such results and then he quoted a number of diverging results from the expert panel on haemoglobinometry's 5 control laboratories.

Dr. von Klein Wisenberg ended the discussion by pointing out to Mr. Moran that the diverging results were obtained with spectrophotometers in routine use in his clinical chemical laboratory and were thus not being used under optimal conditions. Reverting to the W.H.O. query put forward by Dr. Spaander, he stated that work is being done along these lines.

2. Problems with the Cyanmethemoglobin Method in the Laboratory

2.1. General Remarks on Hemoglobinometry

George Brecher, San Francisco, USA

To put our present problems in hemoglobinometry into proper perspective, it might be useful to recall the purpose that led an Ad Hoc Committee of the National Research Council some 15 years ago to recommend a cynamethemoglobin standard which was subsequently adopted with some modifications as an international standard. The Ad Hoc Committee was motivated by rather broad scientific objectives. We wished to insure that we could compare hemoglobin values in different parts of the country and possibly throughout the world over a long period of time. We wished to do so not only for the benefit of the individual patient who might move from one place to another, but also in order to learn whether the range of hemoglobin values of the population stayed the same over a long period of time or whether it may conceivably change, as height and other population parameters have changed in many parts of the world. We also wish to know whether there is a truly universal normal range of hemoglobin values which is only altered by prevalence of disease or whether there are actually differences in the range of hemoglobin values in different populations. The answer to these questions required comparability of hemoglobin values. Such comparability has now been achieved by the cyanmethemoglobin standard. I will illustrate this by data recently collected by the Veterans Administration in 182 hospitals and laboratories. You will note there is complete agreement between the value of the Reference Laboratory that sent out the blood samples and the mean of all 182 hospitals as well as the mean of 17 determinations by one particular V.A. Hospital which happened to be associated with our Medical School in San Francisco. While these results which I believe are representative of the present state of hemoglobinometry certainly speak well for the ICSH standard which has made possible the satisfactory comparability of the means, they also indicate that clinical hemoglobinometry has not improved significantly over the years [1, 2]. The coefficient of variation of the means reported by different hospitals is still 4 % as is the coefficient of variation of the individual determinations in a single hospital. Note that the coefficient of variation of 4 % was not obtained on random samples but rather on reference material which may be presumed to have been handled with special care. The average variation of daily hemoglobin determinations in the same hospitals is probably greater. Fortunately, errors of measurement of this magnitude will seldom be crucial in the care of patients. Physiologic changes between the horizontal and vertical positions, even in perfectly healthy people range from 5-8 % [3]. The variation throughout the day is of similar magnitude [4]. Nevertheless, translating the coefficient of variation of 4 % into 95 % confidence limits, we find that most hospital laboratories cannot do better, and many do worse, than measuring hemoglobin within ± 1 gm. This is certainly an unsatisfactory state of affairs and I will, therefore, devote the rest of my time to a brief survey of the common errors in hemoglobinometry.

The errors in hemoglobinometry include inadequate resuspension of the cells, errors in dilution, and errors in spectrophotometry. Inadequate suspension of red cells is seldom mentioned as a major error primarily because it is rather difficult to isolate it from the dilution error. I suspect, however, that it is an important source of error. This becomes quite obvious when we deal not with freshly drawn blood but with red cells which have been fixed to stabilize them to serve as reference standards for red cell counts. Such cell suspension must be resuspended very vigorously. If one puts them on any kind of shaker and does periodic measurements one finds that one approaches the value of the reference laboratory only gradually as resuspension becomes complete. Resuspension of fresh blood is much easier but it must still be reckoned with as a potential source of error.

Dr. Lewis will deal with problems in dilution for hemoglobinometry. Our own experience with self-filling capillaries and with the Bull-Andersen-Dutcher « aliquanter » [5] has been very satisfactory.

Errors in spectrophotometry are of three kinds. 1. The standardization of the instrument, 2. its stability and 3. the random error of reading a particular sample. It is desirable to be able to distinguish these three sources of error in one's laboratory because instability of the instrument can be corrected if necessary by the purchase of a new instrument. This need not necessarily be more expensive but merely a more stable instrument. Errors of calibration can likewise be remedied. This done, we might be able to reduce the error in hemoglobinometry to the random error of the individual reading. It is at this point that we reach the limits of our conceptual analysis. If we have ascertained that the instrument is stable and that we can read the instrument within 1%, and if we have a flow-through cuvette so that the positioning of the cuvette cannot influence the reading, how is it then possible that aliquots of the same sample put through at different times still give different readings? Certainly these « statistical errors » for which we have no immediate physical explanation are well known to exist and we must deal with them as such, although we should retain a critical eye for any physical variations that can explain them. I wish to illustrate a general approach to this problem. To start with, it is quite useless for determination of stability of the instrument to make up a large volume of blood which has been diluted and converted to cyanmethemoglobin and to measure aliquots. The reading will be the same, unless you have a totally automatic sampling and read-out. This is so, because when an instrument is read visually, particularly one which requires estimates of fractions of a division, it is easy to deceive oneself to obtain the identical answer every time. One must design special methods to ensure true independence of measurement. A very simple and effective means is to pull out 5 or 10 samples after completion of the morning run of samples and re-measure them, preferably after they have been renumbered, both in the afternoon and after refrigeration the next morning. We did such an experiment in two ways (Table 2 and 3): once by rediluting the sample of blood each time and another time by simply remeasuring aliquots of a diluted sample. The fact that the differences between the morning and afternoon measurements average 0 indicates that the instrument was stable, yet an individual standard read differently in the afternoon than in the morning. Since there was no significant difference in the average of 5 determinations, the difference in the reading of a standard of the same lot must represent the unavoidable random reading error. As suspected, redilution of the sample gives slightly bigger errors than remeasuring of aliquots of a single dilution, but please note that the increase in error introduced by repeated dilution is quite small (Table 2 and 3).

In summary, the cynamethemoglobin standard will assure comparability of values provided that we compare means of a large number of determinations as in Table 1. As far as clinical hemoglobinometry is concerned, even the most careful attention to dilution, use of stable

44

Table 1 – 1968 V.A. Survey (182) Laboratories.

Reference Lab.	All V.A. Hospitals	S.F.V.A.
16.4	16.4 ± 0.58	16.4 ± 0.40
8.3	8.3 ± 0.38	8.2 ± 0.41

Table 2 – Samples Rediluted and Remeasured

Morning	Afternoon	Diff.	Next morning	Diff.
10.7	10.7	0	10.7	0
14.7	14.6	− 0.1	14.8	+ 0.2
14.0	13.6	− 0.4	13.8	+ 0.2
14.7	14.6	− 0.1	14.9	+ 0.3
13.7	14.1	+ 0.4	14.1	0
15.2	15.2	0	15.4	+ 0.2
Stand 15.1	15.4	+ 0.3	15.1	− 0.3
Mean Diff.		+ 0.03		+ 0.09

Table 3 – Diluted Samples Remeasured

Morning	Afternoon	Diff.	Next morning	Diff.
10.8	10.9	+ 0.1	11.1	+ 0.2
14.8	14.8	0	14.8	0
13.9	13.7	− 0.2	13.9	+ 0.2
14.8	14.9	+ 0.1	14.9	0
13.7	13.7	0	13.9	+ 0.2
15.2	15.2	0	15.3	+ 0.1
Stand 15.1	15.4	+ 0.3	15.1	− 0.3
Mean Diff.		+ 0.04		+ 0.06

instruments and adequate standardization leaves an apparently irreducible error of the individual determination of about 2%. Without such careful attention, the coefficient of variation is more likely to be 4% or even larger.

References

[1] Sunderman, F.W., « Status of Clinical Hemoglobinometry in the United States », *Amer. J. Clin. Path., 43*, 9, 1965
[2] Skendzel, L.P. and Copeland, B.E., « Hemoglobin Measurements in Hospital Laboratories », *Amer. J. Clin. Path., 44*, 245, 1965
[3] Fawcett, J.K. and Wym, V., « Effects of Posture on Plasma Volume and Some Blood Constituents », *J. Clin. Path. 13*, 304, 1960
[4] Stengle, James M., « Diurnal-Nocturnal Variations of Certain Blood Constituents Normal Human Subjects: Plasma Iron, Siderophilin, Bilirubin, Copper, Total Serum Protein and Albumin, Haemoglobin and Haematocrit », *Brit. J. Haemat., 3*, 117, 1957
[5] Bull, Brian S., Dutchet, T. and Siggaard-Andersen, O., « The Hem-Aliquanter », *Amer. J. Clin. Path., 49*, 295, 1968

2.2. Pipettes and Pipetting in Haemoglobinometry

S.M. Lewis, Royal Postgraduate Medical School, London, W. 12, UK

The international comparability trials have demonstrated that the measurement of haemoglobin is still liable to result in discrepancies in spite of the use of the ICSH haemoglobin standard. Of course, the standard has done much to eliminate the inter-laboratory variation which used to occur when so-called standards themselves varied, and to an extent the use of the standard ensures that haemoglobinometers are set correctly and are functioning properly. But of equal importance is the need for good technique and accurate apparatus to ensure that the blood sample is diluted accurately.

The extent of the errors of technique is illustrated in Figure 1. A fresh blood sample was tested by 20 observers from the same laboratory. They ranged from senior technicians to medical staff who had not carried out a haemoglobin estimation with their own hands since their student days. The cyanmethaemoglobin method was used; all observers used the same photo-electric haemoglobinometer, the same pipettes, and the same standard. The « true » measurement was that obtained by an expert technician who repeated the test several times with identical results. The other observers had a variance of $\pm 3\%$

Figure 1

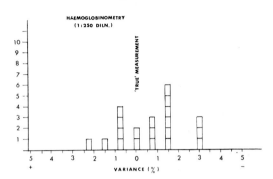

from this measurement. This is the extent of the error of technique independent of instrument error, and it gives an idea of the precision of haemoglobinometry at the routine clinical laboratory level. Essentially it indicates the ability of individual workers to handle the blood sample and to dilute it correctly.

There are several methods by which blood can be diluted. (Table 1). As a rule a dilution of 1 : 200 or 1 : 250 is optimal. This can be obtained by taking a sample volume of 20 mm^3 and a diluent volume of 4 or 5 cm^3. These volumes can be dispensed manually by means of appropriately-sized one-mark pipettes or graduated pipettes. Syringe-pipettes are usually semi-automatic, overflow-type pipettes belonging to the group known as automatic dispensing pipettes. Combined diluters are instruments by which the blood and the diluent are taken up and mixed in a single procedure. They are based on two systems. In the proportioning type the actual volume does not matter, but with the same dispenser one volume of the blood is measured into the requisite

Figure 2

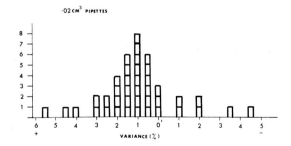

Table 1 – Methods for blood dilution.

BLOOD
(20 - 50mm³)

GRADUATED PIPETTES (contain)
ONE-MARK PIPETTES (contain)
VOLUMETRIC CAPILLARIES
SYRINGE PIPETTES
   Single volume
   Multiple volumes

DILUENT
(1 - 10cm³)

GRADUATED ⎫
ONE MARK   ⎬ (contain or deliver)
SYRINGE PIPETTES
AUTOMATIC (OVERFLOW TYPE) PIPETTES

COMBINED (AUTOMATIC DILUTERS)
(1:100 - 1:500)

PROPORTIONING SYSTEMS
PIPETTE SYSTEMS

Table 2 – Comparison of optical density readings of 0.02 - Ml. volumes of a blood sample (Diluted 1 in 250)

Micropipettes (BSS)	Break-off Capillaries
36.5	36.8
37.5	37.0
36.8	36.8
37.0	36.8
37.0	37.5
38.0	36.8
38.5	37.2
36.8	36.8
37.0	36.8
38.0	37.5
38.0	36.8
36.8	37.2
Mean 37.3 (S.D. ±0.63)	37.0 (S.D. ±0.28)
Maximum deviations:	
+1.2 (3.2%); – 0.8 (2.1%)	+ 0.5 (1.3%); – 0.2 (0.5%)

number of volumes of diluent. In the pipette system the blood and diluent are measured in separate pipettes which have calibrated volumes. 20 mm³ pipettes are the commonest pipettes used in the haematology laboratory. Figure 2 illustrates the accuracy of a batch of such pipettes. Forty single-mark pipettes were taken at random from the departmental stocks and used for haemoglobin measurement of the same blood sample. The diluent was pre-dispensed into tubes by means of a single 5 cm³ pipette and all tests were carried out by the same expert technician. The results show a variance of over 10 %. The correct result was obtained by using an accurately calibrated pipette (see below). The error tended to be due to a greater volume contained in a pipette than nominally marked, leading to results which are up to 6 % higher than they should be.

In several countries national standards organizations have established specifications for pipettes, in which limits of tolerance are defined. Thus, for example, there is a British standard (B.S. 1428 : 1963) in which the limits have been set at ± 2 % on a 20 mm³ pipette [1]. Unfortunately, however, many pipettes are manufactured without regard to these specifications and even when they purport to conform to the standards the reliability of such claims depends upon the adequacy of the manufacturer's quality control, and, of course, this influences the cost of the end products. To attain reasonably priced pipettes we must be realistic in our demand for accuracy but no-one would argue with the modest requirement of B.S. 1428. It is desirable to have a certification scheme whereby the claim to a national standard can be assured by statutory control. This would be in the province of national committees and it would be impracticable for this to be a project of ICSH. Until such control can be instituted, ICSH can play a part by encouraging individual workers to check the pipettes used in their own laboratories. The most convenient method is by colorimetric readings of the colour of an appropriate solution when diluted by means of the pipette under test, as compared with that obtained by a pipette of known accuracy. A more accurate but slightly more laborious procedure is to take up mercury into a pipette and subsequently weigh it. Its weight can then be translated into a measure of volume (20 mm³ of mercury weighs 272 mg). Any pipette found to have an error greater than 1-2 % should be discarded or used with a correction factor. Whether we should accept a tolerance of 2 % or demand greater accuracy is a matter for discussion and for compromise between desirable and practical objectives.

Increasingly, laboratories are using automatic dilution techniques. The problem of pipette accuracy is similar with these instruments. In

Britain the Association of Clinical Biochemists assessed a number of dispensing pipettes [2]. On the basis of accuracy and other criteria only six of the 35 instruments examined could be recommended. For blood counts there are two approaches to the use of semi-automatic diluting procedures. Either a batch of specimens can be diluted for only one investigation at a time, or consecutive dilutions of the same sample can be made for multiple tests. The latter has a number of advantages. The specimen is handled only once and particular care can more readily be taken to ensure adequate mixing — an important aspect of accurate blood counting. For this, the Hem-Aliquanter developed by Bull, Dutcher, and Andersen [3] appears to be a reliable and accurate instrument of value in a busy routine department.

I shall now turn to the simpler methods of dilution which are needed for bed-side blood collection and field surveys by relatively less skilled workers who may be unfamiliar with pipetting technique. Automatic-filling glass-capillary pipettes have been in use for a considerable period of time [4]. They have a limited usefulness mainly to dispense, consecutively, the same volume of blood for serial testing, especially when the exact dilution is of no consequence. They can be used for osmotic fragility and similar studies when a standard is diluted alongside the test specimens, or when the diluted specimens are to be compared one to another.

More recently manufacturers of disposable glass capillaries have improved their process whereby capillaries can be drawn out with uniform bore along their entire length so as to ensure constancy of volume relative to length. The use of such a capillary as a volumetric instrument is illustrated in Figure 3. The capillary is etched at B, and A — B is an accurately calibrated container of 20 mm^3 capacity. The capillary is filled from end C by finger or ear prick blood or by blood already

Figure 3

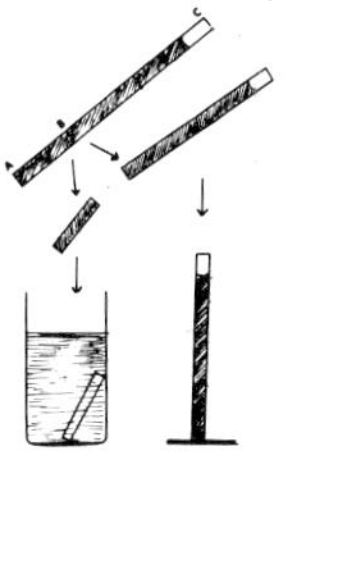

collected into a specimen bottle. The blood is allowed to flow down so as to fill the capillary to at least AB. The tube is easily snapped off where the etch has weakened the glass and AB is dropped into a tube containing diluent. With shaking the blood flows into the diluent and in this way 20 mm³ has been added to diluent without error from contaminant blood on the outside of the capillary. If heparinised, the rest of the capillary can be used for packed cell volume determination by sealing one end with a plastic material.

The accuracy of the break-off capillary is illustrated in Table 2. For haemoglobinometry it appears to be as accurate as pipettes which conform to the British standard [5]. We have used the break-off capillary in surveys and find its precision better than that of pipettes when used by unskilled persons who may experience the difficulties of under and overfilling and of contaminant blood from the outside of the pipette stem being added to the diluent. Moreover, it is easier and quicker to use than a pipette and is particularly suited to field studies and similar population surveys.

In conclusion, I would like to emphasise the fact that there is urgent need for the ICSH haemoglobinometry panel to turn its attention to pipettes and technique, in order to ensure that the enormous strides made by the panel with the development of the reference standard should not be discounted because of errors and deficiencies in these other factors which also influence the accuracy of haemoglobinometry.

References

[1] B.S. 1428 Part D. 4, *Specification for Capillary Pipettes,* British Standards Institution, London, 1963
[2] Broughton, P.M.G., Gowenlock, A.H., Widdowson, G.M. and Ahlquist, K.A., *Automatic Dispensing Pipettes. An Assessment of Thirty-five Commercial Instruments,* Scientific Report No. 3, Assoc. Clin. Biochemists, London, 1967
[3] Bull, B.S., Dutcher, T. and Siggaard-Andersen, O., « The Hem Aliquanter. A Dispenser-diluter for Hematology », *Amer. J. Clin. Path., 49,* 295, 1968
[4] Davie, J.V. and Lewis, S.M., *Practical Haematology,* 4th Edition, p. 168, Churchill, London, 1968
[5] Lewis, S.M. and Benjamin, H., « Break-off Capillary Tube Method for Blood Counts », *J. Clin. Path., 18,* 689, 1965

2.3. On Properties and Stability of Reacting Solutions for Haemoglobinometry

Maria Winkelmann, Edeltraud Mantei and A. v. Klein-Wisenberg, Medizinische Universitaetsklinik Freiburg im Breisgau, Germany

Through the universal adoption of the HiCN-method for determination of haemoglobin, industrially prepared reagent mixtures in solid or solute form have become available for the convenience of laboratories to relieve them from the necessity to prepare in frequent intervals their reacting solutions themselves. As the ferricyanide/cyanide-system is a metastable one [1] it must be feared that decomposed reagent mixtures, no longer apt for their intended purpose, reach the hands of customers. For this reason we think it valuable to report some laboratory observations gained on the stability of reacting solutions for haemiglobinometry.

Out of the many proposed recipes the reacting solutions most frequently used are composed after the recipes of Drabkin [2] (50 mg KCN, 200 mg $K_3Fe(CN)_6$, 1000 mg $NaHCO_3$ per liter) and van Kampen-Zijlstra [3] (50 mg KCN, 200 mg $K_3Fe(CN)_6$, 140 mg KH_2PO_4 and 0,5...1 ml alkylphenolpolyethyleneoxideether-detergent per liter). Thus both have in common a content of 0,768 mMol cyanide and 0,607 mMol ferricyanide. Completeness of haemolysis is attained in the former recipe through a higher pH, in the latter through a lower osmolality. Dissolution of stromata and formed protein elements is being achieved in the Drabkin recipe by higher alkalinity, in the van Kampen-Zjilstra solution by the wetting agent. The components of Drabkin solution can easily be packaged in solid form and thus should keep indefinitely unchanged. Packages for preparation of van Kampen-Zjilstra reagent should take consideration of reproducible dispensing of the highly viscous detergent. Thus it has been attempted to distribute highly concentrated solutions for subsequent dilution. Unfortunately, these concentrates decompose readily.

The criteria for intact reacting solutions therefore are: maintenance of the cyanide- and ferricyanide content, maintenance of the initial pH, and absence of appreciable light absorption at wavelength longer than 500 nm in the concentration and cell path length used for the actual haemoglobin determination.

As the molar absorptivity of ferricyanide is

925 at 420 nm and
742 at 436 nm,

a check for the ferricyanide content is easily performed by a spectrophotometric test: absorbance per cm path length in the ready prepared solution according to the original recipe should be

0,562 at 420 nm,
0,451 at 436 nm and
less than 0,001 at 500 to 800 nm.

As hydrocyanic acid has pK value of 9,3 at room temperature it can be easily separated by steam distillation of hydrogen-carbonate-alkaline solution and subsequently determined according to the well known Liebig-Denigès argentometric titration [4]. Beforehand it may be stated that we did find in all samples analysed accordingly the outlined procedure less than 1/2 of the expected content of cyanide only. Finally we found out that even the a.r. grade potassium cyanide of samples available to us contained only 41...48 % of their theoretical cyanide content, which amounts to a net weight increase through formation of potassium-hydrogencarbonate by uptake of hydrocarbonic acid and loss of hydrocyanic acid of 26...22 %. We do not think this observation unusual and venture to say that one may safely double the amount of cyanide in the recipes in order to obtain the concentration originally intended. The decomposition of reacting solutions by freezing has been discussed in literature recently [5] and should proceed according to

$$CN^- + 2\,Fe(CN)_6^{3-} + H_2O = CNO^- + 2\,Fe(CN)_6^{4-} + 2\,H^+$$

followed by

$$CNO^- + 3\,H_2O + H^+ = NH_4^+ + HCO_3^-$$

to give an overall reaction

$$CN^- + 2\,Fe(CN)_6^{3-} + 3\,H_2O \rightarrow NH_4^+ + 2\,Fe(CN)_6^{4-} + H^+ + HCO_3^- \qquad [1]$$

Figure 1

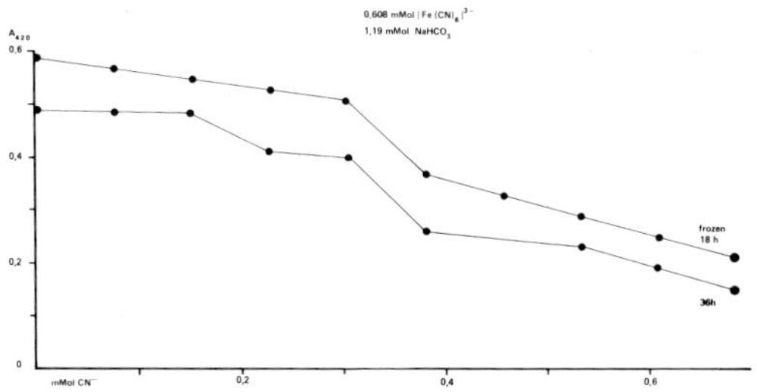

This process is speeded up with increasing concentration of the reactants, therefore decolouration of ferricyanide has been observed upon freezing reaction solutions for haemiglobinometry. Fig. 1 illustrates the sharp decrease in optical density of solutions of frozen and rethawed mixtures of 1,19 mMol $NaHCO_3$, 0,61 mMol $K_3Fe(CN)_6$ and varying amounts of KCN at a molar ratio of ferricyanide/cyanide > 2 and shows the proposed reacting scheme to be valid. Thus, although a reacting solution with excess ferricyanide will not completely decolourize upon freezing, it will nevertheless have lost all its cyanide. Another point of importance is the actinity of ferricyanide solutions. Irradiation, especially ith ultraviolet light, leads to decomposition of ferricyanide and the appearance of turbidity, finally ending — depending on the pH — with the visible appearance of Turnbull's or Prussian blue at pH 7...8 or a sedimentation of iron (III) oxidhydrate at pH $\sim$ 9. This process takes place in clear vessels of glass, quartz, and even in white polyethylene. It is considerably diminished in vessels of brown glass and in polyethylene stained with an ultraviolet protecting pigment. Drabkin's reagent attacks through its alkalinity, van Kampen-Zijlstra's through its content of phosphate and detergent. So a van Kampen-Zijlstra solution stored unopened for 14 months in a 1 l bottle of brown glass of hydrolytical class 3 (common medicine bottle) had lost its cyanide completely, more than 80 % of its ferricyanide and had formed 51 mg of a glittering sediment containing 39 % SiO_2, the rest being $Me_2^{III}O_3$ and $Me^{II}O$.

Details of observation on decolouration, loss of cyanide, change of pH, and other findings occurring upon longtime storage, ultraviolet irradiation together with warming to 35 °C and freezing are listed in complete elsewhere.*

A guaranteed shelf-life for both reacting solutions of a period of more than one month cannot be assured, even if solutions are stored at moderate room temperature, protected from direct incidents of even diffuse daylight by wrapping or painting the bottle, which should be made of polyethylene or glass of hydrolytical class 1. Probably the most suitable containers for reacting solutions for haemiglobinometry are bottles with ground-in glass stoppers made of brown borosilicate glass.

References

* The results reported here make part of the MD thesis of Miss M. Winkelmann.

[1]   von Klein-Wisenberg A. *Bibl. haemat.*, *24*, 150, Basel, 1966
[2]   Drabkin, D.L., Austin, J.A., *J. biol. Chem.*, *98*, 719, 1932
[3]   van Kampen, E.J. Zijlstra, W.G., *Clin. chim. Acta, 6*, 538, 1961
[4 a] Liebig, J., *Am. Chem. Pharm.*, *77*, 102, 1852
[4 b] Denigés, G., *C. r. hebd. Acad. Sci, Paris, 117*, 1079, 1893
[5 a] Mickelsen, O., Woolard, H., Ness, A.F. *Clin. Chem., 10*, 611, 1964
[5 b] Weatherburn, M.W., Logan, J.E., *Clin. chim. Acta, 9*, 581, 1964

54

2.4. *The Use of Haemiglobinazide Instead of Haemiglobincyanide for the Determination of Haemoglobin*

O.W. van Assendelft, E.J. van Kampen and W.G. Zijlstra, Groningen, the Netherlands

In 1966 Vanzetti [5] described a method for the determination of haemoglobin by means of conversion to haemiglobinazide (HiN₃) as an alternative to the internationally accepted haemiglobincyanide (HiCN) method [1]. The author felt justified in presenting an alternative to the latter method because of the danger to analysts when handling KCN, used in preparing the reagent solution. Vanzetti states that, although the use of standard HiN₃ solutions is to be preferred, commercially available HiCN reference solutions may well be used, as HiN₃ and HiCN have identical absorption coefficients at λ = 540-546 nm. The azide reagent to be used is stated to be harmless and to withstand freezing and thawing; the stability of the reagent is claimed to be excellent at 4 °C and satisfactory at room temperature. The purpose of this paper is to give a summary of results obtained while testing the method extensively over the past 2 years.

Properties of HiN₃

Fig. 1 shows a λε curve of HiN₃, with the curve of HiCN drawn in for comparison. HiN₃ is seen to have a well defined light absorption maximum at λ = 542 nm, a secondary maximum at λ = 573 nm and a light absorption minimum at λ = 500 nm. The curve is seen to have a shoulder from λ = 610 to λ = 690 nm. Although the extinction coefficient approaches zero near λ = 750 nm, HiN₃ also absorbs light in the near infra-red.

Table I gives some millimolar extinction coefficients determined using clear solutions prepared from both whole blood and washed erythrocytes. It is clearly seen that, although the extinction coefficient approaches the value of 11.0 at λ = 542 nm, nowhere do the coefficients of HiN₃ and HiCN coincide in this wavelength range.

When excess KCN is added to a HiN₃ solution, the spectrum of HiCN appears shortly, coincidental with a slight rise in the D⁵⁴⁰ value. In a series of 10 measurements, an average increase of D⁵⁴⁰ of 0.9 % was found. This increase is quite consistent with the difference of 0.10 found for the extinction coefficients of HiN₃ and HiCN at this wavelength.

By continuously recording D⁵⁴⁰ from the moment of mixing blood

Figure 1

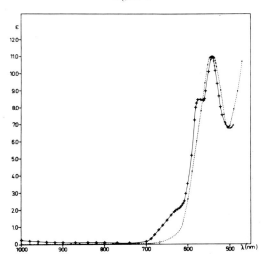

Table 1 – *Quarter millimolar extinction coefficients of HiN₃ determined using both whole blood samples and washed erythrocytes. Beckman DU and Optica CF4 spectrophotometers. ϵ_{HiCN} added for comparison.*

	whole blood			washed cells			
λ (nm)	ϵ	n	$s/\sqrt{n}$	ϵ	n	$s/\sqrt{n}$	ϵ_{HiCN}
538				10.70	5		10.94
540	10.90	37	0.003	10.91	16	0.003	10.99
542	10.95	36	0.003	10.95	16	0.003	10.99
544				10.89	5		10.98
546				10.75	5		10.95
548				10.45	5		10.86
500	6.80	16	0.04	6.78	16	0.03	6.92

$$s = \sqrt{\frac{\Sigma(x - \bar{x})^2}{n - 1}}$$

samples and azide-containing reagent, it was found that the formation of HiN₃ from HbO₂ was complete in some 70 sec. In the case of HbCO, however, complete conversion to HiN₃ proved to take at least 40 min.

Reagent used in the HiN₃ method

The stability of the reagent, which contains 200 mg $K_3Fe(CN)_6$, 30 mg NaN₃, 1 g THAM, 0.5 g monohydrated citric acid and 0.5 ml

56

Sterox SE per liter, has been tested extensively. The results of storing the reagent both at 4 °C and at room temperature are summarized in Table II. Although the results are better when the reagent is stored at room temperature in brown glass bottles than in clear glass bottles, storage at 4 °C should be preferred in all cases as has also been indicated by Vanzetti [5]. When the reagent was frozen and thawed repeatedly, the reagent was seen to begin deteriorating after the third thawing.

As regards toxicity of NaN$_3$, impairment of liver function has been described, among others by Werle and Stücker [6], by Levene [2] and by Vanlerenberghe et al. [4]. Finally, due to the explosive character of NaN$_3$, this substance is not accepted for shipment by many air freight companies unless more or less extensive safety precautions are taken.

Comparison of the HiN$_3$ and the HiCN method

From 24 blood samples obtained during routine heart catherizations, 0.5 ml was diluted to 100 ml with both the azide reagent and the reagent described by Van Kampen and Zijlstra [3]. D^{540} values were measured with an Optica CF4 grating spectrophotometer, half intensity bandwidth 0.13 nm at $\lambda = 540$ nm, and are given in Table III. Although an average difference of around 0.9 %, the D$^{540}_{HiN_3}$ values being lower, was encountered in nearly all cases, considerable positive differences were observed with 3 samples: D$^{540}_{HiN_3}$ + 3.0 %, + 3.7 % and + 14.35 % respectively. A duplicate determination performed the same day gave identical results in all 3 cases. The differences were probably due to turbidity as the light absorption spectra recorded of these samples showed optical density values up to 0.060 in the wavelength range $\lambda = 700$ to $\lambda = 800$ nm.

Conclusion

The HiN$_3$ method cannot find justification as an alternative method to the internationally accepted HiCN method for the determination of blood haemoglobin content on the following grounds.

1. As HiN$_3$ has a distinct light absorption maximum at $\lambda = 542$ nm, either a spectrophotometer or a quite narrow band filter photometer must be used. For accurate results, the use of a HiN$_3$ reference solution is imperative. Purity control of these reference solutions, especially as regards turbidity, is more difficult than in the case of HiCN reference solutions.

Table 2 – Stability of azide-containing reagent on storing at different temperatures.

container	onset of deterioration when kept at	
	$4^{\circ}C$	room temperature
clear glass bottle	16 weeks	1 week
brown glass bottle	17 weeks	3 weeks

Table 3 – Comparison of D_{HiCN}^{540} and $D_{HiN_3}^{540}$ values of 24 blood samples measured using an Optica CF4 spectrophotometer.

sample	D_{HiCN}^{540}	$D_{HiN_3}^{540}$	Δ (%)
1	0.483	0.479	− 0.8
2	0.470	0.468	− 0.4
3	0.466	0.461	− 1.1
4	0.456	0.449	− 1.5
5	0.460	0.458	− 0.4
6	0.467	0.463	− 0.9
7	0.534	0.526	− 1.5
8	0.543	0.538	− 0.9
9	0.566	0.564	− 0.4
10	0.472	0.468	− 0.8
11	0.461	0.457	− 0.9
12	0.503	0.498	− 1.0
13	0.512	0.507	− 1.0
14	0.526	0.541	+ 2.9
14	*0.525*	*0.541*	*+ 3.0*
15	0.452	0.448	− 0.9
16	0.522	0.597	+ 14.3
16	*0.520*	*0.594*	*+ 14.2*
17	0.453	0.447	− 1.3
18	0.543	0.540	− 0.6
19	0.472	0.489	+ 3.6
19	*0.473*	*0.491*	*+ 3.8*
20	0.539	0.534	− 0.9
21	0.548	0.543	− 0.9
22	0.593	0.586	− 1.2
23	0.588	0.587	− 0.2
24	0.612	0.608	− 0.7

58

2. Unexpected gross deviations, probably due to turbidity, may be encountered at any time.

3. The slight advantage of the lesser toxicity of NaN₃ cannot compensate for the necessity of having to store the azide reagent at 4 °C.

References

[1] International Committee for Standardization in Haematology, « Recommendations for Haemoglobinometry in Human Blood », Brit. J. Haemat., 13 (Suppl.), 71, 1967
[2] Levene, C.I., « The Éffect of Lathyrogenic Compounds on the Glycogen Content of the Chick Embryo Liver », Brit. J. exp. Path., 43, 596, 1962
[3] Van Kampen, E.J. and Zijlstra, W.G., « Standardization of Hemoglobinometry. II. The Hemiglobincyanide Method », Clin. chim. Acta, 6, 538, 1961
[4] Vanlerenberghe, J., Guerrin, F., Bar, N. and Bel, C., « Sécrétion de bile par le foie de Rat. VI. Action de l'azide de sodium », C.R. Soc. Biol., 157, 1454, 1963
[5] Vanzetti, G., « An Azide-methemoglobin Method for Hemoglobin Determination in Blood ». J. Lab. clin. Med., 67, 116, 1966
[6] Werle, E. and Stücker, F., « Zur Pharmakologie der Azide », Arzneimittelforsch., 8, 28, 1958

Acknowledgment

We gratefully ackknowledge the assistance of L.M. Zuiderveld, D.H. Dix and J. Leeuwenberg in this investigation.

Comment to the paper of Dr. van Assendelft et al.
G. Vanzetti (Milan, Italy)

1. In our laboratory the azide-methemoglobin method has been used daily since 1965 for specimens of capillary and venous blood: we have never observed the development of turbidity. Before adopting the azide-methemoglobin method, a comparison was made with the cyanmethemoglobin method by performing parallel determination on 50 blood specimens taken from normal subjects or from outpatients; the agreement was always good. Similar control experiments carried out in other laboratories led to similar results There can be some disagreement in a few pathological cases, but in our experience the cyanide reagent is much more likely than the azide reagent to give rise to turbidity, due to floculation of plasma proteins. The pertinent results will be reported elsewhere.

2. I agree on the need to use an azide-methemoglobin reference solution for the azide-methemeglobin method: this solution should be sterilized by means of membrane filtration or Seitz filtration, in order to ensure its stability.

3. We did not find significant differences between the absorbances of

azide-methemoglobin and cyanmethemoglobin solutions of equal concentrations at 542 nm; at 540 nm we found similar values, but we cannot rule out slightly lower values for azide-methemoglobin.

4. Although sodium azide is currently used in many biological laboratories, I am not aware of any explosion or other accident occurring as a result of its use. Many other «explosive» reagents like picric acid and potassium chlorate are widely used in the laboratory without any trouble.

5. According to the data reported by us as well as by others the toxicity of the azide reagent can be estimated to be about 1/10 of that of the cyanide reagent. A preparation of very low toxicity in solid or powder form can therefore be envisaged; Sterox SE should be added separately.

6. Comparative trials have shown that the azide reagent can withstand freezing and thawing, whereas the cyanide reagent deteriorates rapidly; we have also found that the stability of the azide reagent at 4° and at room temperature was at least as good as the stability of the cyanide reagent.

7. The divergencies between our results and Dr. van Assendelft's require further investigation.

Dr. Ferro (Coulter diagnostics).

We have compared the cyanmethemoglobin and azide-methemoglobin methods on several thousands blood specimens, and we have found a good agreement between the two methods.

2.5. Whole Blood Controls and Standards in Hematology

A. Richardson Jones, Director, Research and Development, Dade Reagents, Inch., Miami, Florida, USA

It would seem from an historical viewpoint that the growing recognition of the necessity for adequate controls for the performance of routine hematologic measurements derives, in large part, from the proven value of the use of controls in clinical chemistry.

Prior to 1950 the use of controls in any field of clinico-pathological measurement was virtually unheard of. Those few chemists who used controls did so in a rather tentative and (by today's standards) unsophisticated manner.

I would like to believe without however offering this as a controversial point, that the corporation which I presently have the pleasure of serving was the pioneer in the development of the stable liquid control for clinical chemistry. This liquid control, which today still enjoys a wide sale, is based on a formulation developed nearly 20 years ago. At that time a large-scale study was being performed at the Medical Research Foundation of Dade County in Miami on the nutritional status of certain patients. It was found impossible properly to evaluate the results of this study because it was not known whether the changes observed in the patient were truly a reflection of alteration of his metabolic status or were the result of changes occurring in the reagents, calibration errors in pipets or differences in manual dexterity among different technicians.

The result of raising this question was the development of a stable liquid containing certain biochemical constituents of interest the inclusion of which in the day's run of tests provided an unvarying yardstick by which to judge the influence of other undesirable human, instrumental, or chemical factors which might destroy the validity of the experimental data.

The importance and usefulness of controls in clinical chemistry was further brought home with the introduction of machines for automated chemical analysis. Indeed, without the use of controls one's level of confidence in the results produced by automatic analyzers would be much lower than it is.

There have, of course, been considerable advances in both the technique of manufacture and in the use of controls in clinical chemistry. Today one seeks to provide controls which as closely as possible resemble the unknown serums which are being analyzed. This requirement is generated partly by the increased range and extent of biochemical testing, particularly as regards the biochemist's interest in labile constituents such as enzymes, and partly by the special requirements of automatic analyzers which, generally, do not take kindly to the older (but still useful) quasi-synthetic controls.

One more brief point must be raised with regard to controls in clinical chemistry before proceeding to the matter of controls in hematology. This is the use of controls as calibration standards. Strictly speaking, any analytical method should be calibrated or standardized against a primary standard.

This is a solution of the constituent of interest in an absolutely pure, or at least highly purified form, the concentration of which has been defined by « weighing in » the constituent. Preferably the concentration of the constituent shall be capable of being expressed in terms of some universally accepted definition. A good example of this, and indeed the only example existing in hematology at present, is the primary standard for cyanmethemoglobin measurement which has already been the topic of considerable discussion here. When one considers the practical impossibility of preparing an absolute calibration standard for a constituent such as serum lactate dehydrogenase it is easy to see that calibration must, per force, be made in many analytical procedures by the use of control material which, when used in this manner is dignified by the term « secondary standard ».

The commercial availability of secondary standards grows out of a response by companies such as ours to an expressed need by the profession for an assayed control. In other words as the use of controls grew in popularity it was felt that the long-term stability of control material was, by itself, not enough. It did not enable the user to know whether his method was correct or was merely giving him a consistent invalidity. When an unassayed control is used it tells you that today's results are likely to be as plausible as yesterday's or last week's. It will not, for example, tell you that the total protein results published by the laboratory for the past two years are consistently 0.5 gm/100 ml lower than they should be. An unassayed control, therefore, only detects a change in the quality of the data but does not pin the data back to some absolute point of reference.

I have taken this time to present a brief review of the position of controls in clinical chemistry in order to emphasize the following points.

Firstly, the use of controls in quantitative laboratory procedures as exemplified by chemical analysis, today, is considered to be an essential part of methodology.

Secondly, the widespread use of automated procedures in clinical chemistry has further emphasized the importance of controls and has led to the development of more sophisticated methods of preparation of control material.

Thirdly, much of the credit for the availability of control material must be given to the manufacturers of bioanalytical reagents, such as ourselves, who not only recognize the need for such products but have the plant, personnel and technical facilities necessary for the assurance of high standards of uniformity and consistency from batch to batch of control material and who have the capability of performing highly accurate assays of a wide range of constituents.

In attempting to apply the lessons learned in the manufacture of chemistry controls to the development of control material for use in the hematology laboratory the manufacturer is undertaking, in my opinion, a task of greater magnitude and difficulty than he encounters in the preparation of chemistry controls. This is largely because controls in hematology deal with constituents which depend for their continued integrity upon a continuation of the normal metabolic processes. To a degree, many of these difficulties can be circumvented by offering a variety of control materials, each suitable for controlling the measurement of a specific hematologic parameter.

If this approach is taken one would employ the following different types of controls.

1. *Red Cell Counting Control.* This consists of a suspension of erythrocytes adjusted to yield a predetermined count. These erythrocytes are preserved by a process of fixation of which many methods are available. We ourselves favor the use of osmium tetroxide as a fixative and we have been granted a United States patent to cover this application of osmium tetroxide as a fixative. This method produces an extremely stable suspension of erythrocytes which maintains a count which is consistent within 1.0% over a period of years. Furthermore, the cells maintain a size distribution curve very close to that of the donor from whom they are obtained and this size-distribution also shows excellent stability over long periods of time. We have found that stained films can be made from this material which provide a good representation of the differential white cell count of the donor and therefore it seems possible that this red cell counting control material could also find some application as a differential counting control if one could ever work out a proper procedure for applying control methods to this form of hematologic measurement.

One of the major disadvantages of this type of red cell counting control is that the fixation of the red cells makes it impossible to carry out an accurate hematocrit determination on the material. This is because the fixation process prevents the centrifuged red cells from undergoing the degree of distortion suffered by fresh red cells when packed in the centrifuge. Fixed red cells will give hematocrit values 20 to 25% higher than the hematocrit of the original donor of the blood. This makes it impossible to compute mean corpuscular volume values from fixed red cell suspensions and such information must therefore be obtained from the donor blood prior to the fixation process and confirmed by the use of the cell sizing techniques which are provided by the Coulter Automatic Blood Counter.

One advantage of this method of fixation which we have not yet exploited is the possibility of controlling both the shape and modal point of size-distribution curves by shrinking or swelling the donor

63

cells by manipulation of their osmotic environment at the time of fixation. We have found that we can closely simulate a variety of pathologic size-distribution curves in this manner.

2. *Hemoglobin Concentration Control.* This consists of a solution of purified hemoglobin adjusted to a concentration equivalent to a low normal value. The preparation of purified hemoglobin solutions with good long-term stability is by no means a simple matter. The major problems to be overcome are maintenance of sterility and the avoidance of formation of precipitates on long-term storage under unfavorable conditions. These problems are somewhat lessened by using a concentrated solution of a pigment such as cyanmethemoglobin but this would largely defeat the object and purpose of the control material by bypassing the important step of pigment generation. Parenthetically, it might be noted that hemoglobin control material can be used for checking the accuracy of pipets and for testing the linearity of spectrophotometers and colorimeters in the chemistry laboratory as well as in the hematology laboratory.

3. *White Cell Counting Control.* This is a suspension of fixed avian or reptilian erythrocytes adjusted in concentration to yield a count which is usually set at the upper limit of normal. Fixative techniques similar to those used for human erythrocytes are found to be perfectly satisfactory for this purpose and the stability of such suspensions is equal to that of the fixed red cell counting control. However, in preparing white cell counting controls consideration must be given to simulating as closely as possible the size distribution of human leukocytes. This is achieved by mixing, in the appropriate proportion, the fixed erythrocytes of two or more avian or reptilian species. Fortunately, nature appears to be on our side in providing these animals with an extremely wide range of MCV from species to species. White cell counting controls of this type are quite suitable for revealing errors and inconsistencies in pipetting and diluting and are adequate for pinpointing failures in automatic cell counting instruments. But, of course, they provide no means for controlling the effectiveness of the hemolyzing agent used for the performance of white cell counts on whole blood. In manual counting procedures this, while a disadvantage, is not a serious one but in automated procedures the absence of control of the hemolysis phase of a white count can lead the hematologist into a veritable fool's paradise.

4. *Platelet Counting Controls.* We are not aware, at the present time,

of any satisfactory commercial platelet counting control. Nor does our research and development group consider that there is any immediate likelihood of being able to develop a platelet counting control which satisfies the requirements of the large number of techniques and variance on techniques currently in use. The preparation of suspensions of particles which simulate platelets in size and in concentration is not of itself a difficult matter but the sources of error in platelet counting extend far beyond the two elementary steps of diluting and counting. Indeed, as we all well know, the major sources of error probably lie in the method of specimen collection, transport and storage.

This brings me now to consideration of the original purpose of this communication, namely, a description of some of the specifications and manufacturing aspects of whole blood controls for use in quantitative hematology. I hope that the preceding remarks will have served their purpose in pointing out the fact that the use of individual controls for each constituent leaves many potential sources of error uncontrolled and that these uncontrolled factors are important causes of invalid data.

The whole blood hematology control must satisfy two basic requirements. These are:

1. As close as possible a simulation of all those properties of whole blood which have a bearing and influence upon the performance of quantitative measurement of its constituents.
2. A degree of stability which will allow replicate determinations of the constituents to be reproducible over a specified period of time to within the limits of precision of the techniques being used.

For the sake of simplicity we should limit our control material to be effective as regards red cell counting, hemoglobin measurement, hematocrit measurement, MCV, MCHC, and total white count.

A stable total white count is the easiest specification to achieve. This is done by substituting the original donor white cells by avian or reptilian fixed erythrocytes described earlier. This, of course, necessitates the removal of the donor's own white cells as completely as possible and in our experience such a removal is best achieved by filtering the freshly collected heparinized donor blood through nylon fiber filter columns according to the method of Greenwalt. This removes virtually all polymorphonuclear cells but allows a relatively high proportion of lymphocytes to pass through the filter. Lymphocytes must therefore be removed from the blood by successive differential centrifugation.

In order to preserve the integrity of the red cells for the desired length of time it is necessary to remove their native plasma and resuspend them in a medium which provides a proper electrolyte balance together with a source of colloid osmotic pressure. The exact composition of this medium cannot be revealed at the present time. It allows the red cells to maintain original size and shape and count for a minimum period of five weeks. It will, of course, be appreciated that the design of such a medium does not suffer the same constraints which are imposed upon a medium designed for transfusion purposes since problems of biological compatibility and toxicity do not enter into the picture.

One additional important step in the preparation of red cells for use in this control is the removal of red cells which are already approaching the end of their normal life span. It is well known that such cells do not withstand physical insult with the same fortitude as biologically younger cells. To achieve this separation use is made of the observation by Jandl that approximate distinctions between young and old cells may be made by differential centrifugation. Older cells tend to migrate more rapidly in a centrifugal field than do younger ones.

Thus by combining biologically young red cells with a medium which maintains the structural integrity of the cells without actually going as far as fixation and by then further combining this red cell suspension with a suitable concentration of avian or reptilian erythrocytes one has achieved a material which is eminently suitable for the control of the more important cellular constituents which are most commonly measured in the hematology laboratory.

There is no doubt that much further progress can be made along these lines. For example, polystyrene latex particles of a graded size may be added to this mixture to simulate platelets. Further studies in progress will undoubtedly extend the length of time over which this product will have an assured stability.

Finally I would like to stress again the point that this product and others of a similar nature cannot be economically prepared by the hematology laboratory itself. Only in industry will be found the facilities and personnel together with the capability of meticulous quality control of the product at all stages of its preparation.

2.6. The Mechanism of the Reaction $HbO_2 \rightarrow HiCN$

Takakata Matsubara, Second Department of Internal Medicine, Kumamoto University Medical School, Kumamoto, Japan, and Susumu Shibata, Department of Medicine (The Third Division), Yamaguchi University School of Medicine, Ube, Japan

1. *Dissociation of acid* Hi (Fig. 1)

We have found a pK' value of 8.04 for the dissociation constant of acid Hi (hemiglobin or methemoglobin) at an ionic strength of 0.08 and 25 °C.

The observed dissociation curve deviates slightly but systematically from the simplified theoretical curve, upward on the acid side of the pH of 8.04 and downward on the alkaline side.

This phenomenon can be explained by assuming that the ionic activity is reduced if acid and alkaline Hi subunits coexist in the same Hi molecule.

Figure 1

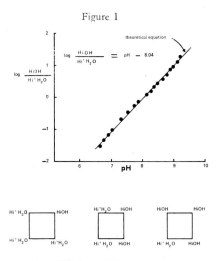

2. *Kinetics of the reaction* $HbO_2 \rightarrow$ Hi

Under conditions similar to those of the clinical Hb determinations the oxidation rate of HbO_2 to Hi fits the experimental equation indicated in Fig. 2.

The values for the velocity constant log k lie on an almost straight line that has a slope slightly steeper than 1 mol^{-1}.l.sec.$^{-1}$ (mol is related to a single of Fe) per pH unit between pH 6 and 8. In the range of pH higher than 8, the values were almost constant.

On the other hand, the exact values of the dissociation constant of $HbO_2 \rightarrow Hb + O_2$ are not yet known at present in the whole range of pH. Previous workers have found, however, that the dissociation of HbO_2 shows a maximum at a pH of about 6.5 and decreases both on the acid and alkaline side of this pH.

Figure 2

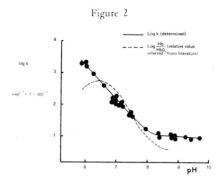

From the above-mentioned data, we conclude that the reaction from HbO₂ to Hi consists of the following elementary reactions (Tab. 1).

The first step is the dissociation of HbO₂ to Hb and oxygen.

The second step is the dissociation of a proton from the first heme-linked acid group, the pK' of which is about 5.25.

Table 1 – Elementary reactions of $HbO_2 \rightarrow Hi$

1     $HbO_2 \rightleftharpoons Hb + O_2$

2     $HHb \rightleftharpoons {}^- Hb + H^+$

    dissociation of the first heme-linked acid group, pK' 5.25

3     $HHb + Fe(CN)_6^{3-} + H_2O \xrightarrow{\text{1a}} HHi^+ \ H_2O + Fe(CN)_6^{4-}$

    ${}^-Hb + Fe(CN)_6^{3-} + H_2O \xrightarrow{\text{1b}} {}^-Hi^+ \ H_2O + Fe(CN)_6^{4-}$

    rate determining step   1a > 1b

4     $Hi^+ \ H_2O \rightleftharpoons HiOH + H^+$ pK' 8.04

The third is the rate determining step, consisting of two simultaneous reactions. It is worthwhile to mention that the velocity constant for non-dissociated reduced Hb is larger than that for dissociated reduced Hb. It is impossible, however, to calculate the values of the constants, because the exact value of the dissociation constant of HbO₂ is not known.

The fourth step is the dissociation of the acid Hi.

68

3. *Kinetics of the reaction* Hi → HiCN

Under conditions similar to those of the clinical Hb determinations the conversion rate of Hi to HiCN fits the experimental equation indicated in Fig. 3.

Figure 3

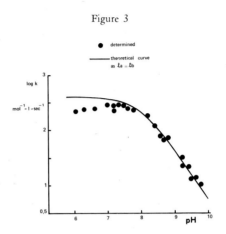

The values found for the velocity constant show a maximum at a pH of about 7.3, and lie on a nearly straight line that has a slope slightly steeper than $1 \text{ mol}^{-1}.\text{l.sec}^{-1}$ per pH unit between pH 8 and 10. On the acid side of pH 7, the values decrease slightly.

The mathematical analysis of these data allows to discuss the mechanism of the reaction.

Theoretically, the four elementary reactions indicated in Tab. 2 are possible, i.e. reactions between acid Hi and HCN or CN^-, and reactions between alkaline Hi and HCN or CN^-.

Table 2 – *Elementary reactions of Hi* ⟶ *HiCN*

1 $Hi^+ \ H_2O + HCN \xrightarrow{\ la\ } HiCN + H^+ + H_2O$

2 $Hi^+ \ H_2O + CN^- \xrightarrow{\ lb\ } HiCN + H_2O$

   $la = lb$
   $= 10^{2.63}$
   $\text{mol}^{-1} - 1 - \text{sec}^{-1}$
   $(25\,^\circ C \ \mu = 0.08)$

3 $HiOH + HCN \xrightarrow{\ ma\ } HiCN + H_2O$

4 $HiOH + CN^- \xrightarrow{\ mb\ } HiCN + OH^-$

   $ma, mb = 0$

Actually, the latter two reactions do not occur. The values of the velocity constant for the former two reactions are equal, $10^{2.63}$ $mol^{-1}.l.sec^{-1}$.

2.7. Evaluation of the Hemiglobinazide Method, in Comparison with the Hemiglobincyanide Method

Takakata Matsubara, Second Department of Internal Medicine, Kumamoto University Medical School, Kumamoto, Japan, and Susumu Shibata, Department of Medicine (The Third Division), Yamaguchi University School of Medicine, Ube, Japan

The absorption spectrum of HiN_3 is similar to that of HiCN (Fig. 1). The concentration of hemoglobin can be calculated from the optical density of HiN_3 at the maximum wavelength 542 to 543 nm. The millimolar extinction coefficient of HiN_3 was 1.032 times as much as that of HiCN.

Figure 1

	$Hi N_3$	HiCN
λ min	501 ∿ 502	503 ∿ 504
λ max	542 ∿ 543	540 ∿ 542
Quotient	1.62 ∿ 1.64	1.60 ∿ 1.62
$\varepsilon HiN_3 / \varepsilon HiCN$	1.032	1
pH range	where optical density is constant 6.2 ∿ 7.5	6.2 ∿ 9.8

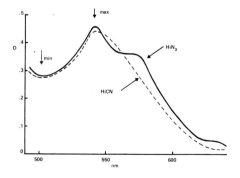

The purity of HiN₃ can be checked by measuring the ratio $D^{\lambda\,max}/D_{\lambda\,min}$. The value lies between 1.62 and 1.64. The pH range where the optical densities are constant is 6.2 to 7.5, narrower than that of HiCN (6.2 to 9.8).

Our experiments showed that the affinity of Hi (hemiglobin or methemoglobin) for azide is smaller than that for cyanide (Fig. 2). The equilibrium constant pK for azide was 5.60 mol^{-1} (mol is related to a single atom of iron) while that for cyanide was 6.26 (pH 7.1, ionic

Figure 2

Equilibrium constant   pH 7,1   μ 0,08   25°C

total Hi + N₃ ⇌ Hi N₂   total Hi + total CN ⇌ Hi CN

pK = 5.60 mol⁻¹·l   pK = 6.26 mol⁻¹·l

100% = 4 x 10⁻⁵ mol·l⁻¹
(64.5 mg/dl)

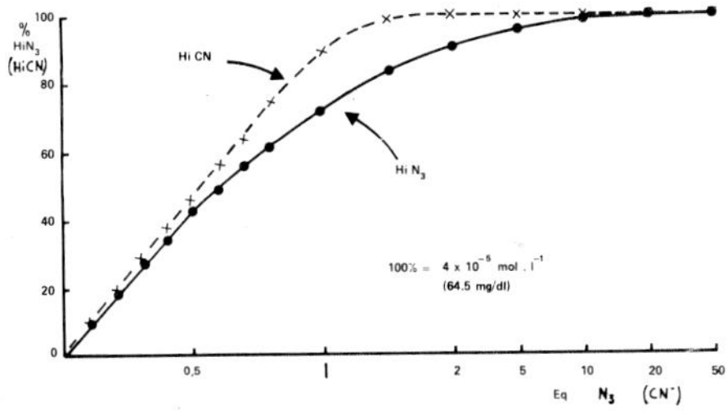

Figure 3

Velocity constant   pH 7,1   μ 0,08   25°C

reagent	Na N₃	K C N
reaction	Hi + N₃ → HiN₃	Hi + total CN→HiCN
forward constant	250	217
	mol⁻¹·l·sec⁻¹	
backward constant	25.4	2.89
	sec⁻¹	

Hi, NaN₃, KCN 4 x 10⁻⁵ mol·l⁻¹

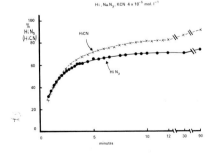

strength 0.08, 25 °C). Consequently, the conversion of Hi to HiN₃ required a larger excess of the anion. For example, to convert 0.04 millimol per liter of Hi completely 20 equivalents were required with NaN₃, while 2 equivalents were sufficient with KCN.

The velocity constant (Fig. 3) for the forward reaction $Hi \rightarrow HiN_3$ was 250 $mol^{-1}.l.sec^{-1}$, slightly larger than that HiCN (217). On the other hand, the velocity constant for the backward reaction of the former was 25.4 sec^{-1}, about 10 times as much as that of the latter (2.89 sec^{-1}).

Our conclusions are summarized in Table 1. The azide method is superior to the cyanide method, as is well known, on the points of stability on freezing and toxicity. On the other hand the cyanide method is superior on the points of breadth of the maximum band, degree of affinity between Hi and CN^- and wide range of pH.

Table 1 – Comparison of HiN₃ method with HiCN method

item	H_1N_3		HiCN
breadth of λmax		<	superior
complete coversion		≪	superior
pH range		≪	superior
velocity	superior	≧	
stability on freezing	superior	≫	
toxicity	superior	≫	

in short

HiCN – superior in accuracy
HiN₃ – superior in practicality

2.8. Discussion

After a short discussion between Drs. Lewis, Zettner, Brecher and Helleman regarding different types of pipets, Dr. Richardson Jones informed the meeting of the difference in « calibrated as to volume » and « calibrated to deliver ».

Dr. Zettner asked Dr. van Assendelft, whether detergents were used in the determination of $\varepsilon_{540}^{HiN_3}$

O.W. van Assendelft. « Yes, they were. What did surprise us, by the way, was the excellent agreement between the extinction coefficients determined using washed cells and using whole blood samples ».

Dr. Zettner answered that he believed plasma proteins themselves to play but a slight role in turbidity. Dr. Matsubara then presented his comparison results of the HiCN and the HiN_3 method.

W.G. Zijlstra. « While in Washington last week during the congress of physiological sciences I ran across an exhibit by Coulter Electronics. They stated that they had found a new reagent and could now perform a reliable and accurate haemoglobin determination in 7 to 10 sec. When I asked for further particulars I was told that the people present did not know, and even if they had known they would not have told because the whole process was secret ».

Dr. Brecher answered to this that it might be possible that e.g. 95 % conversion takes place and that, because the machine always measures with exactly the same time lag, more or less reliable results could perhaps be obtained. Mr. Moran stated that he had for years asked that the HiCN spectrum should be judged by looking for a hump at $\lambda = 578$ nm. If present this would indicate incomplete conversion. He finally urged more frequent and intensive contacts between manufacturers and scientists, especially European scientists.

Dr. Zettner answered by saying that he had already advised Mr. Moran some years ago that the method of acquiring contacts was for the manufacturers to also publish in scientific journals. Mr. Ferro (Coulter diagnostics) then said that manufacturers can only publish after they have made their money out of a new product.

*Symposium of the International Committee
for Standardization in Hematology
Moderator: G. Brecher
3. Hematology of Normal Man*

3.1. Standardization of Haemoglobinometry: Establishing the Reference Point

W.G. Zijlstra, E.J. van Kampen and O.W. van Assendelft, Groningen, the Netherlands

Establishing the reference point in haemoglobinometry is to a certain extent a matter of choice. This, however, does not imply that the point of reference can be chosen arbitrarily. Establishing the reference point primarily involves a double decision on the soundness of which its value and durability depend. The first decision concerns the selection of a physical or chemical property of haemoglobin, which can be measured both easily and accurately. The second one is to adopt one or more methods to exactly correlate the result of the physico-chemical measurement with a certain amount of haemoglobin. Theoretically, it would seem that these decisions involve a choice from a multitude of possibilities. Most of these possibilities, however, are either unreliable or unpractical or both.

Among the few physico-chemical properties of haemoglobin, which can be measured easily and accurately, the absorption of visible light has been the one most widely used. With modern spectrophotometers the optical density of a haemoglobin solution can be measured to within $\pm 0.5 \%$. It needs little argument that in the solution to be measured all haemoglobin must be converted into one and the same derivative, or at least into types of haemoglobin which are photometrically indistinguishable at the wavelength of measurement. As to the haemoglobin derivative most suitable in this respect, there is little difference of opinion. Haemiglobincyanide (HiCN) is almost universally recognized as the most suitable compound. It is the most stable of all known haemoglobin derivatives, it has a favourable absorption spectrum with a flat maximum around $\lambda = 540$ nm, it follows Lambert-Beer's law over a wide concentration range and the haemoglobin derivatives commonly present in human blood can, by simple means, be completely converted into HiCN. The first decision thus can be made without evoking much controversy. The quantity to be measured is the optical density of HiCN solutions at $\lambda = 540$ nm (D_{HiCN}^{540}).

The second decision is a little more difficult. First it should be decided whether to choose either a method based on some functional property of haemoglobin, e.g. oxygen or carbon monoxide binding capacity, or an analytical method based on the chemical composition of the haemoglobin molecule. Although from a physiological point of view standardization of haemoglobinometry on the basis of the oxygen binding capacity may seem to be desirable, both the existence of temporarily inactive haemoglobin — e.g. haemiglobin, which in human blood is continuously being formed and again reduced to haemoglobin — and the technical difficulties and uncertainties in blood gas analysis, favour the use of an analytical method aimed at the chemical composition of haemoglobin. Moreover, the complete elucidation of the composition of the haemoglobin molecule [1, 2] has added a strong argument in favour of chemical analysis.

Having chosen for chemical analysis, the next step is to choose the most suitable atomic species among the six (C, H, O, N, S and Fe) contained in the haemoglobin molecule. Although N has been proved suitable [10], Fe appeared to be the atom of choice. This brings about the last, perhaps the most crucial, certainly the most debated choice to be made. Which method(s) should be selected to determine haemoglobin iron?

In this connection it should be noted that the determination of « absolute » chemical values must ultimately be based upon a direct method of analysis, i.e. a gravimetric or volumetric one. Indirect methods are not suitable for the determination of chemical quantities, unless properly prepared standard solutions based on weight analysis are used and all possible interfering factors have been thoroughly studied, preferably by repeated comparison with a direct method of analysis. These safeguards having been taken, the spectrophotometric iron determination using α,α'-dipyridyl [19] and the haemoglobin iron determination by X ray emission spectrography [6] have been developed into reliable technics. Atomic absorption spectrophotometry, on the other hand, has been shown to be inadequate for the « absolute » determination of haemoglobin iron, mainly because of the influence of the method of sample preparation upon the results [12].

As an example of a practical direct method for the determination of haemoglobin iron the titrimetric method with titanous chloride [19] may be mentioned. To 1 ml of a haemoglobin solution in a digestion tube 1 ml concentrated sulphuric acid and 250 mg potassium sulphate is added and intensive electric heating started. After 30 min heating is interrupted for 5 min and 1 ml of sulphuric acid and 0.5 ml of 30 % hydrogen peroxide added. The addition of peroxide is repeated twice, after 1 and 2 h, the total digestion time thus amounting to 3 $\frac{1}{2}$ h. After cooling 10 ml water and 1 ml 20 % potassium thiocyanate are added and the titration with titanous chloride is carried out in the digestion tube at room temperature in a CO_2 atmosphere. The $TiCl_3$ solution is frequently standardized against an iron stock solution of ferric ammonium sulphate. The iron content of the ferric ammonium sulphate is repeatedly checked by gravimetric analysis and the salt is stored in an atmosphere corresponding to the water vapour pressure of the crystals (6 mm Hg).

After measuring D_{HiCN}^{540} of a clear solution of exactly known millimolar concentration of haemoglobin in a calibrated 1.000 cm glass cuvette by means of a spectrophotometer of which wavelength and optical density scales have been checked using mercury emission lines and a NBS carbon yellow or similar reference filter respectively, the millimolar extinction coefficient can be calculated. $D = \varepsilon\, cl$ and, since $l = 1$, $\varepsilon = c/D$. Table 1 shows the results of 16 series of determinations of the quarter-millimolar extinction coefficient by 10 research groups in 7 countries (Germany, France, the Netherlands, U.K., Italy, U.S.A. and Sweden). In all but two series of measurements adult human blood was used. One research group used horse blood, another one human foetal blood. In a few series whole blood was used, in others the haemoglobin solutions had been more or less purified by various methods. All but one series of determinations were based on iron analysis, only Tentori et al. [10] resorted to N analysis.

From the data of Table 1 a total mean value and corresponding standard error of the mean have been calculated using the equations

$$x_g = \frac{1}{n_{tot}} \cdot \Sigma_i\, n_i \cdot x_i$$

$$\frac{s^2}{n_{tot}} = \frac{1}{n_{tot} \cdot (n_{tot} - 1)} \cdot \Sigma_i\, (n_i - 1) \cdot s^2_i + n_i \cdot (x_i - x_g)^2$$

where x_g = mean value of all determinations

x_i = mean value of the i-th series of determinations

76

Table 1 – ϵ 540 HiCN as reported by different authors, based on iron or nitrogen determination.

author	material	ϵ 540 HiCN	$s/\sqrt{n}$	n	method
Meyer-Wilmes and Remmer (4)	horse Hb	11.0	0.04	12	Fe; o-Phenantrolin
Remmer (7)	horse Hb	11.0	0.04	12	Fe; TiCl$_3$
	human whole blood	11.09	0.03	11	Fe; TiCl$_3$
	human whole blood	11.19	0.065	4	Fe; complexon
Minkowski and Swierczewski (5)	foetal whole blood	11.15	–	5	Fe; o-Phenantrolin
Zijlstra and Van Kampen (19)	human Hb, toluene	10.99	0.01	123	Fe; α, α'-dipyridyl
	haemolysis	10.94	0.03	35	Fe; α, α'-dipyridyl
		11.05	0.02	101	Fe; TiCl$_3$
Wootton and Blevin (17)	human Hb, toulene haemolysis	10.68	0.04	14	Fe; ferric perchlorate
Van Oudheusden et al. (15)	human whole blood	10.99	0.05	10	Fe; α, α'-dipyridyl
	human whole blood	11.06	0.08	8	Fe; α, α'-dipyridyl
Salvati et al .(8)	human Hb purified on CMC column	10.95	0.03	46	Fe; α, α'-dipyridyl
Tentori et al. (10)	human Hb purified on CMC column	10.90	0.05	55	N analysis
Morningstar et al. (6)	human whole blood	11.02	0.03	10	Fe; X ray emission spectrography
	human washed cells	10.97	0.07	6	
Stigbrand (9)	human Hb purified on CMC or Sephadex column or by dialysis against Na$_2$–EDTA	11.00	0.02	55	Fe; sulfosalicylic acid

$s/\sqrt{n}$ – standard error of the mean; n – number of determinations

n_{tot} = total number of determinations
n_i = number of determinations in the i-th series
s_i = standard deviation of the i-th series of determinations
s = standard deviation of all determinations

When the work of Minkowski and Swierczewski [5], who did not publish their standard deviation, is excluded, a mean value of 10.98 is obtained for ε_{HiCN}^{540} $n = 502$, $s/\sqrt{n} = 0.009$. The result of one series of determinations, that of Wootton and Blevin [17], differs more than 3 times the standard error of the mean from the total mean value. Exclusion of this series brings ε_{HiCN}^{540} at 10.99, $n = 488$, $s/\sqrt{n} = 0.009$.

The quarter-millimolar extinction coefficient thus having been determined, standardized haemoglobinometry may be performed by means of any spectrophotometer, provided proper wavelength calibration and absorption checks have been made.

When the spectrophotometer does not fulfill the necessary requirements or when a filter photometer is used, a HiCN standard solution [13] of exactly known concentration is necessary for calibration. As clear HiCN solutions follow Lambert-Beer's law, a single concentration of the standard solution is sufficient for establishing a reliable calibration line. To enable manufacturers of HiCN standard solutions to check their products as to conformity with the requirements put forward by ICSH [3], an international reference solution is prepared on behalf of ICSH by the Dutch Institute of Public Health (R.I.V., Utrecht, the Netherlands). Each batch is tested at regular intervals by laboratories in Germany, the Netherlands, Sweden, the U.K. and the U.S.A. The control data collected from November 1964 till March 1967 have been published recently [11].

The concentration of HiCN standard solutions is usually given in mg/100 ml. This is possible since the molecular weight of haemoglobin (64500 for Hb4) has been calculated exactly from the completely known molecular composition [1, 2]. The same exact value for the molecular weight is also used to convert concentrations in mmol/1 as derived from spectrophotometric measurements based on the millimolar extinction coefficient, into g/100 ml.

Although some technical points, especially concerning clinical haemoglobinometry (methods of obtaining blood samples, calibration of pipettes, stability of reagent solutions etc.) are still under discussion, the fundamentals of standardized haemoglobinometry have now been firmly established. The extinction coefficient of HiCN, the molecular weight of haemoglobin and the international reference solution are in our opinion the solid basis upon which in the forseeable future haemo-globinometry should rest.

As to the nature of future fundamental research in this field, two rather resistant problems present themselves. The first one could be considered to be one of the technical points mentioned above, but its more fundamental character justifies special consideration. Mixing a blood sample with the reagent solution provides a crude HiCN solution, which may display slight turbidity. Of this solution the optical density is measured, either spectrophotometrically on the basis of ε_{HiCN}^{540} or by means of a filter photometer calibrated with a clear HiCN standard solution. The turbidity of the diluted blood sample thus may cause a slight positive error, the magnitude of which depends on the reagent solution used. Using Drabkin's solution the error may be as high as 6%, but also with the reagent recommended by Van Kampen and Zijlstra [14] errors of 1-2% frequently occur. So it is not yet possible to strictly come up to the requirement of ICSH, that the reagent « must be of such a quality that after dilution of the blood there is no turbidity » [3]. Future research should provide a stable reagent solution giving perfectly clear solutions in the shortest possible time (preferably < 3 min).

The second problem results from the decision to determine ε_{HiCN}^{540} on the basis of the composition of the haemoglobin molecule, instead of its functional capability. Theoretically, each iron atom binds one molecule of oxygen, the oxygen binding capacity thus amounting to 1.39 ml O_2 per gram Hb. As a small amount of « inactive » haemoglobin, i.e. haemoglobin derivatives unable to combine with oxygen, is always present in human blood, the actual oxygen binding capacity of human haemoglobin *in vivo* will be less than 1.39 ml/g. It is worthwhile to determine the actual oxygen capacity per gram haemoglobin as accurately as possible, because the relationship between oxygen capacity and haemoglobin concentration is of prime importance in human physiology. In a pilot investigation Zijlstra et al. [18] used the Van Slyke-Neill method [16] for the determination of the oxygen content of blood samples equilibrated with gas mixtures containing 40% O_2, and the spectrophotometric HiCN method based on ε_{HiCN}^{540} to determine the haemoglobin concentration of the samples. An average value of 1.31 ml/g was found in this series, with a standard error of 0.0033 ml/g (n = 20). Thus it would seem that the red cell contains an appreciable amount of haemoglobin derivatives which cannot combine with oxygen. Speculation as to the nature and cause of this inactive haemoglobin, however, should certainly be postponed until these data have been confirmed in a larger series of experiments performed in several laboratories, using various technics for the determination of the oxygen capacity.

References

[1] Braunitzer, G., Gehring-Müller, R., Hilschmann, N., Hilse, K., Hobom, G., Rudloff, V. and Wittmann-Liebold, B., « Die Konstitution des normalen adulten Humanhämoglobins », *Hoppe-Seylers Z. physiol. Chem.*, 325, 283, 1961

[2] Hill, R.J., Konigsberg, W., Guidotti, G. and Craig, L.C., « The Structure of Human Hemoglobin. I. The Separation of the α and β Chains and Their Amino acid Composition », *J. biol. Chem.*, 237, 1549, 1962

[3] International Committee for Standardization in Haematology, « Recommendations for Haemoglobinometry in Human Blood », *Brit. J. Haemat.*, 13 (Suppl.), 71, 1967

[4] Meyer-Wilmes, J. and Remmer, H., « Die Standardisierung des roten Blutfarbstoffes durch Hämiglobincyanid. I. Mitteilung. Bestimmung der spezifischen Extinktion von Hämiglobincyanid », *Arch exp. Path. Pharmacol.*, 229, 441, 1956

[5] Minkowski, A. and Swierczewski, E., « The Oxygen Capacity of Human Foetal Blood », In : *Oxygen Supply to the Human Foetus* (Editors : J. Walker and A. Turnbull), Blackwell, Oxford, 1959, pp. 237-253

[6] Morningstar, D.A., Williams, G.Z. and Suutarinen, P. « The Millimolar Extinction Coefficient of Cyanmethemoglobin from Direct Measurements of Iron by X-ray Emission Spectrography », *Amer. J. clin. Path.*, 46, 603, 1966

[7] Remmer, H., « Die Standardisierung des roten Blutfarbstoffes durch Hämoglobincyanid. II. Mitteilung. Eisengehalt und O_2-Bindungsvermögen von menschlichem Blut », *Arch. exp. Path. Pharmakol.*, 229, 450, 1956

[8] Salvati, A.M., Tentori, L. and Vivaldi, G., « The Extinction Coefficient of Human Hemiglobincyanide », *Clin. chim. Acta*, 11, 477, 1965

[9] Stigbrand, T., « Molar Absorbancy of Cyanmethaemoglobin », *Scand. J. clin. Lab. Invest.*, 20, 252, 1967

[10] Tentori, L., Vivaldi, G. and Salvati, A.M., « The Extinction Coefficient of Human Haemiglobincyanide as Determined by Nitrogen Analysis », *Clin. chim. Acta*, 14, 276, 1966

[11] Van Assendelft, O.W., Holtz, A.H., Van Kampen E.J. and Zijlstra, W.G., « Control Data of International Haemiglobincyanide Reference Solutions », *Clin. chim. Acta*, 18, 78, 1967

[12] Van Assendelft, O.W., Zijlstra, W.G., Buursma, A., Van Kampen, E.J. and Hoek, W., « The Use of Atomic Absorption Spectrophotometry for the Measurement of Haemoglobin-iron, with Special Reference to the Determination of ε_{HiCN}^{540} », *Clin. chim. Acta*, in press

[13] Van Assendelft, O.W., Zijlstra, W.G., Van Kampen, E.J. and Holtz A.H., « Stability of Haemiglobincyanide Reference Solutions », *Clin. chim. Acta*, 13, 521, 1966

[14] Van Kampen, E.J. and Zijlstra, W.G., « Standardization of Haemoglobinometry. II. The Hemiglobincyanide Method », *Clin. chim. Acta*, 6, 538, 1961

[15] Van Oudheusden, A.P.M., Van de Heuvel, J.M., Van Stekelenburg, G.J., Siertsema, L.H. and Wadman, S.K., « De ijking van de haemoglobinebepaling op basis van ijzer (Calibration of the haemoglobin determination based on iron) », *Ned. T. Geneesk.*, 108, 265, 1964

[16] Van Slyke, D.D. and Neill, J.M., « Determination of Gases in Blood and Other Solutions by Vacuum Extraction and Manometric Measurement », *J. biol. Chem.*, 61, 523, 1924

80

[17] Wootton, I.D.P. and Blevin, W.R., « The Extinction Coefficient of Cyanmethaemoglobin », *Lancet, 434,* 1964 II
[18] Zijlstra, W.G., Van Assendelft, O.W. and Rijskamp, A., « Oxygen Capacity of Normal Human Blood », *Acta physiol. pharmacol. neerl., 13,* 229, 1965
[19] Zijlstra, W.G. and Van Kampen, E.J., « Standardization of Haemoglobinometry. I. The Extinction Coefficient of Hemiglobincyanide at $\lambda = 540$ mμ: ε_{HICN}^{540} », *Clin. chim. Acta, 5,* 719, 1960

3.2. Problems of Conducting an Hemoglobin Survey in Latin America

Joginder G. Chopra, Adviser on Nutrition Research, Pan American Health Organization, Regional Office of the World Health Organization, Washington, D.C., U.S.A.

Introduction

One of the most widely used methods in appraisal of nutritional status is the determination of hemoglobin in the blood. The mean level of hemoglobin and the percentage of persons with value below the accepted range of normal have been considered good indices of the general health of the population [1]. Impaired nutrition should be suspected if more than three per cent of an adult population has hemoglobin levels of 12 gm per 100 ml or less at sea level [2].

Many adverse environmental conditions, numerous pathologic states, particularly infections and diseases associated with blood loss, and several dietary factors are important in the production of anemia.

Iron deficiency is the most common dietary factor leading to anemia but deficiency of protein, folic acid or other less well defined nutrients such as the extrinsic factor may be of etiologic importance.

I deal in the paper with the problems of conducting hemoglobin surveys in Latin America. Suggestions have also been made for the solution of some of the problems frequently encountered in undertaking these investigations.

Hemoglobin Field Survey

This is a cross-section study seeking to determine the number of cases of anemia present at a particular time in relation to the size of the population in which they occur. Technically, it is a prevalence study. The objectives are variable, sometimes to determine the occurrence of anemia, or to assess the effects of supplying specific hematinic in known dosage to those individuals in an area whose evidence of deficiency has been recorded before therapy [3]. The approach in a field survey can be laboratory or clinical. Usually the two combine to advantage, adding precision to the study.

To make the hematological information meaningful, certain basic facts about the subject must be obtained, such as: age, sex, occupation, activity, height, weight, history and so forth. The specific items may vary with the hypothesis to be tested. All auxiliary data needed in the interpretation of the hematological data should be anticipated and obtained at the time when data is collected [4]. There should be a realization of the time cost, cooperation, and the degree of precision necessary to obtain a picture of the hematological status of an individual.

Surveys of various types in localized areas of many countries of Latin America and on special groups are by no means new. Dietary and clinical studies have been made quite frequently. Except for the ICNND surveys and WHO collaborative studies on nutritional anemias, laboratory investigations have been fragmentary and limited to a few surveys of red blood cell and hemoglobin determinations on special groups as pregnant and lactating women and rural and urban school children. Most of these were done in the central area of the country and, therefore, may or may not reflect conditions prevalent all over the country.

Field Reconnaissance and Organization of the Survey

The first step in any field study is to assure the support and cooperation of governmental authorities in the region where the work is done, especially those responsible for public health. After discussion on objectives and study plan, field reconnaissance determines the practicability of operation in what is judged as suitable area.

During the pre-survey period the objectives, scope, and need for collaboration and assistance (including financial and personnel), are discussed with those governmental, university and research organizations of the country that are vitally involved in public health activities. These include Ministries of Health, governmental and private research organizations, organizations assisting the country through bilateral agreements or in collaboration with the United Nations agencies such as FAO, WHO and UNICEF. In the initial briefing, guidance and advice should be obtained from all these agencies regarding data and information that will be required for preparing the background report and for the development of preliminary plans for the survey. This includes information concerning the various ethnic and population groups which have unique hematological problems.

A review of literature at this stage on what has been done will tell of successes and failures in relation to the particular problem and in the general field. Facilities of a library for the review are often lacking in several countries. Under such circumstances, consultation with colleagues or visits to contemporary studies may prove to be helpful. Preliminary assessment of the place where the work is to be done is one principle in field investigation, never to be violated. There is no substitute for personal observation.

The first obligation is to establish working relations with local health and administrative authorities and through their introduction to consult with physicians who have been working in the field. Omissions have been the source of future difficulties or even failure of the project.

It is good sense to start with national or state health authorities and through them with administrative departments, but not to the neglect of local officials. That is where the work is to be done and it is sound investment to establish solid understanding of what is proposed, to enlist the desired cooperation, and to assure the importance attached to the community contribution.

Technically, now is the time to start a field diary. Details escape, especially names, titles and addresses, information of much value in the eventual planning of the study.

In regions unfamiliar to the investigator, and especially in another country, personal knowledge of people, language, terrain, and facilities within the study area enter strongly into planning. Professional colleagues of the country scarcely can reflect the reactions to strangers or the effect of customs, habits and traditions on the results.

The time required to effect a going organization varies with the locality, the project and plan of operation. A month may suffice, six to eight weeks is more likely, especially in another country.

It is peculiar and yet almost invariable circumstance that this phase in the development of a field study always seems to take longer than anticipated. Still the future flow of operation and the satisfaction with results obtained are strongly influenced by the time given to preparation.

Sampling Procedures

In most surveys, an attempt is generally made to obtain a stratified sample of the entire population for inclusion in the survey.

Often this is not possible as much more advanced planning is required and also because census and the Vital Statistics Bureau data are incomplete and recognizably inaccurate. Furthermore, data may not be available for all the sites to be included in the survey [5]. Because of these and other logistical problems, this goal is considered unpractical for several areas of Latin America.

The proportion of the sample families that are generally seen by the survey team vary from 17-45 per cent with an overall average of 30 per cent [6].

The other survey sampling procedure frequently employed with success is not designed to obtain a true cross sectional sample of the country's population properly weighed to give balanced representation of various economic, ethnic and geographical groups. This is designed to place the major emphasis of the study upon those groups in which the problems of anemia might be expected to be of the greater importance, namely the low income group, both rural and urban, pregnant and lactating women, and children. However, it should never be concluded that the results of these studies represent the average hemoglobin levels of the population as a whole, but rather that they reflect the major problems which confront a large and significant segment of the people [7, 8, 9, 10].

Additional factors that may influence the sampling procedures and should be considered are the heavy concentration of the population groups in certain areas of the country, and the presence of sparsely inhabited and relatively isolated community groups in several parts of Latin America.

An unexplained circumstance which occurs sometimes, is that a large number of people present themselves at survey sites as volunteers [6-11]. The age and sex structure of the volunteer population, when compared to that of the random population, is seen to differ. The volunteer population has generally a higher proportion of children aged 5-14 and male adults, but smaller population of women and of children under five, than the random population. This tendency is more marked in urban areas.

In order to determine if the volunteer population was representative of the random population, the following study was carried out. In two locations a comparison was made of hematocrit values obtained from those coming voluntarily to the field center with those from a random subsample of the households in which the hemoglobin studies were made. It was seen that variations by age and sex grouping between those checked at home and those seen at the center was minimal. Thus, it would appear that the volunteer population is representative of the random population when evaluated within the specific age groups 5-14 and 15 plus [11].

In some instances, larger than expected number of families may result from situations where more than 50 per cent of the dwelling units are found to be occupied by more than one family [12]. Often, the sample consists chiefly of pre-school and school age children and women. Very few adults present themselves for examination as they cannot frequently be induced to come for an examination because of the need to pursue their daily occupation [9].

Another major problem that is difficult to overcome is that in the majority of instances not all the members of the family are seen. This is illustrated by the fact that a total of 1696 persons from 734 families were examined, 2.3 persons per family. This is lower than the 3.6 persons per family obtained during the pre-survey census [6]. The persons that are left behind are usually non-ambulatory, such as the pre-scholars, malnourished, and the aged.

In order to obtain the desired sample and maximum cooperation, families on the sample blocks should preferably be visited once and often twice by a group of social workers who precede the survey team by one to three days. Each family should be given an appointment slip for a specific time. Newspaper, radio and television coverage of the survey activities are valuable as a propaganda in a few « barrios ». Neighborhood committee and extra encouragement by the local health center personnel are of great help in convincing people to participate [13-14].

On occasions a sound truck can be used for 2 or 3 days prior to the date of proposed examination to announce to the people the time of the examination and its purpose. On the day of the examination a repetitive announcement of similar nature may be made.

Inter-personal Relationships

The willingness and ability of the subject to cooperate is necessary in any field survey and especially in those where blood samples are a requisite. It is not easy to obtain cooperation from people who have been subjected to visits by health teams but who, on the contrary, have learned from previous experience to avoid outside visitors [19]. It is felt that progress might be most rapidly brought about in certain areas by working with leaders and that a thorough knowledge of their habits and attitudes would be essential for such efforts [15-16]. However, despite working through the leaders, it is sometimes found impossible to carry out fully the planned procedure on most of the more « traditional groups », where the attitude is of suspicious uncooperativeness.

Modern medicine including chemotherapy are not wanted for even severe illnesses, a situation quite understandable if related to the totally different concepts of disease existing in the local culture. In addition, fear is expressed that the team's efforts would result in the sore arms that have been the result of previous vaccination and TAB campaigns. Under these circumstances, the only possible course is house-to-house examination [17].

The effectiveness of various methods used in hemoglobin surveys depend greatly on the type of population involved. Some of the techniques for the more developed countries are obviously impractical for under-developed areas. When working in less sophisticated societies in which illiteracy and poverty are general characteristics of most of the groups, the classic methods of organizing surveys are inappropriate and the skill of the field worker becomes more important in order to obtain the cooperation of the subjects.

Field and Laboratory Sites

A health center operated under the state or federal health agencies serves effectively as the center for survey activities in the field. Assembly of family groups at the survey site is largely accomplished by the local public health complement of workers.

Under the existing field conditions in Latin America, most of the laboratory examinations can only be carried out satisfactorily at the base laboratory. The base of operations should preferably be a university, a hospital, a research institute or an official health agency, having several of the following functions: It should provide administrative direction, it should be the source of staff and supplies and also furnish central laboratory and statistical services. Sound policy is to separate research from general activities by establishing a special unit.

The laboratory space should be equipped with running water (preferably hot and cold) and a large sink for washing glassware. A constant source of electricity capable of a 100 ampere load is necessary to ensure the proper functioning of the laboratory's electrical equipment. During preliminary planning for the survey, the exact nature of the electrical supply at the prospective laboratory site should be determined so that proper electrical equipment, transformers and adapters can be purchased. A telephone and refrigeration facilities are required.

Recruitment and Training of Local Personnel

Other considerations include available number, competence and reliability of local recruits to the technical staff, with bilingual ability sometimes a feature. The field staff should be recruited and trained with a clear definition of responsibilities.

The use of the laboratory methods for the estimation of hematological levels necessitates the training of laboratory technicians in these procedures. The demand of such trained personnel has exceeded the supply and at the termination of the survey many of these technicians may become permanent members of the laboratory staff in the hospitals and health departments.

Perhaps more important, however, than the training of technical personnel is the incentive which the survey provides for the biochemists to develop methods which may be applicable in mass studies and the opportunity to test these methods in practice.

Requirements for field staff are obviously a function of the problem under study and the volume and complexity of the data to be collected. The field director, ordinarily a physician, recruits his key staff members. Large scale and particularly foreign projects also require an assistant director to ensure satisfactory direction. A laboratory worker with qualifications suited to the problem is a primary member of the staff. The statistician of a field study group departs from his usual status of an office worker. He may be stationed wholly in the field or divide his time between base and field station but under any arrangement he should participate in active field work, sufficiently to evaluate quality of record keeping, completeness of collected information, and methods used.

Another key person is the supervisor of field workers, who is responsible for directing the work of the day on data collection. This is a most consequential position, and in our experience no one quite equals a public health nurse. Recruiting general-trained field workers is often quite a problem. The first choice is again the public health nurse, as trained field workers are often unavailable in several countries of South America.

A command of the country's language and familiarity with the environment, aims and outlook of the people make persons of local origin highly desirable. For some areas, male and female workers are required in order to obtain maximum community cooperation.

Hemoglobin and Hematocrit Determinations

There are many methods for the determination of hemoglobin, none of which are ideal under field conditions. The field laboratory for the determination of hemoglobin and hematocrit should be located, if possible, in the detailed clinical examination area. If field conditions do not permit, the samples of necessity have to be transported to the base laboratory for analyses. The most important feature of collection is to have a free movement of the samples to avoid confusion and duplication of responsibility. Each technician must clearly understand his responsibilities and must be taught to appreciate the virtues of teamwork. If the supervisory technician can be free to move in where needed, much time can be saved and the free flow of the samples can go on unimpeded. The number of biochemical samples to be collected depends upon the number of persons that present themselves for examination, the satisfaction of statistical requirements for a sufficient sample size, and the ability of the laboratory to handle a given number of samples. The collection of the blood should be planned so as to ensure that a minimum of time will elapse between the collection and transportation of the samples to the main laboratory. When possible, a 3-5 ml sample of blood should be taken in oxalated or EDTA vacutainer tubes [8].

After water-proof labelling and packaging for shipment, they should be immediately stored at ice-box temperature (not frozen). For the bulk of field work, disposable vacutainer needles give highly satisfactory results. This procedure avoids the usual problem of maintaining functionally clean, sharp and sterile needles that are often a source of difficulty, although it is possible to obtain perfectly satisfactory sanitary and handling procedures with the regular non-disposable vacutainer or syringe-type needles. For the routine field surveys, the disposable needles are superior because precautions are not always taken with regular equipment.

Two difficulties that are often encountered with the blood procedure are the following:

a) a tendency to clotting traceable to inadequate mixing of the samples;
b) hemolysis of some samples.

The first is easily rectified by stopping the flow of blood before the tube is completely full and immediately mixing the sample by gentle multiple inversions of the tube.

The second is in part traceable to vigorous mixing in the field and it has also been observed that after storage and transit to the laboratory, the red cells became sufficiently more friable to cause a slight hemolysis upon performing the necessary mixing to ensure an homogeneous sample for the aliquot for hematocrit and hemoglobin determinations [8].

Some degree of hemolysis is best prevented by making sure that centrifuge tubes are dry, that the needle is removed from the syringe before blood is introduced gently down the side. In the West Indies survey [12], it was found that a large number of hemolysed samples were obtained with oxalate and especially if the samples stood for a long time before analysis. On the other hand, similar tubes containing EDTA (ethylene diamine tetra acetic acid) as an anticoagulant, gave excellent unhemolysed supernatant and, therefore, this procedure for collection was highly recommended by this group.

It is often not possible [9, 8, 18] to do venipunctures on small children and some adults. Under these circumstances, Sahli hemoglobin pipet and small heparinized capillary tubes for hematocrit determinations should be filled with blood from finger tip puncture.

The method of choice for hemoglobin determination is the cyanmethemoglobin and, for hematocrit, the Wintrobe technique [19]. When insufficient amount of blood is available, microhematocrit may be used. Although these methods have been selected for reliability, the experienced biochemist knows that any analytical procedure is subject to numerous possible errors. In surveys where wide variations of even constant abnormal values may result, it is not possible to judge a method merely by the appearance of results. It is essential that a laboratory control program be included in order to obtain a measure of precision and accuracy. Day by day quality control of hemoglobin determination is difficult because of a lack of stable biological standard; some estimate of precision can be obtained by measuring every fifth sample in duplicate.

Furthermore, the standard hemoglobin solutions should be read each day. The standard deviation in this case represents instrument variability and the ability of the operator to read the scale in a reproductive manner.

Regardless of the method chosen, photoelectric instruments are preferable to the older visual colormeters for measurements of intensity of color. All instruments should be calibrated with one of the several accurate methods.

Interpretative Guides

These should be prepared to permit, within limits of knowledge and methods, the realistic interpretation of data collected in hemoglobin surveys.

Because of the sample structure often obtained, clinical and bio-chemical findings are more representative when discussed under separate age and sex groupings. Overall prevalence figures may reflect the situation in male adults and school-age children to a disproportionate extent [20].

Laboratory Equipment and Supplies

Requirements for field operations would depend upon the study plan. When the field station is at a great distance from the base laboratory field, facilities are necessarily elaborate. When the base is a few miles away as in some surveys [11] in Central America· much of the work otherwise done in the field could be accomplished centrally.

Equipment for sampling and pre-survey visits is relatively simple. Large scale maps locating all households of the study area are the first requirement. Governmental sources occasionally have such maps but usually the field staff prepares them.

The equipment and supply list should be completed during the planning stage. It should include supplies for the micro and macro methods for blood analysis and recording cards both for the use in the field and the base laboratory.

In most cases it will be convenient to prepare all of the sterile syringe and needles needed in the main laboratory rather than attempt the sterilization in the field.

The field laboratory equipment should be prepared and packed in the main laboratory in such a manner as to facilitate its use in the field. As nearly as possible, the supplies and the method of packing should be standardized. The containers used for the transportation should be such that they can be used over again, and of course they must be convenient to handle.

Transportation

This is a factor of great importance and cannot be disregarded in the planning of a survey. The sample to be studied should by necessity be limited to those areas which the field team could reach and from where they could return to their base within a reasonable period of time. Thus, the details of logistics and transportation of team members throughout the survey and the shipment of biological sample to the headquarters laboratory must be given careful attention at the onset of the planning. Time schedules must be set for shipment of biological samples back to the laboratory. In all cases schedule should recognize the need for flexibility and alternate possibilities in the itinerary due to delays caused by weather, travel problems or local holidays. Despite prior planning, transportation always poses a greater problem than expected. When the study area is rural with a relatively large population, substations may be needed on a village basis.

The samples are usually best carried by commercial flights, and where air transportation is not available [9], specimen should be brought to the bases laboratory by commercial bus or rail and, on some occasions, samples may have to be brought from outlying districts by military vehicle [7, 8, 19]. Under normal survey conditions, the blood is from 12 to 24 hours old before it can be analyzed.

If roads are good there is no difficulty in getting from headquarters to the local study areas or sub-stations, but in some areas, due to rains and other seasonal difficulties, even jeep travel is hard going; bicycle is sometimes more suitable.

Where house-to-house visiting is the basic procedure and the population is urban or centered in villages, as in many rural parts of the world, travel is by foot.

Field surveys these days are usually a team effort employing a variety of ancilliary skills in support of the principal investigator. Modern methods of machine tabulation, computer analysis and statistical manipulation have obvious advantages in dealing with extensive projects with much data, but the interpretation of results remain rooted in the valued judgment of the worker in the field.

Record forms should comply with individual features of the survey with special attention to precision in terminology and the inclusion of an explanatory code stating what information is wanted and defining technical terms for every form put into field use. A noteworthy technical consideration is to prescribe methods of assembly and recording data which permit mechanical sorting and tabulation.

Analysis of results is more than an obligation of the statistician; in varying degrees, it is a responsibility of all staff members. Analysis is a three-level function, the first is a concurrent function of regular field activities, the second is the periodic examination of results and a third is final analysis for the interpretation of results.

Preparation of Reports

The report combines clinical and laboratory results with field observations.

The three steps that should be considered in reporting are as follows:

Firstly, an initial report which outlines the activities carried out during the pre-survey, the sites visited, contacts made and pilot studies undertaken. Secondly, a preliminary report based upon considered analysis of the data. This report should combine clinical and laboratory results with field observations, and lastly, the final report including recommendations for prevention and control, and suggestions for follow-up studies. Here it may be useful to note institutions that are considered cooperative, capable and interested in conducting future research programmes.

Conclusions

Considerable progress has been made in biochemical evaluation of nutritional anemias.

However, most diagnostic methods have been developed for use in private or hospital practice and some of them are slow, cumbersome and expensive for use on a public health scale. Some of these methods are subject to wide range of interpretation. Apparently such difficulties have discouraged many health officials from attempting appraisal work. New tests are needed and experiments under carefully controlled conditions with existing methods should yield valuable data. The development of simple methods will greatly facilitate their application to mass examination and should assist in solving many existing problems.

Low hemoglobin concentrations alone should not be the criterion for diagnosis of iron deficiency without further charcterization of the anemia. Much iron deficiency in tropical regions is induced by blood loss associated with intestinal parasitism and the possibility of conditioned deficiency must always be considered. Other factors such as race, climate and customary altitude may also play a role.

In general it may be stated that determination of the concentration of hemoglobin in the blood is a valuable procedure in appraising nutritional status, if the method is carefully applied and its limitations are sufficiently appreciated and if findings are interpreted with full realization of the variability consistent with normal health.

References

[1] Stott, Gordon, MRCP, D.T.M., S.H., « Anaemia in Mauritius », *Bulletin Org. Mond. Santé, Bulletin World Health Organization*, 23, 781-791, 1960
[2] Interdepartmental Committee on Nutrition for National Defense, *Manual for Nutrition Surveys*, 2nd Edition, 1963
[3] Bulletin of the National Research Council, « Nutrition Surveys - Their Technique and Value », *117*, May 1949

[4] Young, Charlotte M., Ph. D., Fapha and Trulson, Martha F., D. Sc. Fapha, « Methodology for Dietary Studies in Epidemiological Surveys - Strengths and Weaknesses of Existing Methods », *American Journal of Public Health*, 5, 6, 803-816,

[5] Interdepartmental Committee on Nutrition for National Defense, *Report on the Nutrition Survey of Northeast Brazil*, Washington, D.C., 1965

[6] Interdepartmental Committee on Nutrition for National Defense, *Report on the Nutrition Survey of Uruguay*, Washington, D.C., 1963

[7] Interdepartmental Committee on Nutrition for National Defense, *Report on the Nutrition Survey of Bolivia*, Washington, D.C., 1964

[8] Interdepartmental Committee on Nutrition for National Defense, *Report on the Nutrition Survey of Venezuela*, Washington, D.C., 1964

[9] Interdepartmental Committee on Nutrition for National Defense, *Report on the Nutrition Survey of Colombia*, Washington, D.C., 1961

[10] Interdepartmental Committee on Nutrition for National Defense, *Report on the Nutrition Survey of Paraguay*, Washington, D.C. (Unpublished)

[11] Interdepartmental Committee on Nutrition for National Defense, *Report on the Nutrition Survey of Pakistan*, Washington, D.C., 1966

[12] Interdepartmental Committee on Nutrition for National Defense, *Report on the Nutrition Survey of West Indies*, Washington, D.C., 1962

[13] Interdepartmental Committee on Nutrition for National Defense, *Report on the Nutrition Survey of Peru*, Washington, D.C., 1959

[14] Gordon, J.E., The American Journal of the Medical Sciences, « Preventive Medicine and Epidemiology », *Field Epidemiology*, 246, 3, 354-374, September 1963

[15] Scrimshaw, N.S., Guzman, M.A., Kevany, J.P., Ascoli, V., Bruch, H.A., Gordon, J.E., « Nutritional and Infection Field Study in Guatemalan Villages. 1959-64 », *Archives of Environmental Health, 14*, 6, 787-801, June 1967

[16] Scrimshaw, N.S., Morales, Julio O., Salazar, Alfonso, Loomes, Charles P., « Health Aspects of the Community Development Project, Rural Area, Turrialba, Costa Rica, 1948-1951 », *American Journal of Tropical Medicine and Hygiene, 2*, 583-592, 1953

[17] Jelliffe, D.B., M.D., Pelliffe, E.F.P., S.R.N., « The Children of the San Blas Indians of Panama. An Ecologic Field Study of Health and Nutrition », *The Journal of Pediatries, 59*, 2, 271-284, August 1967

[18] Interdepartmental Committee on Nutrition for National Defense, *Report on the Nutrition Survey of Ecuador*, Washington, D.C., 1960

[19] Interdepartmental Committee on Nutrition for National Defense, *Report on the Nutrition Survey of Chile*, Washington, D.C., 1961

[20] Interdepartmental Committee on Nutrition for National Defense, « Suggested Guide for Interpreting Dietary and Biochemical Data », *Public Health Reports*, 75, 687, 1960

3.3. Normal Hemogobin Values Versus Observed Values: Problems of Establishing the Normal Haemoglobin Values in a Community

S.M. Lewis, Department of Haematology, Royal Postgraduate Medical School, Ducane Road, London, W. 12, U.K.

The range of so-called normal haemoglobin has been a matter of controversy for a long time. The difficulty in establishing the levels of haemoglobin and related haematological parameters in health has been due to a number of factors. In the past, variation in technique and lack of an international haemoglobin standard have been blamed for the discrepancies in the data from different laboratories. When, not so long ago, results were expressed in percentage, the use of the Haldane scale (100 % = 13.8 g/100 ml), enabled the Englishman to appear truly red blooded, and to be so much better off than the pale Europeans whose haemoglobin was measured by the Sahli method (100 % = 17.3 g/100 ml). Although this problem has now been clarified, variations in technique and instruments still seem to be a factor of some significance. There is, however, little excuse for it, now that the international haemoglobin standard has been adopted and accuracy and precision can be ensured by intralaboratory quality control and interlaboratory comparability trials.

It is because of the lack of precision that haematologists have tended to discount minor fluctuations in haemoglobin measurement. But there is need to establish the value for normal haemoglobin with precision if we are to assess intelligently the significance of variations from the normal.

It is my intention not to discuss the method of haemoglobinometry, but to review the factors which cause difficulties in our attempts to establish the normal range.

Haemoglobin fluctuates in normal subjects, and apart from this physiological variation one must also consider sampling variations. Capillary blood has approximately 5% higher concentration of red cells than does venous blood, and stasis by a tourniquet before taking a sample of venous blood will also cause haemoconcentration.

Muscular activity, if at all strenuous, raises the haemoglobin level, either because of re-entry into the capillaries, or due to loss of circulating plasma. Posture, too, causes transient alterations in red cell concentration: Mollison [12] demonstrated an increase of about 10% in a normal adult male when he changed from a recumbent to a standing position. Eisenberg [3] has shown that alteration in the position of the arm alone during sampling, that is, whether dependent or at the atrial level, affects cell concentration.

Diurnal variations, sometimes of considerable extent, have been reported [10, 17], and it has been suggested that seasonal variations also occur, although evidence for this has been conflicting, and this question requires further study [13, 16].

Altitude results in an increased haemoglobin, the magnitude of which depends on the degree of anoxaemia [7]. Thus, at an altitude of 2 km (6500 feet) the haemoglobin is about 1 g higher than at sea level, and at 3 km (10,000 feet) it is 2 g/100 ml higher. This appears

94

to be in part a true increase because of increased erythropoiesis, but a secondary factor is a decrease in plasma volume which occurs at high altitudes [9].

Age and sex are other important factors. This is, of course, well known, but it is less clear what is their significance.

Is the lower haemoglobin that occurs in women due entirely to hormonal differences, or do women invariably have a degree of iron deficiency sufficient to affect their haemoglobin concentration? Hallberg [6] has found that a loss of 60-100 ml of blood with each period results in low serum iron with a high iron-binding capacity, but no significant decrease in the haemoglobin concentration even when the loss is 100 ml per month. Burton [1] noted that oral contraceptives given to healthy women result in an increase in serum iron and iron-binding capacity, but do not affect the haemoglobin level. He suggested that iron-binding capacity is controlled partly by circulating oestrogen and/or progestogen, and that lower serum iron of women does not necessarily betoken iron deficiency. On the other hand, it is of interest to note a report that there was no difference in the haemoglobin level between men and women in a group of Australian aborigines where the women have a very low menstrual loss [2]. The significance of the volume of blood loss in relation to a developing iron depletion and lowering of haemoglobin has been further studied by Fielding [5], who showed that iron depletion without anaemia can occur in male blood donors who donate two or more bottles of blood per year, and thus lose the equivalent of 80 ml of blood per month. These observations suggest that iron depletion is a continuing process in menstruating women, but that it is unlikely that iron therapy could increase the haemoglobin concentration to that found in man. Would women benefit from a higher haemoglobin? For that matter, is there a haemoglobin concentration for men or women, which is optimal on the criteria of physiological efficiency, exercise tolerance, physical health and mental well being? The criteria of normality are so difficult to establish that my question is, perhaps, imponderable.

It is also necessary to consider environmental differences. There have been a number of studies of population groups in different areas of the world, and some of these have been the subject of papers in this symposium. Recent studies have included that of Miall et al [11] in Jamaica, Robson [15] in Tanganyika, Kilpatrick and Hardisty [8] in Wales, Elwood [4] in Ireland etc. etc. Indeed, the list of countries where such surveys have been carried out forms a directory of the membership of the United Nations. In general, the surveys have shown that haemoglobin is lower in the less highly developed countries, and mild to severe anaemia is so prevalent in some areas that a range which is considerably lower than that generally accepted is sometimes taken as the normal in such areas. This emphasises the need for clearer thinking on the subject of normal range, and indicates the need to distinguish between normal and mean or modal. The mode may not be normal, and there is, thus, need to set adequate criteria for selection of subjects from whom normal data can be derived.

I should now like to tell you about a study which illustrates this point particularly well.

Tristan da Cunha is an isolated island in the South Atlantic half-way between South America and Africa. It has an area of less than 100 km², and as it is dominated by a volcanic mountain the only inhabitable area is a narrow plateau leading from the seafront in one small part of the island. On this island lived a group of 268 persons in 70 family units with seven surnames. Life on the island was primitive and hard. Nonetheless, or perhaps because of it, the islanders had been reputed to enjoy a high standard of health, free from the ills of modern civilization. As a result of a volcanic eruption the entire community was evacuated to Britain in 1961, and an opportunity was presented, sponsored by the Medical Research Council, for an intensive study of their health pattern, and for the determination of various parameters of a normal population. The investigations included haemoglobin and plasma protein studies. The assumption that this was a remarkable healthy normal population was soon shown to be false. The first investigations were carried out shortly after their arrival in Britain, and haemoglobin was again measured after three to four months and again one year later. The first series of measurements showed that the range and means of haemoglobin were low by British standards. The mean haemoglobin increased significantly within three months of arrival in Britain, and there was a further increase thereafter (Fig. 1).

An analysis of the data in individual cases shows, as might be expected, that the greatest increase in haemoglobin occurred in the most anaemic persons while those who initially had higher haemoglobin levels showed little or no change on the occasion of the re-testing.

On the first examination in most cases the red-blood cells were normocytic and normochromic or slightly hypochromic (MCHC ranged between 28 and 33 %). Serum Vitamin B_{12} was determined in only a few randomly-selected subects, in whom it was normal. There were no abnormal haemoglobins.

What is the significance of these findings? As I have already re-

96

Figure 1

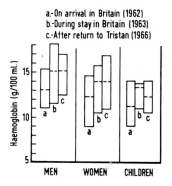

a.-On arrival in Britain (1962)
b.-During stay in Britain (1963)
c.-After return to Tristan (1966)

marked, there is need to distinguish « normal range » from « average range », in other words, can a lower range be considered « normal » if everybody in a community falls within it? This becomes a question of practical importance in deciding whether such a community should be regarded as unhealthy.

Table 1 — Incidence of infestations in an apparently «healthy» population.

		%
Trichuris Trichiura	..	72
Ascaris Lumbricoides	..	23
Endolimax Nana	..	27
Entamoeba Histolytica	..	11
Entamoeba Hartman	..	0.8
Toxoplasma Antibodies	..	80

The present study show, clearly, that this was the case with the Tristan Islanders. There was a high incidence of asthma, chronic bronchitis, infestation with intestinal parasites (Table I). Their teeth were in a bad state and dental caries was rife. The change of environment from an under-developed community to one where there is continuous medical care resulted in an increase in haemoglobin to the higher range normally found in the more advanced country. When indicated, medical treatment was given, for example, for intestinal worms and oral hygeine was improved but in no case was iron therapy specifically given.

Plasma proteins were studied in 21 randomly selected islanders [19]. In all cases there was an abnormal pattern, consisting of low albumin and high globulin. The gamma globulin fraction especially was increased (Table 2). In many tropical communities the presence of anaemia and an abnormal protein pattern consisting of low albumin and high gamma-globulin is frequently due to malaria, filariasis, leishmaniasis or other tropical infections. In view of the absence of these factors in the Tristan group it might be presumed that the abnormality was due to some other form of infection or to a dietary deficiency of protein or a combination of these factors.

Table 2 – Plasma protein findings in random-sample study of Tristan Islanders.

	Range (g%)	Mean (g%)
Albumin	0.90 – 3.54	2.48
Globulin	3.52 – 6.40	5.08

I have already mentioned the high incidence of infestations with intestinal parasites and upper respiratory tract infections. With regards to diet, the community had depended on products of the island. The staple diet had been fish and potatoes and to a much lesser extent milk, meat, seabirds and eggs. In a survey [18] one year after arrival in England it was found that they had settled down on modest incomes which enabled them to enjoy all the necessities and some of the luxuries of life. However, their dietary customs had not changed radically; they ate less fish but relatively large quantities of meat, especially stewing mutton.

A typical main meal would include a sort of Irish stew which consisted of corned beef hash, together with potatoes and cabbage but no other vegetables and no salads. They ate canned fruit but no fresh fruit. Tea was the most popular drink, taken very sweet with evaporated milk. Analysis showed that the total food intake was still less than that of an average British sample, with a mean intake of about 1600 kcal, as compared with the National food survey average of 2660 kcal per person per day. They did not appear to be in a negative calorie balance and they were apparently not losing weight, but it was thought that they were relatively lethargic [18].

The proportion of protein, fat and carbohydrate appeared to be similar to that in the average British diet, as was iron and vitamin B, although the intake of vitamins A and C was low. The children's diet was considerably re-inforced by school milk and the midday school meal.

It appears that the increase in haemoglobin was not due to dietary improvement alone, but from the improved health which resulted from medical care, with diet playing only a secondary role.

After 2 years in Britain the Islanders returned home, but now with facilities for improved sanitation and public health and with an adequate medical service. Two years after their return to their homeland their haemoglobin was again measured, as part of a general nutritional survey by Miss Margaret Chambers of the Medical Research Council (Fig. 1). The adults have retained their higher levels; the children have shown a reduction, possibly because of their growth rate, possibly because of the loss of school meals. Living conditions have certainly improved and the Islanders remain free of infestation and infections, although dental caries has again become a problem.

The Tristan picture is similar to that seen in other immigrants to Britain from tropical countries and of course there have been several reports of this pattern of morbidity and normocytic anaemia in the tropics. What is interesting in the Tristan story is firstly that this South Atlantic island might be regarded as a tropical community at least with regards to the pathogenesis of the anaemia which was so prevalent; secondly, that the so-called nutritional anaemia was essentially an anaemia of chronic ill health and treatment of the causes of the ill health rather than dietary improvement led to the improvement in the anaemia. Finally, the presence of chronic ill health in an entire community results in the acceptance of that state as normal until it is shown in its true perspective by comparison with a higher standard of health. This is the important point to be remembered when we establish a normal range for clinical measurement of health.

But even within an apparently homogeneous, developed, community there are pitfalls in our search for a normal population. Dr. G. Discombe of the Central Middlesex Hospital, London studied a group of hospital workers, ranging from physicians to porters, and a comparable group of factory personnel in the same district of London. These people were of similar socio-economic status, they were all apparently healthy but the hospital workers had to walk about much more· and were

99

noted to be, as a group, of a more cheerful disposition. The hospital
group had significantly higher haemoglobin (Fig. 2).

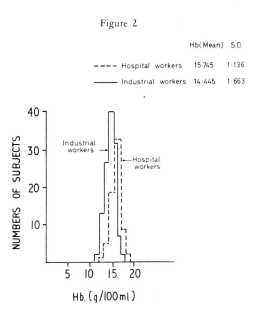

Figure 2

This emphasises the difficulty in establishing the truly normal group
even within a normal population.

Finally, the method by which the data is expressed is also an
important aspect of the problem. The concept of a range to include
all apparently normal subjects, and the use of an arithmetical mean
is of little value. The bias of selection can, to an extent, be discounted
by applying statistical principles, and using a small random sample to
represent the parent population. A distribution curve provides useful
information. Pryce [14] has suggested that by taking the modal
value as the point of reference, and super-imposing a gaussian curve
on the mode, a normal range can be defined, without being influenced
by outlying data (Fig. 3). A mean can then be estimated with reasonable accuracy, even when there is skewness of the distribution curve.
There is little doubt that the use of a mode and 2 standard deviations
around the mode will provide a better guide to the probable significance
of an individual measurement than the use of a wide range of « normal
values ». But even so, it is important to remember the difficulty in
defining a normal population, and it is a question of careful balance

100

between selecting a suitable population for measurement in order to
obtain the data and prejudging the whole issue of what is the normal
level by statistical manipulation.

Figure 3

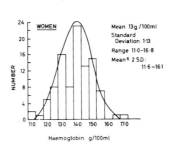

References

[1] Burton, J.L., *Lancet, 1*, 978, 1957
[2] Casley-Smith, J.R., *Australian J. exp. Biol. med. Sci., 36*, 23, 1958
[3] Eisenberg, S., *J. Lab. clin. Med., 61*, 755, 1963
[4] Elwood, P.C., *Brit. J. prev. soc. Med., 18*, 81, 1964
[5] Fielding, J., Karabus, C., Brunström, G.M., *J. clin. Path., 21*, 402, 1968
[6] Hallberg, L., Högdahl, A.M., Nilsson, L., Rybo, G., *Acta med. scand., 180*, 639,
1916
[7] Hurtado, A., Merino, C., Delgado, E., *Arch. int. Med., 75*, 284, 1945
[8] Kilpatrick, G.S., Hardisty, R.M., *Brit. med. J., 1*, 778, 1961
[9] Levin, N.W., Metz, J., Hart, D., van Heerden, P.D.R., Boardman, R.G., Farber,
S.A., *S. Afr. J. med. Sci., 28*, 132, 1960
[10] McCarthy, E.F., van Slyke, D.D., *J. biol. Chem., 128*, 567, 1939
[11] Miall, W.E., Milner, P.F., Lovell, H.G., Standard, K.L., *Brit. J. prev. soc. Med.,
21*, 45, 1967
[12] Mollison, P.L., *Blood Transfusion in Clinical Medicine*, 4th edn, p. 121, Blackwell
Scientific Publications, Oxford, 1967
[13] Natvig, H., Bjerkedal, T., Jonassen, O., *Acta med. scand., 174*, 351, 1963
[14] Pryce, J.D., *Lancet, 2*, 333, 1960
[15] Robson, J.R.K., *J. trop. Med. Hyg., 67*, 282, 1964
[16] Saunders, C., *Lab. Pract., 14*, 1390, 1965
[17] Stengle, J.M., Schade, A.L., *Brit. J. Haemat., 3*, 117, 1957

[18] Taylor, E.C., Hollingsworth, D.F., Chambers, M.A., *Br. J. Nutr.*, 20, 393, 1966
[19] Woodruff, A.W., Pettit, L.E., *Trans. roy. Soc. trop. Med. Hyg.*, 59, 356, 1965

Acknowledgements

I wish to thank the Secretary of the Medical Research Council Tristan Working Party (Dr. H.E. Lewis) and Miss Margaret Chambers for providing some of the data; also Dr. G. Discombe for providing the data of Figure 2.

3.4. *Normal Hemoglobin Values Versus Observed Values: Selecting the Population Samples*

Miguel Layrisse, Instituto Venezolano de Investigaciones Científicas, Apartado 1827, Caracas, Venezuela

In 1958 the report of the W.H.O. [1] study group on iron deficiency anemia called the attention to the scanty information on the prevalence of anemia in the world. The W.H.O. and other Institutions interested in the problem have made a special effort in the last years to fill this gap; however, this information in still insufficient for the mapping of the world distribution of anemia. Data on the prevalence of anemia is even smaller in countries where this type of information is urgently needed in order to organize thoughtful programs for its prevention.

Perhaps the most handy and exact laboratory procedure to be used in surveys on anemia in both urban and rural communities, is hemoglobinometry. The cyanmethemoglobin method [2] modified by the addition of 1 drop of 0.1% sodium azide to the Drabkin solution [3] permits also to collect samples in the field during several days and then read in the laboratory center of the region, when the sampling is finished.

The setting up of the basis for a survey on hemoglobin values is undoubtly very useful as preliminary step for the study of the distribution of anemia. The results of this survey would be the background for a second step, in which thoughtful studies on the etiology and pathogenesis of anemia would be performed in selected areas.

The examination of a large number of subjects from a population requires time, and it is not necessary in many cases. However, when the sample is small, attention should be paid to all possible variants which could modify the results. In the special case of hemoglobin survey, several considerations should be kept in mind before the sampling is taken; they are as follows:

a) *Source of the samples*

It is a common habit to report frequency of anemia in a population from the values obtained in patients which are either hospitalized or attending dispensaries. Information obtained from this type of survey may distort the true prevalence in the locality. In the University Hospital of Caracas, for instance, hemoglobin values below 8 g % are very often observed in hospitalized subjects coming from rural areas where hookworm infection is endemic. The examination of the areas where these patients come from, reveals surprisingly that less than 4 % of the population carry such hemoglobin values [4]. These discrepancies can be explained by the fact that only the very anemic subjects leave the region in order to attend dispensaries and hospitals for treatment. The sampling of patients for a survey is permissible only when they are attending clinics as normal subjects, such as pregnant women and infants attending pre-natal and nursery clinics.

b) *Sampling the subjects*

A suitable method of sampling which could be applied as a general pattern for any population has not been developed yet. The method may vary in some respects from one population to another. Perhaps the most accurate method would be randomizing family groups in their local geographical area. This encounters several inconveniences such as: slowing down the progress of the survey and the recruiting of all members of the family. It is more suitable to randomize segments of the population located in different places, for example: pregnant women at pre-natal clinics, infants and lactating women in baby and child clinics, pre-school children in pre-natal clinics, children over 7 years of age in schools and adult people in industries [5].

c) *Stratification of the population*

As normal hemoglobin values vary according to the age and physiological status of the individuals and according to their environmental conditions, it would be advisable to make a stratification of the population prior to the survey. The major stratification to be considered is that concerned with age and physiological status of the individuals. In this connection, the following groups could be included:

1. Infants (below 2 years of age);
2. Pre-school children of both sexes (from 2 to 6 years)
3. School children (from 7 to 13 years)
4. Menstruating women (over 20 years)

5. Pregnant women
6. Lactating women
7. Post-Menopausal women
8. Adult men
9. Aged group

Since the most frequent cause of anemia is nutritional, especially iron deficiency type, a second sub-division could be made according to the socio-economic status of the individual.

Additional sub-groups may be considered according to the population density (urban, sub-urban, rural), geographic altitude and other climatic conditions. Further details on this aspect can be consulted elsewhere [6, 7].

d) *Size of sample*

In order to obtain a true representation of the universe under study, subjects must be selected at random from the population without discrimination. When the sample is small, special attention should be paid to randomize the subjects from the same stratum rather than from the total population. This would prevent the disproportion of individuals from different strata.

Unless the total population is examined, there is always an error in the sampling of a population. This error is a function of the affected individuals in the population and the number of individuals tested [7]. If we want to study the proportion of anemic individuals in a population, the standard error can be calculated according to the formula:

$$\sqrt{\frac{pq}{n}}$$

Where p is the proportion of the anemics in the population, q the proportion of non-anemic and n the number of individuals tested. This standard error can be expressed in percentage of the frequency of anemic subjects as follows:

Anemic subjets		S.E. expressed in percentage of anemic subjects $\frac{\text{S.E.} \times 100}{p}$
p %	S. E.	
90	3.0	3.0
80	4.0	5.0
50	5.0	10.0
20	4.0	20.0
10	3.0	30.0
5	2.2	44.0

104

According to this figure, in rural agricultural areas of Venezuela, where more than 30 % of non-pregnant women are anemic [4], about 100 samples would be representative of the universe of this population with a margin of 15 % error. If we study non-pregnant women living in the United States, where the frequency of anemia is about 12 % [8, 9], 300 samples would be necessary to have a representative sample with 13 % error.

In conclusion, the sampling of a population for hemoglobinometry encounters various problems inherent to the origin of samples and to the peculiar physiology of hemoglobin in human and the proportion of anemic subjects. It is recommended therefore, to stratify the population, according to the physiological hemoglobin variations before the survey is under way and select the number of individuals according to the expected prevalence of anemia.

References

[1] World Health Organization, *Report of a Study Group on Iron Deficiency Anemia*, Technical Report Series No. 182, Geneva, 1959
[2] Crosby, W.H., Munn, J.L. and Furth, F.W., « Standardizing a method for clinical hemoglobinometry », *U.S. Armed Forces M.J., 6*, 693fi 1954
[3] Layrisse, M. and Lopez-Calzon, G. Hemoglobinometry in the Field. In preparation
[4] Layrisse, M. and Roche, M., « The relationship between anemia and hookworm infection », *Amer. J. Hyg., 79*, 279-301, 1964
[5] U.S. Interdept. Com. on nut. for Nat. Def., *Manual for Nutrition Survey*, 1963
[6] Organization Mundial de la Salud, « Los métodos de muestreo de las encuestas sobre morbilidad y en las investigaciones sobre salud pública », *Informe técnico, 336*, 1966
[7] World Health Organization, *Immunological and Haematological surveys. Inform from the Study Group*, 1959
[8] Hervey, G.W., McIntire, R.T. and Watson, V., « Low hemoglobin levels in women as revealed by blood donor record », *J.A.M.A., 149*, 1127-1128, 1952
[9] Bothwell, T.H. and Finch, C.A., *Iron metabolism*, Little, Brown and Co., Boston, 1962

3.5. Hemoglobin Level: Normal and Observed Values Interpreting the Results of Surveys

P.C. Elwood, Cardiff, Wales, U.K.

The usual clinical concept of anaemia implies a dicotomy of subjects into those who are « normal » and those who have levels of circulating haemoglobin indicative of disease. Circulating haemoglobin however is best considered as a continuous quantitative variable and if it is, then any so called lower limit of normal is seen as an arbitrarily chosen point in its distribution. In any case, the definition of any single level of haemoglobin as a criterion of anaemia is unreasonable in view of its significant associations with other variates such as age, bodyweight and phase within the menstrual cycle.

The symposium is unusual, in that it is concerned with haemoglobin level and not simply with « anaemia », however defined. However it would not seem to be unreasonable to suggest that circulating Hb. level is only of importance if it is shown that low levels significantly often indicate disease or ill health. Furthermore the difference between the values observed in any population and « normal » values, however these are defined, is only of importance if there is valid evidence that this difference in indicative of an increased morbidity. In our own investigations we found no evidence of such increased morbidity. « Normal » values defined in the absence of such evidence would seem to be of little meaning.

The original data which will be presented were gathered during community surveys. All these surveys have been of total communities or of random samples of communities in South Wales. All have been of adult, non pregnant women, all estimations of circulating Hb. were on venous blood, usually in triplicate, using cyanmethaemoglobin and a photo-electric colorimeter and packed cell volumes (P.C.V.) were estimated by a microhaematocrit method. Unfortunately the studies have been small and most of them should be regarded as pilot studies only; they are not put forward as exhaustive nor the results from them as conclusive. They indicate a line of argument however, which is basic to the whole concept of « Normal » values.

Underlying Disease

It is commonly believed that in addition to any importance low levels of circulating haemoglobin may have in themselves, their detection is often of value because they frequently indicate the presence of serious underlying disease. In order to examine this belief, we recently screened 1,000 women in the community. Of these 44 had haemoglobin levels below 10.0 g and of these, 37 who were not already under treatment were referred to a hospital for further investigations. In eight cases further investigation led to action of possible relevance to iron deficiency: one woman had haemorrhoids injected, six had uterine dilatation and curettage, and one, who could not tolerate oral iron was admitted for blood transfusion. One hundred and twenty women were found to have haemoglobin levels below 12.0 g. These were all asked to supply 3 specimens of faeces for testing for occult blood. In order to enable the results of these tests to be evaluated a representative sample of a similar number of women with levels above 12.0 g were also screened in the same way. Of the women with low haemoglobin levels, 16 % gave at least one positive test. This is higher figure but not significantly so, than the proportions in women who had haemoglobin levels above 12.0 g (8 %). However, in the women with haemoglobin levels below 12.0 g there was no evidence of a significant association between the proportion of positive results and haemoglobin level, and on re-testing, only four of the fifteen women who had given a positive result on the first occasion did so again. These results give little support to the not uncommonly expressed belief that anaemia is commonly a sign of a serious underlying pathological condition, and that this is « all too frequently » (Harris, 1963) a malignant tumour of the gastro-intestinal tract.

Symptomatology

In order to further assess the importance of low levels of circulating haemoglobin we have examined the associations between haemoglobin level and both symptoms and cardio-respiratory function, and the effects of iron therapy on both.

In the survey of 1,000 women the grade of a variety of symptoms were ascertained by questionnaire. The symptoms chosen included those commonly believed to be caused by iron deficiency and included a set of questions from which the degree of neurosis of each subject could be ascertained. Table I shows the correlation coefficients between the severity of a variety of symptoms and haemoglobin level. All the coefficients are small and clinically unimportant and the only one which is statistically significant (palpitations) is positive, and implies that the higher the haemoglobin level the more severe the palpitations. The data on neurosis (Table I) suggests that the severity of these symptoms in the community is quite unrelated to the level of circulating haemoglobin, but is closely related to the degree of neurosis of a subject.

The effect of a change in haemoglobin following iron therapy appears to confirm that in the community, symptoms are not caused to any important extent by iron deficiency. From the survey of 1,000 women, 100 with levels of circulating haemoglobin below 12.0 g were given oral iron or placebo tablets at random. Although this led to a rise in haemoglobin levels in those given Fe which was almost 2 g/100 ml greater than the change in those given placebo, there was no significant difference in the change in the severities of the various symptoms (Table II).

Table 1 – Correlation coefficients («r») of symptom grades and haemoglobin level, and symptom grades and «neurotic» grade (see text) in a population sample.

Symptoms	Correlation coefficients of symptom grades	
	With Hb. level	With «neurotic» grade
Irritability	0.01	0.21*
Palpitations	0.16*	0.26*
Dizziness	-0.05	0.36*
Breathlessness	-0.02	0.24*
Fatigue	0.03	0.30*
Headache	-0.01	0.28*

* Statistically significant at P   0.05

Table 2 – Mean changes in symptoms and in haemoglobin level in 90 women given, at random, either iron or placebo for eight weeks.

Symptom	Given Iron	Given Placebo
Irritability	- 0.03 ± 0.37	-0.78 ± 0.30*
Palpitation	- 0.37 ± 0.34	0.03 ± 0.35
Dizziness	- 0.79 ± 0.25	- 0.65 ± 0.34
Breatlessness	- 0.11 ± 0.18	0.19 ± 0.20
Fatigue	- 0.13 ± 0.27	0.30 ± 0.22
Headache	- 1.05 ± 0.37	- 0.97 ± 0.38*

Note: If a rise in haemoglobin level is associated with an improvement in a symptom then the sign will be negative.

* Statistically significant at P   0.05

These data therefore give no evidence of any association in the community between circulating haemoglobin level and symptoms, nor of a beneficial effect of iron on symptoms. The only one who would seem to feel better following a haematological survey is possibly the doctor who conducted it.

Cardio-respiratory function

To assess the associations between circulating haemoglobin level and cardio-respiratory function, the distribution of haemoglobin level in almost 3,000 women in a community sample was defined. The lowest 1 % approximately were referred to Dr. J.E. Cotes and his colleagues for detailed tests of cardio-respiratory function and these results were compared with those found in a further random sample of 80 women with normal levels of circulating haemoglobin. Table III shows that the two samples were similar with regard to age, height and weight, and shows that there was no evidence of any clinically important difference in transfer factor, exercise ventilation or exercise cardiac frequency. Having said that it should be admitted that the women with anaemia were more reluctant to exercise than the normal women. However this is almost certainly a reflection of their attitude to the investigation. The control women knew they were normal, whereas the iron deficient women had beed told they had severe anaemia· and the tests on which these results are based were only part of a fuller evaluation which included a clinical interview and examination.

The effects of iron therapy on cardio-respiratory function is shown in Table IV. Unfortunately the numbers involved in the trial were very small. However despite a marked effect of the Fe on circulating haemoglobin and on total body haemoglobin there is very little evidence of any effect on cardio-respiratory function. Transfer factor has increased by about 14 % in those given iron, but this is to be expected as this index is derived from a variety of factors one of which is circulating haemoglobin level itself. In any case a change of this magnitude is of doubtful clinical importance. Cardiac frequency and exercise ventilation shows no important change with treatment in either group.

The original search in all this work was for a meaningful definition of anaemia in terms of symptomatology or function. It was felt that if a level of circulating haemoglobin could be defined below which symptoms or effects occurred which would respond to iron, then this would be a useful and meaningful diagnostic criterion of anaemia, and

Table 3 –   Lung function and response to exercise; mean values in female subjects with low haemoglobin concentrations compared whith controls.

Index	Subjects	Controls
Number	20+	79
Age in yrs.	44.8	48.4
Weight in Kg.	63.38	62.65
Height in m.	1.58	1.59
Haemoglobin conctration (g/100 ml).	8.6	14.0
Total body haemoglobin (g)	338	–
Forced expiratory volume ($FEV_{1.0}$ in l)	2.29	2.43
Forced vital capacity (l)	3.09	3.14
Transfer factor (diffusing capacity in ml/min/mm/Hg).	21.2	25.9
Exercise ventilation (1/m)*	27.1	26.9
Exercise cardiac frequency (per/min)*	133	131

+ 16 for exercise studies and 11 for total body haemoglobin
* standardized to oxygen uptake 1 l/min.

Table 4 –   Lung function and response to exercise: change after 2 months of treatment with iron or control tablets.

Index	Treated	Controls	P
Number	12+	8+	
Haemoglobin Concentrazion	+ 4.4	− 0.6	< 0.01
Total Body Haemoglobin	+ 104	− 21	< 0.05
Transfer Factor (Diffusing Capacity)	+ 3.4	− 0.4	< 0.01
Exercise Ventilation*	+ 1.6	− 0.3	NS
Exercise Cardiac Frequency	− 6	− 7	NS

+ 9 and 3 respectively for exercise studies: 6 and 5 for total haemoglobin
*standardized to oxygen uptake 0.75 l/min.

110

hence would lead to a reasonable definition of «normal» values. In fact we have found no evidence of any harmful effect whatever in terms of symptoms or cardio-respiratory function of anaemia in communities in South Wales. While the results presented are of direct relevance only to communities in South Wales, the aspects considered seem to be essential to the concept of «normal» values and indeed should be considered in every survey. It seems to be of little value in work of this nature, simply to give a mean level of a haematological, or any other variate, or the proportion of subjects found to have levels below an arbitrarily chosen «lower limit of normal».

3.6. Normal Hemoglobin Values versus Observed Values: Comparing the Results of Surveys

George V. Mann, Vanderbilt University, Nashville, Tennessee, U.S.A.

The fundamental necessity in both clinical hematology and in the interpretation of surveys is for a frame of reference which will allow a clinical judgment of health status. This is not a statistical problem but rather a medical problem because the significance of level of hemoglobin is determined by medical events. It is distressing that medical scientists have been so slow to buttress their judgments in scientific terms.

« The Second World War may be regarded as the great divide, after which it was no longer possible for the clinician, however distinguished, to discuss the prognosis and treatment of disease unless his words were supported by figures » (L.J. Witts in *Medical Surveys and Clinical Trials*, Oxford University Press, 1964).

If Witt's estimate is correct we are now 25 years past the great divide and yet it is still necessary to insist that science ought to be scientific, not anecdotal and colloquial. Few laboratory measurements are simpler than that of hemoglobin. The reference substances is crystallized, stable and its physical constants are adequately characterized. The tools are available for the procedure and they are simple enough and yet hemoglobin is often badly measured.

Maxwell Wintrobe begins the section on hemoglobinometry in his *Clinical Hematology*, Lea and Febiger, 6th Edition 1967, with this sentence, page 427: « In spite of the fact that it is one of the most useful procedures in clinical medicine the measurement of hemoglobin has been one of the least satisfactory ».

He goes on to say this is because of Hayem's proposal at the turn of the century that results should be expressed as percentage of some arbitrary standard. While Wintrobe and others have effectively diminished this practice there is still a fondness of certain investigators to evaluate their surveys or clinical results by reference to a local set of standards. That practice has been eloquently defended by Professor Alexander R.P. Walker of Johannesburg and in the same place criticized by me [1, 2].

When a scientist reads a scientfic report there are four automatic questions asked. A good reporter answers them because these answers are the key to the usefulness of his data.

1. Whom did they measure? To be useful, measurements must be related to age, sex, ethnic and cultural characteristics. In the instance of hemoglobin the altitude at which the subjects live is important. If they were volunteers this must be known before one risks generalizations.

2. How did the workers do these measurements? Were the number of samples sufficient to answer the questions posed and to support the conclusions? Was the data obtained without distortion of the material measured? This means attention to tourniquets, glassware cleanliness and refrigeration. Were there damaging delays between sampling and measurement?

3. How did the method perform? There are now entirely adequate ways of characterizing the specificity and reproducibility of methods for hemoglobin. These are not sufficient if they are applied only at the beginning of a study. They should be systematically repeated under the serial study conditions. It is not enough to ask technicians to « run some duplicates » or « throw in a few duplicates » or even to « run this reference standard every morning ». Technicians soon begin to convey their own ideas of what the method performance should be. An effective measurement of specificity in hemoglobinometry is achieved through the use of reference standards which are available from the American College of Clinical Pathologists or the World Health Organization. An effective way to measure reproducibility is by the introduction of blind replicates in the daily work load. Let one sample collector (not engaged in the analysis) obtain double specimens each day from 3 to 5 % of the subjects. Process these with names or identities not distinguishable from the usual run of samples. When they are measured and decoded the technical error of the measurement * gives a useful measure of method perfor-

mance. This will include the entire error including that of mislabeling, measurement, computational and recording but this sum of technical error is what is needed. This is a generally useful way to measure the bias introduced by laboratory error.

4. What are the criteria for interpretating these data? There are two options. One, which is the more defensible, would be to use a unitary, international reference based on accurate measurements of a population of human being living in near optimal conditions as judged by health performance. This method has the advantages of stability with time, freedom from distortion by local conditions of nature, i.e. genetics, and nurture, i.e. environment. The use of one international frame of reference has the other advantage of making comparisons between groups possible.

The other option, advocated by Walker, is the use of colloquial experience as a frame of reference. Thus the Congolese Pygmies ought to be evaluated on a Pygmy table of heights and the Watutsi ought to be interpreted on their table of heights. This is a return to the confusion of Hayem because each survey will have the intricate problem of a moving denominator in its interpretation. The reference is unstable because, as environment changes and gene pools are mixed the reference characteristics change also. This local reference wrongly incorporates into the concept of normal the measurements made on populations which are straining to adapt to their challenging environment. In the context of inter-survey comparisons the practice will lead to pandemonium.

The problem of a frame of reference has two faces. One, the statistical side, appears to consist of matters of sampling and distribution. This view tends to ignore the crucial question of meaning. What does a low level mean? What is a low or a high level? Suppose the entire distribution is pitched so high or so low that morbidity is a consequence. The medical face of the problem over-emphasizes the complications. If a physician says that children with low levels of hemoglobin are prone to infection, ignoring now the validity of this opinion, what does he know about the health of children with equally low hemoglobin who do not develop infection and so do not come into his surveillance. The statistician is handicapped often by his ignorance of consequences, the clinician is misled by the biased sample he sees. The surveyor is in a position to serve them both.

The problems of measurement and interpretation of hemoglobin levels do have solutions. These are not always easy or at first attractive, but they are possible to a greater extent than for most other measurements. In the interests of international comparison and in addition to the presently available reference solutions for standardizing laboratory methods for facilitating comparisons and judging the optimum we need an international reference population. From this reference population the more controversial sub-references for optimal levels of hemoglobin in childhood, or pregnancy or at the several adult ages could be readily derived. Nutritionists have found it expedient to devise a standard man. He is 25 years old, he weighs 70 kg, he requires 2 mgm of nitrogen/ basal kcal daily energy expenditure, he lives in a mean environmental temperature of 20 °C, and he has a number of other useful attributes. Not unexpectedly he has a standard mate who also has defined dimensions. For survey work we need a standard population which has no race, color, or continental abode. It is a group of human beings which lives on this planet Earth and enjoys superior health. Such a population could be readily « constructed » from existing information. Its assigned characteristics, like the iridium bar in Paris, would serve all our surveys as a reference. I propose this is the logical next step beyond the standardization of hematological laboratory methods.

$$ \text{T.E.} = \sqrt{\frac{\Delta^2}{2P}} \qquad \text{where } \Delta = \text{duplicate difference} \\ P = \text{number of pairs} $$

References

[1] Walker, A.R.P., « Interpretation of Biological Data on One Ethnic or Regional Group May or May Not Be Equally Applicable to Other Groups », *Am. J. Clin. Nutr.*, 30, 1025, 1967
[2] Mann, G.V., « Interpretation of Human Measurements », *ibid.*, 20, 1040, 1967

3.7. International Haematological Trial [1]

A.H. Holtz, Rijks Instituut voor de Volksgezondheid (National Institute of Public Health), Utrecht, the Netherlands

In March-May 1968 an international haematological trial was organized by the Rijks Instituut voor de Volksgezondheid (National Institute of Public Health), Utrecht, the Netherlands. Its purpose was to provide information on the reproducibility of and the methods used for the haemoglobin determination and the red-cell count in laboratories in different countries.

The announcement was sent to 293 laboratory specialists (mainly haematologists) in 43 countries; 198 of them applied for the samples and of these 158 submitted their answer. The spontaneous cooperation was very gratifying.

The testing material for the haemoglobin determination consisted of two fresh blood samples,[2] a glycerol-containing haemolysate[3] and an aqueous haemiglobincyanide solution.[4] For the red-cell count the same two fresh blood samples and a stabilized red-cell suspension[5] were used.

Previous trials had shown that the blood samples would retain their original values long enough to reach laboratories all over the world, provided those outside Europe would not lie too far from international airports (Coster, 1964, 1965). In view of their nature the other preparations could be regarded as stable in any case.[6]

In addition, packed cell volume measurement was included in the trial in order to get some information on the condition of the blood samples at the time they were analysed in the various laboratories.

Most samples reached their destination within five days after dispatching. A few were delayed due to local delivery problems. Contrary to expectation, in a number of samples some haemolysis was observed. The reason for this could not be traced. In any case the absence or presence of haemolysis was not correlated with the distance between the receiving laboratory and Utrecht or the time elapsed between dispatching and receiving the sample.

The « correct » values, specified below, were determined by the Rijks

Figure 1

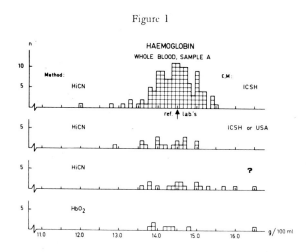

Instituut voor de Volksgezondheid in conjunction with four reference laboratories.

Haemoglobin determination

The reference values of the samples (± standard deviation) were as follows:

blood sample A   14.5 ± 0.2 g/100 ml
blood sample B   14.1 ± 0.2 g/100 ml
haemolysate   13.6 ± 0.2 g/100 ml
HiCN solution (as Hb)   14.2 ± 0.1 g/100 ml
(method and standard as recommended by ICSH)

The results of the participating laboratories are summarized in Figures 1-4. Each result is represented by a square.

Figure 2

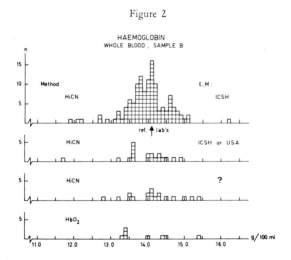

Nearly all (95 per cent) determinations were done using the haemiglobincyanide (HiCN) method and for the majority of these a standard was used based on the ICSH recommendations for the millimolar extinction coefficient (ε) of HiCN and the molecular weight (M) of Hb. In a few cases not sufficient information or no information at all was given concerning the basis of the standard.

The oxyhaemoglobin method was used in only a few laboratories.

116

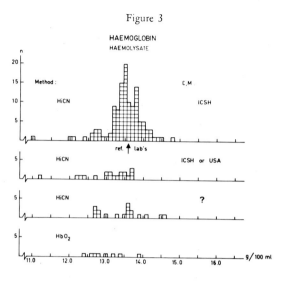

Figure 3

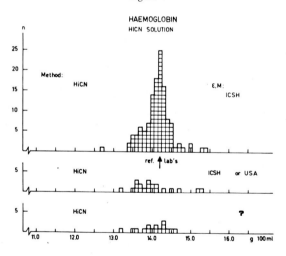

Figure 4

Details on its standardization were often insufficient or completely lacking.

The variation of the results around the reference values is rather large for all samples: plus and minus 1.0 - 1.5 g/100 ml. Even wild results deviating as much as 2.5 g/100 ml occur.

In Figure 5 the HiCN - ICSH results are combined for better comparison. It is easily seen that the variation increases in the order HiCN

Figure 5

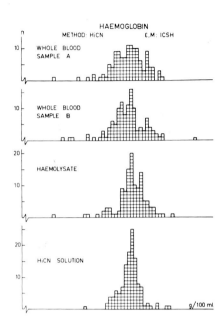

solution — haemolysate — blood, which is due to the introduction in each step of a new factor which contributes to the over-all variation (diluting + conversion and homogeneization, respectivily). It is, however, evident that the basic measurement, i.e. the optical density measurement (in turn dependent on the calibration of the photometer), contributes most to the over-all variation. Generally speaking, it seems to be this step of the haemoglobin determination that will need most attention if better results are to be obtained.

Red-cell count

The reference values of the samples (± standard deviation) were as follows:

blood sample A	$4.59 \pm 0.07 \times 10^6/\mu l$
blood sample B	$3.64 \pm 0.10 \times 10^6/\mu l$
suspension	$4.11 \pm 0.12 \times 10^6/\mu l$

(electronically counted)

118

The results of the participating laboratories are summarized in Figures 6-8. Those obtained with counting chambers, which were to be stated to one decimal place, are represented by rectangles; those

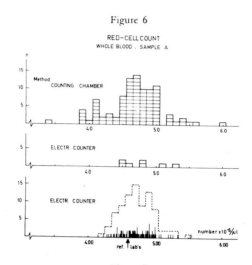

Figure 6

RED-CELL COUNT
WHOLE BLOOD . SAMPLE A

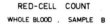

Figure 7

RED-CELL COUNT

WHOLE BLOOD . SAMPLE B

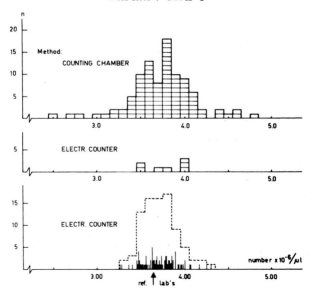

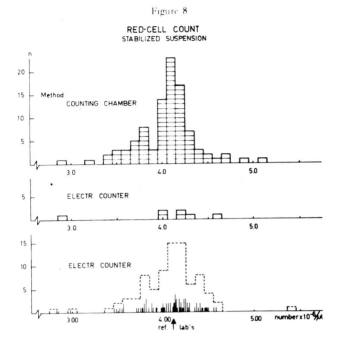

Figure 8

RED-CELL COUNT
STABILIZED SUSPENSION

obtained with counters by vertical lines of the same height as the above rectangles if they were stated to two decimal places (as had been asked), or by rectangles if they were stated to one decimal place only.

For a better comparison of the counter results with those of counting chambers, the former were also grouped in tens around the values to one decimal place and using these numbers the dashed curve was obtained.

The variation of the counting chamber results around the reference values (plus and minus about $0.7 \times 10^6/\mu l$) is only slightly larger than that which can be expected on theoretical grounds (Poisson distribution). The variation of the counter results is not much smaller; here, however, the theoretical limits are far exceeded. It is to be expected that the availability in the near future of a reference preparation in the form of a stabilized red-cell suspension, on which steady progress is being made, will bring improvement.

---

[1]) Report presented at the ICSH Assembly, New York, September 4, 1968. Not all data obtained had been fully evaluated at that time.

120

2) Prepared using EDTA as anticoagulant, 140 mg/100 ml, without further additives.
3) Prepared according to a method received from Marguerite L. Candler, M.D., National Communicable Disease Center, Atlanta (Ga), USA, personal communication.
4) Prepared according to Holtz, 1965.
5) Prepared according to Lewis and Burgess, 1966.
6) As regards the haemiglobincyanide solution, see for instance: van Assendelft et al., 1966.

Conclusions

An international trial on haemoglobin determination and red-cell count is described, in which 158 laboratories in 43 countries participated.

Although most haemoglobin determinations were performed in accordance with the recommendations of the International Committee for Standardization in Haematology, the results are still far from satisfactory. Apparently it is the inaccuracy in the optical density measurement (in turn dependent on the calibration of the photometer) which is the main cause of the variance.

For the red-cell counts, counting chambers and electronical counters were used in about equal proportion. Here too the results leave much to be desired, particularly as regards the counters.

References

Coster J.F., Bibl. haemat., 18, 92, 1964
Coster J.F., Bibl. haemat., 21, 7, 1965
Holtz A.H., Bibl. haemat., 21, 75, 1965
Van Assendelft O.W., Zijlstra W.G., van Kampen E.J. and Holtz A.H., Clin. chim. Acta, 13, 521, 1966
Lewis S.M. and Burgess B.J., Lab. Pract., 15, 305, 1966

4. Reports of Proceedings of 7th Board Meeting and 5th General Assembly of ICSH

4.1. Presidential Address

S. Watanabe, Research Institute for Nuclear Medicine and Biology, University of Hiroshima, Japan

As President of the International Committee for Standardization in Hematology I have great pleasure in opening this meeting of the Board, and in reviewing the activities of ICSH since our last Board Meeting.

Outstanding among the panels, the activity of the hemoglobinometry panel has been, I believe, most successful and fruitful so far; this owes its success to the diligent and practical efforts of the members, as we have seen in the symposium and panel discussion held yesterday and on the day before. I believe the first international approach for « Hematology of Normal Man » is one of the epoch-making events in hematology.

The reports of other Panels have been circulated, and I think that the activities and results obtained in the various fields for the standardization in hematology all owe much to the efforts of the members of ICSH as well as those of the Secretariat and the Board.

One of the prominent aspects in the progress of ICSH is, I believe, the establishment of national committees in individual countries as registered or affiliated organizations throughout the world. This will urge further development and play an important role in each country.

Another significant thing, I believe, is the establishment of a cooperative liaison with other international organizations such as WHO, IAEA, ISO, International Federation of Clinical Chemists, International Society of Clinical Pathology, International Society of Blood Transfusion.

Lastly, but not least, we extend our sincere gratitude to the Secretariat members, without whose diligent and earnest activities this meeting will not have been realized.

4.2. Report of Chairman of Secretariat

J. Spaander, National Institute of Public Health, Utrecht, the Netherlands

Since the previous assembly in Sydney in 1966 there have been three meetings of the Secretariat, the minutes of which were circulated to the Board. During this period ICSH has continued to be active in several fields. Foremost, the hemoglobinometry panel has continued its activities. It has maintained control of the international reference standard of cyanmethemoglobin and has considered a number of problems relating to hemoglobinometry. Some of these problems have been the basis for the scientific session of the panel on 3rd September 1968, during the 12th Congress of the International Society of Hematology.

The Council of Europe has supported the activities of the haemoglobin panel by a grant to RIV and the distribution of the haemoglobin reference standard has been a project of the Council. National delegates are reminded that ampoules of the standard are available free of charge for use by National Committees; application should be made to Dr. A. H. Holtz, Sterrenbos 1, Utrecht, Netherlands. The standard has now been established by WHO as the International Haemoglobincyanide Reference Preparation (20th Report of WHO Expert Committee on Biological Standardization, WHO Technical Report Series No. 384, Geneva, 1968).

The Panel on Terminology has worked out more than 100 definitions which are now being prepared for presentation to ICSH as a first recommendation. This panel has also become established as the Nomenclature and Glossary Committee of the International Society of Hematology.

The Panel on Documentation has been active along two lines — standardization of haematological data and of haematological literature.

The Panel on Sedimentation Rate has prepared a draft recommendation which will be completed shortly. The Panel on Iron has had several meetings and has made significant progress towards development of reference preparations.

At a meeting of the Sub-Committee of Specialists on Blood Problems in May 1968 it was proposed that the Council of Europe should extend its interest in standardization to include parameters for haemocytometry. On behalf of RIV and ICSH Dr. A.H. Holtz proposed a project for developing a stabilized red-cell suspension as an international standard. This proposal was considered with interest and Dr. Holtz has been invited to present a report to the Council of Europe on this subject.

Other panels have been variably active; their progress reports will be published as available.

With the cessation of the European Society of Haematology ICSH required amendment to the Constitution. The Board and Assembly in Sydney in August 1966 authorized the secretariat to amend the Constitution

123

appropriately. Subject to Board approval this will be presented for acceptance by the Assembly, with whatever further amendments as may be proposed by the Board at its meeting prior to the Assembly. It was decided that discussions should take place with the International Society of Hematology in order to establish a relationship with that Society when formed.

As an interim measure it was essential to register the Secretariat as a legal body (Foundation). This has been achieved in the Netherlands and the registration has been recognised officially by the Dutch Ministry of Justice.

Contact has been established with WHO by several panels. These include the Panels on Terminology, Haemoglobinometry and Iron. IAEA and ISO have endorsed the proposal for mutual contact and collaborations between their organizations and ICSH. Cooperation has also been established with the Committee on Standards of the International Federation of Clinical Chemists, Standards Committee of the International Society of Clinical Pathology and the International Society of Blood Transfusion.

National contacts at an individual level have been urged to develop committees and national committees have been urged to establish themselves as registered organizations or to be affiliated with registered organizations in their own countries. Since the 1966 assembly, national committees have been established in the following countries: Argentine, Brazil, Chile, France, Greece. A regional committee has been established in Malaysia and Singapore.

The proceedings of the Symposium on Automation in Haematology was published as a supplement to British Journal of Haematology (Vol. 13, 1967), together with report of ICSH and Recommendations on Haemoglobinometry. It is planned to publish the Symposium on *Haematology of Normal Man: Haemoglobin Concentration* and the scientific activities of the Expert Panels.

The following Board Members are due to retire: Alexeieff, Crookston, Crosby, Eilers, Rewald, Walsh and Watanabe. Crosby was confirmed as President-elect to take office as President in September 1968 and Spaander as Vice-President, to follow Crosby as President in 1970.

It is noted that in accordance with our rules and the decision of the Sydney Meeting there are two Vice-Presidents, one of whom becomes the next President. To clarify the position the following scheme is proposed by the Secretariat.

	President	(President-elect) Vice-President	Vice-President
1966	Watanabe	Crosby	Spaander
1968	Crosby	Spaander	(1)
1970	Spaander	(1)	(2)
1972	(1)	(2)	(3)

(1) Preferably from Asian-Pacific Area
(2) Preferably from American Area
(3) Preferably from European Area

124

4.3. Report of Treasurer
G. Astaldi, The Blood Research Foundation Center, Tortona, Italy

The chairman of the ICSH-Secretariat has mentioned in his report, the generous financial contribution that the Council of Europe has given to support our Committee for Standardization in Hematology, with the specific goal to support studies on Haemoglobinometry and in particular, the preparation and distribution of a Haemoglobin Standard Preparation. However, this support has been given as a grant to the RIV, the Netherlands, and therefore, it could not be put into the ICSH-Treasury.

Minor contributions have been supplied from several different Firms, first of all for the Iron Expert Panel, and a lesser amount for the Working Group on the Standardization of Documentation of Haematological Findings. For this reason, it became necessary to open a bank account in a place where a member of the Secretariat is living, but that was not very easy to do in Italy because of the local bank regulations. In fact, it is not possible to have a bank account in foreign currency, so that the incoming money should be transferred to Italian lire, and the outgoing money from Italian lire to American dollars, or other handy currency. This would have caused a loss of money and therefore, the Secretariat during its meeting in Bilthoven on June 5-6, 1967 unanimously decided to open a bank account in dollars in Bilthoven, the Netherland. This was arranged with the Algemene Bank Nederland N.V., and Coster was asked to accept the task of handling matters in connection with the new situation. He has carried out his duties ably, and I believe he will kindly report here the financial situation. Again, also in the name of the other members of the Secretariat, I would like to recommend to the Board to officially nominate Coster as Treasurer of our Committee.

4.4. Report of General Assembly

1. The meeting was attended by national delegates and observers from the following countries: Argentina, (E. Rewald,* G. C. Vilaseca); Austria (F. Gabl); Brazil (G. Hoxter); Canada (P. H. Pinkerton, C. D. Greifeneder); France (C. Sultan); Germany (Ch. G. de Boroviczeny,* L. Heilmeyer,* A. Klein-Wisenberg); Israel (G. Izak *); Italy (G. Astaldi,* L. Tentori); Japan (T. Abe,* T. Matsubara, K. Takikawa, S. Watanabe *); Netherlands (J. Coster,* P. W. Helleman, A. H. Holtz, J. Spaander,* O. W. van Assendelft, E. J. van Kampen, W. G. Zijlstra); Sweden (B. Thorell *); United Kingdom (S. M. Lewis *); U.S.A. (W. H. Crosby,* R. J. Eilers,* A. Warren, L. R. Weintraub); Yugoslavia (A. Milosavbjevic).

* Board Member.

Apologies were received from Czechoslovakia, Poland, Roumania, and the U.S.S.R.

2. Crosby was installed as President. In his inaugural comments he thanked Watanabe for his active contributions to ICSH as previous president during the past two years, and especially commended him and his colleagues of the Japan Society of Hematology for the successful symposium on standardization which they held in April 1968. He commented on future scope of ICSH activities, and emphasised that progress could be made along several lines, including organisation of symposia, publications, international trials, accumulation of bibliography, evaluation of data. Investigational work should however, be left to individual workers and other independent agencies.

3. The report of the secretariat was adopted. The proceedings of the board meeting were reviewed by the Chairman. Matters arising therefrom are dealt with below. The nominations of Spaander as President in 1970 and Izak as incoming Vice-President were endorsed.

4. Seven Board members were due to retire (Alexeieff, Crookston, Crosby, Eilers, Rewald, Walsh and Watanabe). All retiring members were re-elected with the exception of Crookston and Walsh, who did not wish to seek re-election. To replace Crookston, Pinkerton (Toronto) was elected as a Board Member. It was agreed in principle to have a second Board member from Latin America, to be filled when a formal proposal is made to the Board.

5. The national committees of Argentina, Brazil, Chile, France, Greece and the regional committee of Malaysia and Singapore were accepted as members of the Assembly. It was agreed also to accept Bolivia, Peru and Venezuela as members when their national committees become established. There are now 26 Assembly members and in addition contacts have been established with individuals in 7 other countries and regions.

6. Reports of several national committees were received. They indicate considerable activity in hematological standardization at national levels, and active collaboration with ICSH. A special symposium on standardization was held by the Japan Society of Hematology in April 1968 and the Italian Committee for Standardization of Hematological and Laboratory methods (CISMEL) held a symposium in November 1967 during the National Congress of the Italian Association of Clinical Pathologists. CISMEL is planning an international symposium on standardization in Hematology at the Carlo Erba Foundation, Milan in November 1968. In several countries committees have been formed with representatives of general clinical pathologists, chemists, blood transfusionists and other groups. The Assembly emphasised the need for such a broad basis of representation in National Committees in order to pursue the aims of ICSH as laid down in the Constitution.

7. The proposed amendments to the Constitution were accepted and the Constitution as set out was adopted.
8. The Treasurer's report was adopted. Astaldi's proposal that Coster be appointed as Treasurer was approved.

Coster presented a 1969 budget estimate of $ 5,600 for the administration of the committee with the requisite meetings of Secretariat, Board and Assembly. To help meet this budget it was proposed that national committees be asked to make an annual voluntary contribution to ICSH. It was agreed to, without any formal objections, and a sum of $ 200 was suggested as a suitable contribution from each national committee. The treasurer was authorised to contact national committees to request their co-operation in this.

9. A preliminary report of the recent international trial was presented by Holtz. The final report will be distributed to all members of ICSH and will be published.
10. A report by the Panel on Terminology was distributed. The report will be completed, during the next few months; its recommendations will then be circulated to all ICSH members for a postal vote.
11. The Board had accepted an invitation by Heilmeyer to meet in Munich in 1970 on the occasion of the XIIIth Congress of the International Society of Hematology. It was agreed that this would also be an appropriate occasion for the next Assembly of ICSH.

It was proposed that the symposia on Haematology of Normal Man should be continued with a suitable subject at the XIIIth Congress of ISH. The enthusiastic co-operation offered by the organising committee was noted with appreciation. It was agreed that ICSH business meetings and Panel meetings (other than symposia within the framework of the Congress) be held prior to the Congress, and that ICSH activities be co-ordinated by collaboration with Boroviczény and Dr. W. Stich Secretary of the Congress Committee.

4.5. Relationship of ICSH with International Society of Hematology

The following resolution was moved, seconded and agreed to in principle at the Business meeting of the International Society of Hematology in New York on 5th September, 1968.

The members of the International Society of Hematology:

Considering the aims to promote standardization as laid down in the Constitution of ISH,
having regard to the aims and the Constitution of ICSH,
taking into account the results achieved by ICSH,

a) empowers the Council of ISH to establish a working relationship with ICSH,

b) authorises ICSH to act as the official agency of ISH for the standardization of laboratory methods and procedures in the field of hematology.

It was agreed that ISH Secretariat General should meet with ICSH Secretariat in order to work out a scheme for implementation of the resolution (a)* and that a mail vote of the Council will subsequently be taken to decide on acceptance of resolution (b).

4.6. Constitution of the International Committee for Standardization in Hematology

1. The Standardizing Committee of the European Society of Hematology was founded in Lisbon on 31st August, 1963 at a session attended by representatives of the European Society of Hematology, of national hematological societies, of clinical pathology societies and of other national, international and supranational societies and corporations. At the subsequent Assembly in Stockholm on 29th August, 1964 it was agreed to enlarge the representation of the committee and to amend the rules of procedure. With the merging of the European Society of Hematology with other regional societies to form the new International Society of Hematology the Committee's parent-body went out of existence. The Secretariat was registered legally as an independent Foundation in the Netherlands on the 29th April 1968. The constitution as further amended was confirmed by the General Assembly of Members in New York, on the 4th September, 1968.

2. The Committee will be known as « International Committee for Standardization in Hematology ». Its shortened title will be ICSH. Its aim is to achieve reliable and reproducible results in laboratory analysis, primarily in diagnostic hematology.

3. The Standardization Committee is directed by a Managing Board, of whom a President, Vice-Presidents, an Archivist, Secretaries and a Treasurer are named. The Managing Board is elected for four years by the Assembly of members and members may be re-elected. The Board will appoint specialists who will attend meetings and participate in discussion without voting rights. The Board will appoint a Secretariat formed by the named secretaries, the treasurer and the archivist. From its members the secretariat will appoint one who will act as Chairman of the Secretariat, and another as Vice-Chairman.

* Immediately after this meeting contact was established with Dr. T. Arends, Secretary General of ISH and an informal meeting took place between representatives of ISH and ICSH, in order to consider methods for implementation of this resolution.

4. Membership of the Committee is open to all national and regional hematological standardizing committees or test boards; or, in case no such body is established, to national hematological societies or clinical pathology societies, or, in exceptional cases, to an individual hematologist as representative of his country or region. National committees should be registered in their countries, in accordance with local law, either as an independent organisation or as a constituent part of a registered organisation. Any national or regional body wishing to have representation on the Committee will present credentials to the Board, who will have the right to reject or to recommend for election. Such election will be by an open vote at the Assembly. There will be no limitation of number of members.

5. Members will be invited by the Board to send one accredited representative, delegated for one session only, to the Assembly of the Committee. This Assembly will be convened at regular intervals, on the occasion of hematological congresses at the international level. The activity report of the Managing Board will be read; new members of the Board and of the Committee will be elected when necessary, and standardizing decisions will be made. Decision will be made by simple majority and through open voting. Each delegate and each member of the Board has one vote. A memorandum of the proceedings of the Assembly will be circularized by the Secretariat to all members as soon as possible after the meeting and members not able to attend the meeting may vote by post within six weeks of the memorandum being sent out. The Assembly will also be open to invited observers from national, international and supranational societies and corporations. Such observers may participate in discussion, but without voting rights. Assembly proceedings will be confined to non-technical matters. Scientific subjects will be discussed at symposia or meetings of specialists.

6. The Managing Board will meet at intervals as necessary, and when possible on the occasion of Hematological Congresses at the international level. Members of the Board may be represented at the meeting by a proxy or, alternatively, may submit their views by letter and may exercise a right to postal vote on any proposal. Such vote most be received within six weeks of the date on which the memorandum of the meeting is circularzed by the Secretariat. No answer within this period will be taken as an acceptance of the proposal.
The Secretariat will meet when necessary, by decision of its chairman. Board documents and a copy of all correspondence will be lodged in a central file kept by the archivist. No quorum will be necessary for Assembly or Board Meetings; Secretariat Meetings require a quorum of four members of the Secretariat.

7. The Managing Board will make enquiries into methods and apparatus of hematological analysis, will deliberate on standardizing possibilities, will elaborate standardizing proposals and will stimulate and co-ordinate

scientific work in this connection. A prime activity of ICSH will be the conduct of international comparability trials. When opportune for the promotion of discussions and propagation of standardizing procedures the Board may decide, instead of convening the Assembly, to choose a subsidiary procedure by inviting National Standardizing Committees and individual experts to attend or be represented at Expert Panels held in conjunction with congresses or as special conferences. The Board will also appoint specialists and working parties.

8. Conclusions at a scientific level will be reported to the Board and to Members of the Committee or their accredited delegates for consideration. The Board will take note of comments by the Committee and will prepare specifications for standards. These will be presented to the Assembly. Ample time will be given for their consideration. When they are approved they will be circulated by the Secretariat to the Members of the Committee, to international bodies, to national standards organizations, to national hematology and allied societes and as widely as possible to individual hematologists. The Board will take responsibility for the production and distribution of standard solutions for international reference.

9. The International Standardization Committee works in co-operation with any international organization with allied interests in order to promote the goals of the Committee.

10. Bodies represented on the Committee are requested to translate the decisions of the Committee into the language of their respective countries, to have them published in their professional journals and to ensure that the decisions are put into operation in their countries. National or regional standardizing Committees or Test Boards are requested to remain in contact with the Secretariat and to support the work of the International Committee.

11. All documents issued or published by, or on behalf of ICSH will remain the copyright property of ICSH, unless this right is waived.

12. Accounts will be produced annually by the Treasurer and shall be audited by an independent auditor appointed by the Board.

4.7. *Rules of Procedure for Board Meetings and Assembly Meetings* *

1. Meetings will be conducted by the President. In his absence, one of the Vice-Presidents will take the chair.
2. An agenda will be circulated by the secretariat in advance of the meeting.

* In accordance with the revised Constitution and various decisions of Assembly and Board, as documented in reports of Board Meetings and General Assemblies.

The following items may be contained in the agenda for a Board Meeting.
1. Opening remarks by President.
2. Report of secretariat.
3. Treasurer's report.
4. Nominations for Board membership.
5. Nomination for Vice-President (President-elect).
6. Nomination for Vice-President.
7. Election of New President.
8. Recommendations for membership of Committee.
9. Nominations for expert panels.
10. Report of expert panels.
11. Arrangements for Meetings of Board and Assembly and for scientific symposia.
12. Appointment of Auditors.
13. Changes in rules and Constitution.
14. Other business.

3. At the Meeting the agenda will be confirmed.
4. Resignation of Members of Board and/or Secretariat will be received. Any new appointments to Secretariat will be made on a formal proposal by a member of the Board, duly seconded and voted by the Members. The same procedure applies for the removal from office. Decisions will be based on a simple majority vote; a two-thirds majority vote will be required for removal from office.
5. The Board will nominate a Chairman for an Expert Panel in a field which has been agreed to by the Board. This nominee will propose other members for his panel. The Board will confirm the names of these members and may nominate additional members. The Board will nominate a liaison member of the Panel from amongst the members of the Board. The Board member so serving on the Panel will report to the Board on the proceedings of the Panel. The Panel will remain in existence until a Board decision to disband the Panel. Individual members may resign or be removed from office by a two-thirds majority vote of the Board. The Panel will conduct its work in accordance with the rules of procedure for Expert Panels.
6. No quorum shall be required for a Board Meeting. A Board member may submit any reports or comments in writing or may delegate a proxy to attend on his behalf. After the meeting absent members will be notified of the proceedings and may participate in decisions by writing to the secretariat within 6 weeks. No answer within this period will be taken as acceptance.
7. There will be an ordinary Board Meeting at intervals as necessary, and when possible on the occasion of a congress at the international level.
8. The Board will convene assembly meetings at intervals, and all national committees will be notified at least four months in advance. Committees

will be asked to nominate their delegates who will attend the assembly. All correspondence will be sent to the named delegates. Appropriate international organisations will be invited to send observers who will be entitled to participate in the discussion but will have no voting rights.

9. The following items will be contained in the agenda of an assembly.
    1. Register of attendance.
    2. Opening remarks by President.
    3. Report by Secretariat.
    4. Committee elections.
    5. Board elections.
    6. Report of National delegates.
    7. Report of Expert Panels.
    8. Recommendations on standardization.
    9. Other business.
    10. Closing remarks by President.

10. No quorum shall be required for an assembly. A memorandum of proceedings will be circulated to all members after the meeting.
    Members of the committee who were not represented at the assembly have the right to express their views on any items contained therein, by correspondence with the Executive Secretary within six weeks of the memorandum being sent out. If deemed appropriate such items will be referred to the Board and the Assembly, but in general decisions will be based on a simple majority vote. No answer within the prescribed period to any specific question circulated to members will be taken as acceptance.

4.8. *Rules of Procedure for the Expert Panels*

1. Expert Panels are established by the Managing Board in order to work on specific questions and they continue in existence until the work with which they have been charged is completed or the Panel is disbanded by the Board. Terms of reference are set out by the Board. They include (a) Preparation of specifications for standard reference materials; (b) Preparation of recommendations for standard methods; (c) Assessment of suitability of an item for standardization or for review for action at a future time.

2. Each Expert Panel consists of a Chairman, a Secretary and Members. The Chairman will be appointed by the Board on the basis of eminence in the field. The Board will also appoint one of its members to serve on the Panel ex-officio, as liaison between the Panel and the Board.

3. The Chairman will appoint the Panel Secretary and will establish the composition of the Panel. Experts in the proposed subjects from all over the world will be invited to participate and collaboration may be

sought with other international bodies with similar interests. If various views prevail regarding the question under discussion, representatives of these various views should be invited whenever possible. It is' desirable that on an Expert Panel each continental group should be represented by one, preferably two experts. So as to avoid bias, not more than one quarter of the members of an Expert Panel should come from the same country. An Expert Panel should have at least 5 members. Working groups may be established within the Panels.

4. The list of names of an Expert Panel must be placed before the Board Members, whenever possible at a Board meeting but alternatively by correspondence. Only when this list has been approved by the Board can the Expert Panel officially begin its task.

5. The members of the Expert Panel can be appointed for a specified or non-specified period. In the latter case membership ceases on the dissolution of the Expert Panel or on the retirement or death of the member. The Board can pass a resolution by a two-thirds majority calling for the dismissal of a member of the Panel or the premature dissolution of the Expert Panel.

6. The Chairman of the Expert Panel is entitled, at his discretion, to invite the co-operation of further experts but he must notify the Board Members not later than the next Board Meeting..

7. The Expert Panels carry on their work in general by correspondence, but should also meet when opportune, and, if possible, especially on the occasion of international congresses.

8. An annual report will be presented to the Board by the liaison member, and to the Assembly by the liaison member or by the Chairman or Secretary of the Panel at the discretion of the Chairman of the Panel.

9. The resolutions and proposed recommendations prepared by the Expert Panel must be submitted to the Board. They can be accepted by the Board or referred back for further deliberation, but not altered.

10. After acceptance by the Board, all proposals are presented to the Assembly for consideration and are then published. After ample time has been allowed for their consideration and for comments by any interested parties, the Expert Panel will prepare a definitive Recommendation which will be submitted to the Board and to the Assembly for final acceptance.

11. Expert Panels are authorized to act on behalf of ICSH in obtaining funds from foundations, commercial firms and other possible sources. To avoid overlap between panels it is highly desirable that the Treasurer be kept informed of proposed approaches. All funds are payable to ICSH, and their receipt will be acknowledged by the Secretariat; 10 % of the funds will be retained for secretariat administration; the remaining 90 % will be delivered by the Treasurer to the Panel. The Chairman of the Panel will send a detailed account of expenditure of the funds to the Treasurer at the end of each year, for that calendar year.

4.9. *Rules of Procedure for the Secretariat*

1. The Secretariat consists of members of the Board and is composed of an archivist, secretaries and a treasurer. It acts as a unit. One member is elected by the Secretariat as its chairman and one as its vice-chairman to serve in that capacity for the remainder of their current tenure as members of the Secretariat. One of the secretaries shall act as an executive secretary in order to co-ordinate the activities and correspondence of the secretariat.

2. The Secretariat will meet when necessary. The meetings are convened by the Chairman, who prepares the agenda of the meeting.
   Items for the agenda can be proposed by all members of the Secretariat, and shall be precirculated wherever possible. Members of the Board have the right to attend the meeting, and the Chairman may invite experts. Every meeting requires a quorum of 4 members of the Secretariat.

3. The purpose of the meeting is to enable the Secretariat to review all the activities since the previous Secretariat meeting, prepare minutes of previously held Board and Assembly meetings, send letters to the correspondents of the Committee, draw up agendas for subsequent Board and Assembly meetings, initiate and develop projects as previously decided by the Board, prepare financial statements. Any difficulty or controversy which cannot be resolved in the meeting of the Secretariat will be referred back to the Board for amplification.
   Reports of the meeting of the Secretariat will be prepared and agreed by all members of the Secretariat present before the conclusion of the session.

4. If any subject-matters cannot be postponed until the next Secretariat meeting, any member of the Secretariat may send preliminary letters. Copies of these letters will be sent directly to the Executive Secretary who will circulate them to the rest of the Secretariat as required. Official confirmation or further discussions of the preliminary correspondence will take place in the next meeting of the Secretariat.

5. Any controversy interfering with the Secretariat acting as a unit will be brought before the Board.

6. The Archivist will maintain a central file of ICSH records. Copies of all official correspondence of the Board, the Secretariat, expert panels, working parties, etc., will be sent to Executive Secretary for filing.

7. The Executive Secretary will be allocated an annual budget for the administration of the office of the Secretariat. He will submit an annual statement of expenditure to the Treasurer.

8. Agenda and reports of Secretariat meetings will be circulated to all Board members for information.

134

4.10. List of Members of the ICSH: 1969

President

Dr. W.H. Crosby, New England Medical Center Hospitals, Boston, Mass 02111, U.S.A.

Secretariat

Dr. G. Astaldi, The Blood Research Found. Center, Ospedale Civile, Tortona, *Italy*.
Dr. Ch. G. de Boroviczeny, Medizinische Universitatsklinik, 78 Freiburg, *W. Germany*.
Dr. J.F. Coster, National Institute of Public Health, Sterrenbos 1, Utrecht, *Netherlands*.
Dr. R.J. Eilers, University Kansas Medical Center, Kansas City, Kansas 66103, *U.S.A.*
Dr. G. Izak, Hadassah University Hospital, P.O. Box 499, Jerusalem, *Israel*.
Dr. S.M. Lewis, Royal Postgraduate Medical School, London, W. 12, *England*.
Dr. J. Spaander, National Institute of Public Health, Sterrenbos, Utrecht, *Netherlands*.

Other Managing Board Members

Dr. T. Abe, University of Tokyo School of Medicine, Bunkyo-bu, Tokyo, *Japan*.
Dr. G. Alexeieff, Postgraduate Medical Institute, Place Vosstania, 1/2, Moscow D. 242, *U.S.S.R.*
Dr. G. Brecher, Division of Clinical Pathology, San Francisco Medical Center, University of California, San Francisco, California 94122, *U.S.A.*
Dr. J.B. Chatterjea, School of Tropical Medicine, Calcutta, *India*.
Dr. L. Heilmeyer, Medizin-Naturwissenschaftliche Universität, Steinhovelstr 9, D 79/ Ulm, *W. Germany*. Deceased, September 1969.
Dr. P.H. Pinkerton, Sunnybrook Hospital, 2075 Bayview Avenue, Toronto 12, Ontario, *Canada*.
Dr. E. Rewald, Fundacion Hematologica, Mar del Plata, *Argentina*.
Dr. B. Thorell, Karolinska Sjukhuset, Stockholm 60, *Sweden*.
Dr. S. Watanabe, National Cancer Institute, Tsukiji 5-1-1, Chou-ku, Tokyo, *Japan*.

National Hematology Standardizing Committees

Argentina. Dr. G.C. Vilaseca, Comite Argentino de Estandarizacion, Angel Gallardo 899, Buenos Aires.
Bolivia. Dr. Mario Ergueta, Casilla No, 2301, La Paz.
Brazil. Dr. G. Rosenfeld, Institute Butantan, Caixa Post 65, Sao Paulo.
Chile. Dr. C. M. Arrau, Estado 360, Santiago.
Czechoslovakia. Dr. J. Libansky, Institute of Haematology and Blood Transfusion, U Nemocnice 1, Praha 2, Nové Mëste.
Denmark. Dr. K. Jørgensen, Rigshospitalet, 9 Blegdamsvej, Copenhagen.
France. Dr. C. Sultan, Hopital Henri Mondor, 94-Creteil.
East Germany. Dr. K. Ruckpaul, Inst. Pharmakologie, Lidenbergerweg 70, Berlin-Buch.
West Germany. Director, Standardisierungsinstitut, Hugstetterstrasse 55, D-78 Freiburg/Br, (Dr. Ch. G. de Boroviczeny).
Greece. Dr. H. Tsevrenis, 1st Regional Transfusion Center, Hippokrations Hospital, Athens.
Hungary. Dr. E. Kelemen, Orvostovábbképzó Intézet, Szabolcs utca 33, Budapest XIII.
India. Dr. S.J. Baker, Christian Medical College Hospital, Vellore.
Israel. Dr. G. Izak, Dept of Haematology, Hadassah University Hospital, P.O. Box 499, Jerusalem.
Italy. Dr. A. Fieschi, Ist. Clin. Med. Università di Genova, Genova.
Japan. Dr. S. Watanabe, National Cancer Institute, Tsukiji 5-1-1, Chuo-ku, Tokyo.
Malaysia and Singapore. Dr. K.S. Lau, Dept of Pathology, University of Malaysia, Kuala Lumpur.
Netherlands. Dr. F.J. Cleton, Academisch Ziekenhuis, Leiden.
Norway. Dr. A. Schrumpf, St. Joseph's Hospital, Porsgrunn.
Poland. Dr. S. Pawelski, Instytut Hematologii, Ulica Chocimska 5, Warsaw.

Rumania. Dr. I. Bruckner, Inst. Medicina Intern, 19 SosStefan cel Mare, Bucharest.
South Africa. Dr. J. Metz, South African Institute for Medical Research, P.O. Box 1038, Johannesburg.
Spain. Dr. J. Triginer, Instituto Nacional de Prevision, Ciudad Sanitaria de la Seguridad Social « Francisco France » Servicio de Hematologia y Hemoterapia, Barcelona - 16.
Switzerland. Dr. H.R. Marti, Kantonsspital, 5001 Aarau.
Turkey. Dr. F. Reimann, Inst. Med. Research, Istanbul-Capa.
U.S.S.R. Dr. G.V. Derviz, Inst. of Haematology and Blood Transfusion, Novosikovsky pr. 4, Moscow A 176.
United Kingdom. Chairman, British Committee for Standards in Haematology, King's College Hospital, London, S.E.5 (Professor W.M. Davidson).
U.S.A. Chairman, Standards Committee of College of American Pathologists, 230 N, Michigan Avenue, Chicago, Ill. 60601 (Dr. R.J. Eilers).
Venezuela. Dr. T. Villalobos Capriles, Avenida Los Proceres 34, Ed. Esmeralda 1-A San Bernadino, Caracas.

Other National Contacts

Austria. Dr. F. Gabl, Medizinische Universitatsklinik, Anichstrasse 35, Innsbruck.
Belgium. Dr. R. Verwilghen, Universiteitsklinieken « St. Rafael », Kapucijnenvoer 35 Leuven.
Finland. Dr. H.R. Nevalinna, Fin. Red Cross Blood Transfusion Service, Tehtaankatu 1, Helsinki.
Kenya. Dr. H. Foy, Wellcome Trust Research Laboratories, Box 30140, Nairobi.
Portugal. Dr. F. Parreira, Facultade de Medicina, Ave Professor Egas Moniz, Lisboa 4.
Sweden. Dr. B. Gullbring, Blood Transfusion Service, Karolinska Sjukhuset, Stockholm 60.
Yugoslavia. Dr. I. Crepinko, Bolnice « Dr. O. Novosel », Zajceva 19, Zagreb.

International Organisations

Council of Europe
Mr. H. Pfeffermann, Public Health Division, Secretariat General, Council of Europe, Strasbourg, *France.*

International Atomic Energy Agency
Dr. H. Belcher, Section of Nuclear Medicine, IAEA, Kartnerring 11, Vienna, *Austria.*

International Federation of Clinical Chemistry (Committee on Standards)
Dr. A.H. Holtz (Secretary), Rijks Instituut voor de Volksgezondheid, Sterrenbos 1, Utrecht, *Netherlands.*

International Society of Clinical Pathology Standards Committee
Dr. Bradley Copeland, New England Deconess Hospital, 195 Pilgrim Road, Boston 15, Mass., *U.S.A.*

International Society of Haematology
Dr. T. Arends, Inst. Venezolano de Investigaciones Cientificas, Caracas, *Venezuela.*
Dr. H. Braunsteiner, Med. Universitats Klinik, Innsbruck, *Austria.*
Dr. S. Hibino, Nagoya National Hospital, Nagoya, *Japan.*

International Society of Blood Transfusion
Dr. J.P. Soulier (Secretary General) 6 Rue Alexandre Cabanel, 75 Paris XVe, *France.*

International Standards Organisation
Director of Technical Coordination, 1 Rue de Varembe, Geneva 20, *Switzerland.*
Secretary, ISO Technical Committee TC 76, BSI, 2 Park Street, London, W.1, *England.*

136

International Union of Pure and Applied Chemistry
Director General Dr. R. Moss, C/O F. Hoffmann - La Roche & Co., Basel 2, Switzerland.
League of Red Cross Societies
Dr. Z.S. Hantchef, Medical Director, Petit Saconnex, Geneva, Switzerland.
World Health Organization
Dr. M.G. Candau, Director General, WHO, Avenue Appia, 1211 Geneva, Switzerland.

Expert Panels (with contact addresses)
1. Blood Collecting Procedures
   Convenor - Dr. S.M. Lewis, Royal Postgraduate Medical School, London W.12, England.
2. Cell Counting
   Chairman - Dr. J.W. Stewart, Bland-Sutton Institute of Pathology, Middlesex Hospital, London, W.1. England.
3. Cytochemistry
   Chairman - Dr. B. Thorell, Karolinska Sjukhuset, Stockholm, Sweden.
4. Documentation
   Chairman - Dr. G. Astaldi, Ospedale Civile, Tortona, Italy.
5. ESR
   Chairman - Dr. E. Rewald, Fundacion Hematologica, Mar del Plata, Argentina.
6. Folate and Vitamin B_{12}
   Chairman - Dr. B. Cooper, Royal Victoria Hospital, Montreal, Canada.
7. Haemoglobinometry
   Secretary - Dr. A.H. Holtz, Rijks Instituut voor de Volksgezondheid, Sterrenbos 1, Utrecht, Netherlands.
8. Iron Assay
   Secretary - Dr. J. Fielding, Paddington General Hospital, Harrow Road, London, W.9., England.
9. Isotopes
   Chairman - Dr. L. Szur, Dept of Radiotherapy, Royal Postgraduate Medical School, London, W.12. England.
10. Normal Values
    Chairman - Dr. S. Watanabe, National Cancer Institute, Tsukiji 5-1-1, Chou-ku, Tokyo, Japan.
11. PCV
    Chairman - Dr. L.R. Weintraub, New England Medical Center Hospitals, Boston, Mass 02111, US.A.
13. Serology
    Chairman - Dr. K.L.G. Goldsmith, Blood Group Reference Laboratory, Lister Institute, Gatliff Road, London, S.W.1, England.
14. Terminology
    Secretary - Dr. Ch. G. de Boroviczeny, Medizinische Universitatsklinik, 78 Freiburg, West Germany.
16. Coagulation
    Convenor - Dr. R.J. Eilers, University of Kansas Medical Center, Kansas City, Kansas 66103, U.S.A.

Part II

Proceedings of the International Symposium on Standardization of Hematological Methods (Milano, November 9-10, 1968)

Editors:

G. *Astaldi,* Director, The Blood Research Foundation Center, Tortona, Italy

A. *Fieschi,* President, Italian Committee for Standardization of Hematological and Laboratory Methods, Genova, Italy

C. *Sirtori,* President, Carlo Erba Foundation, Milano and General Director, G. Gaslini Institute, Genoa, Italy

G. *Vanzetti,* Director, Center Analytical Biochemistry, Ospedale Maggiore, Milano, Italy

139

Welcoming Address by the President of the
Carlo Erba Foundation Prof. Carlo Sirtori

Dear friends and colleagues:

The Carlo Erba Foundation is proud of having you as its guests and wishes to express particular thanks to Prof. Fieschi, the President of CISMEL and a prominent clinician; to Prof. Vanzetti, who promoted and organized this meeting; to Prof. Astaldi, the Coordinator of CISMEL; to Dr. Lewis, who also represents Dr. Spaander; and to the speakers and all of you, Ladies and Gentlemen.

This Symposium comes as a booster to my hopes, since I've always looked with a good deal of apprehension at doctors mixing, pouring, centrifuging, and counting things in their laboratories—that is, fighting a losing battle, because machines can do these jobs much better than men. Nervous stimuli travel at a speed of only 100 meters a second in the human body, as contrasted with hundreds or thousands of kilometers in a machine. Today the only test that calls for a human mind in the laboratory is histological and cytological observation; and even this is giving way to the advance of more and more refined cytoanalyzing machines.

See how widely the evaluation of a carcinoma in situ can vary from one diagnostician to another—and the same is true of tricky cytological and histological examination. I have attended several meetings of the WHO dealing with the classification of tumors: some of these tumors had been diagnosed in ten or fifteen different ways! We hope that the machine will make good the incapacity of man.

The Vickers machines (four-hundred of them, with as many doctors) could make histological diagnoses for 19 million people a year. The TICAS machines have already proved cleverer than man: fed 30 histiocytes, 30 normal endometrial cells, and 30 cells form endometrial carcinoma, they gave only one wrong answer.

Look at the « social contribution » we can reasonably expect of machines that can do a complete blood examination in 40 seconds. Think of the possible large-scale applications of such machines, when 30 per cent of young women have iron-deficiency anemia and therefore hyperkeratinized epithelia, sometimes with binuclear cells, and enzymatic defects, and present the typical passive behavior of « stale » women.

I also envisage the possibility of examining human behaviors with the help of machines. For example, if we had a machine that could assay adrenalin (the hormone of aggressiveness) in the saliva, we would certainly have much to gain.

Working with machines, the busy doctor will have more free time. Freed of these menial jobs of counting and measuring, he will have more time for cultivating his intelligence. «Never was my mind so active as in repose», said Plato. Leisure is a time for renewing one's ideas and remedying one's errors.

But who is going to pay for the machines? The hospital? The university? The government? Industrial outfits can afford to renew their mechanical equipment, because machinery is a source of profit. Man thinks more about industry than about his own health. So the burden of thinking about health is dumped upon the State. But look at what happens in Italy: the State makes 570 billion lire a year selling cigarettes—and we know that one person out of every ten dies because of cigarette smoking; on the other hand, the socialized medicine program is afflicted with a deficit of 470 billion lire a year. My point is, why don't they use the 570 billion from the tobacco business to pay for the socialized medicine program?

This Foundation, which is an agape for the doctors, hopes that the advent of laboratory machines will bring grace, objectivity, certainty, and freedom from debatable diagnoses.

Welcome by the President of the CISMEL,
A. Fieschi

First of all I would like to thank Professor Sirtori and the Carlo Erba Foundation for the hospitality and the support to this meeting of the Italian Committee for the Standardisation in Hematology. I would also like to thank Dr. W.H. Crosby, President of I.C.S.H. for sponsoring our meeting. I welcome all foreign guests who will give important contributions to the solution of the problems which will be discussed here, and on behalf of the organizing Committee I thank all contributors and partecipants to this Symposium.

Few words on the importance of the standardisation of methods in hematology: in medical practice and in research, we need reliable methods and reproducible ones. The field of routine tests which are being performed on patients is broadening every day and has expanded from the more common ones (hematocrit, hemoglobin, retics, white cell count, etc.) to the more complicated (red cell enzymes etc.). Sometimes it is difficult to compare results obtained in different laboratories. Thus the importance of setting up reproducible and reliable methods, to work in national and international teams for this purpose, to persuade all labs to use the recommended techniques. In Italy CISMEL has already done some good work on the standardisation of hemoglobin determination and we are now coming to grips with other techniques. I am sure that the contributions in this meeting will be extremely important, and opening this international meeting, I wish you all good work and plenty of sport.

Opening Remarks by President-Elect of ICSH
J. Spaander *

In the Constitution of ICSH it is stated that « National Standardizing Committees are requested to be in contact with ICSH Secretariat and to support the work of ICSH ». In the present meeting this contact between the central body and a national committee is very well shown.

CISMEL is to be congratulated on the initiative for this meeting, for which they have found the Foundation Carlo Erba prepared to be a sponsor. The Italian Committee could be an inspiration to other national committees to achieve similar co-operation and collaboration.

It is from this type of meeting that the material comes, from which ICSH Expert Panels can start working. The subjects in the programme indicate how this material can be a basis for the work of the Panels.

We can be thankful that we meet here in the home of the Carlo Erba Foundation. The work of the Foundation is well know. Its publications are in medical libraries all over the world. They are well produced and one can be proud to be associated with these elegant publications.

We, as the people coming from abroad, thank our Italian colleagues and the Foundation Carlo Erba for their hospitality, especially at this present time when it is appreciated by us how much anxiety has been caused by the floods so near to this region.

The traditional friendships of medicine can nowhere better be seen than amongst those of us working in the field of standardization, for standardization is to us a shared hobby rather than career work; however, this hobby is of great importance. It gives us our mutual aim to advance the standard of the haematological practice by means of improved and more precise methods and instruments. Moreover standardization will enable inter-laboratory collaboration, and by this means international

* Because of family circumstances, Dr. J. Spaander was not present and these remarks were made for him by Dr. S. M. Lewis (Secretary of ICSH).

exchange will become more meaningful and will increase our friendship and opportunities for an exchange of views and ideas. We are grateful that WHO is represented here by Dr. Sansonnens. The interest of WHO in the standardization work is shown in its recognition of the cyanmethaemoglobin reference standard. The improvement of quality, and the foundation of adequate laboratories, especially in underdeveloped countries, is one of the big aims to which Dr. Sansonnens and his coworkers strive. I give you this thought for consideration, that one of our aims should be to help WHO develop simple methods of sufficient accuracy for this purpose, in addition to the development of the more sophisticated methods which we are mainly concerned with at this meeting and which is a main interest of ICSH activities.

I have already given thanks to the Carlo Erba Foundation, but I would like to mention specifically the President of the Foundation Professor C. Sirtori, who has assisted us greatly by his personal interest in the meeting.

Of CISMEL I would like to thank especially its President Dr. A. Fieschi and, as conveners of the symposium, Dr. G. Vanzetti and Dr. G. Astaldi. Dr. Astaldi has been the link between the ICSH and CISMEL. Thank you all for the work you have done for this symposium; its papers will cover a wide range of subjects and the large audience here gathered is a demonstration of the ever increasing interest in our work.

ICSH is very happy that it has been invited to participate in your activities and wishes you a very great success in this symposium.

1st Session

Chairmen: A. Fieschi, A. Giovanardi, J. Spaander

1.1. *Statistics in the Evaluation of Analytical Methods*

G.A. Maccacaro of Department of Biometrics and Medical Statistics and G. Zambon Center for Biomedical Applications of Electronic Calculus, University of Milan, Italy

The role of the clinical laboratory in modern medicine is often viewed from different angles by the patients, the analysts and the clinicians; some clinicians feel that its function is mainly that of a checking or monitoring device, whereas others lean heavily on laboratory data in diagnosis and even in therapy. All, however, agree that in today's medicine the clinical laboratory occupies an eminent position and fulfils a unique role.

As a statistician, I would say that the laboratory is a mediator of signals designed for transforming into comprehensible messages the chemical, physical, and biological signals that the patient emits at a level below the threshold of human perception. In the word « mediator » I would include a number of functions, such as selection, transduction, conversion, amplification, and others.

Mediation as just defined presents two essential features. Firstly the signals elicited by the laboratory do not constitute information until they are received, interpreted, and integrated by the physician; and secondly, the laboratory, as any other signal mediator, adds its own « noise » to the signals.

The clinical laboratory, therefore, is a mixer of signals and noises, and the data delivered to the doctor invariably contain both, in unknown proportions. As a rule, the doctor utilizes the datum as a pure signal without evaluating the role of noise.

One of the possible contributions of statistical analysis to the improvement of the clinical laboratory is that of measuring the background noise on which the signal is inscribed, identifying its sources, and exercising some sort of control over it. This is no easy task. The Ospedale Maggiore of Milan alone does over 30,000 physiocardiological examinations in one year, 270,000 microbiological tests and 400,000 biochemical tests. In a city like Milan, where in addition to this very large hospital there is a complete set of University Departments, about a dozen more hospitals, and some fifty private clinics, we have counted sixty private laboratories that carry out clinical analyses.

We also know that the work load of clinical laboratories doubles approximately every five years. And it is interesting to learn from the published data of INAM (the National Institute for Insurance against Disease) that while the number of radiological or laboratory examinations in O.D. patients has increased from 18 to 48 for every 100 enrolled patients from 1956 to 1965, and total enrolment has gone up from 20 to 26 million in the same period, the overall increase of laboratory examinations was 250 %. The total expenditure per annum of our largest socialized medical institution is in the region of dozen of billion lire (INAM, 1967). This great expenditure for a commodity of prime necessity is certainly justified, but has two peculiar aspects. Firstly, the consumer has no direct or indirect control on the quality of the commodity. And secondly, if the quality of the product is poor, there will be an increased demand for the same commodity.

The former characteristic is anachronistic; the latter is only apparently paradoxical, since according to a well-known law of the theory of information, the immediate antidote to noise is redundancy. The doctor applies this law unconsciously when, being unconvinced of a platelet count or blood bilirubin assay, he sends his patient back to the laboratory for a repeat test.

So far, the only people who have shown concern about the quality of their work, for ethical or professional reasons, have been the analysts themselves. An outstanding example is Prof. Giulio Vanzetti, the promoter of this Symposium; and with him many others who have been devoting their time and money to research aimed solely at raising the standard of performance of our analytical laboratories.

One of these investigations was planned and coordinated in my Department by Dr. Rodolfo Saracci; I should like to show you the results and discuss its conclusions. A detailed paper is going to appear in print in the next few weeks (Saracci, 1968). A total of 1775 Italian

145

laboratories were asked to take part in a quality control experiment. Of these, 421 accepted. This represented about one-fourth of the original statistical population; and it constituted a self-selected sample, which is obviously not nearly so representative as a random sample. Besides, a scrutiny of the response list suggests that these were the more efficient laboratories, eager to improve further their standards of performance.

Each of these laboratories was sent two specimens of the same lyophilized serum, packed differently so as to suggest that they originated from different patients.* Along with this material, each laboratory received a volumetric pipette, an ampoule of distilled water for reconstitution of the serum, and a form on which to record their findings for: glucose, urea, total protein, and total cholesterol.

The completed forms were collected by a public notary, who noted the sender's name and address and then turned them over to us as anonymous forms for elaboration.

From the same batch of lyophilized serum vials, 60 specimens were taken at random and sent to the Department of Pathology of the Englewood Hospital (Englewood, New Jersey) as reference laboratory.

While referring to Dr. Saracci's paper for further details I should like to point out that our study was mainly concerned with three problems, namely:

a) the distribution of imprecision;

b) the distribution of inaccuracy; and

c) the factors of imprecision and inaccuracy.

For precision, we measured the absolute variance of the two values given by the same laboratory for each of the assays. An example concerning glucose is shown in Fig. 1. Since this was a distribution of ranges, one might expect it to be practically triangular for maximum frequencies and minimum values, and vice versa. Alternatively, one might figure that the distribution is a composite of at least two other distributions, one for high-precision laboratories and one for those of lower precision. Resolution of the first part of histogram *1 a* in histogram *1 b* seems to corroborate this impression.

By inaccuracy we mean the variance between the observed value and the « true » value, this being the average value given by the reference laboratory. Fig. 2 also shows the value of the average of all determina-

(*) The serum, prepared by the Warner-Chilcott Company in the United States, was supplied to us by the Angiolini S.p.A. Company of Milan — to whom our thanks are hereby extended.

Figure 1 - *Frequency distribution of the imprecision (for the determination of glucose) in the sample of 404 laboratories. In abscissa is the absolute difference between the two replicates made in each laboratory (SARACCI, 1968).*

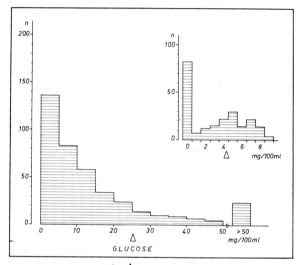

Figure 2 - *Frequency distribution (showing inaccuracy) of the 808 determinations of glucose:*

x_o = *mean of the 808 determinations made in the 404 laboratories*
x_r = *mean of the 60 replicates made in the external laboratory*
x_e = *true value (SARACCI, 1968)*

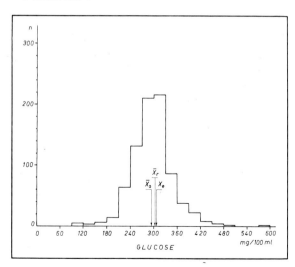

tions made in the 404 laboratories, for glucose, and the glucose level determined by weighing at the time of preparation of the serum.

The difference between the average of all the laboratories, and the other two values just mentioned, may be taken as indicative of the overall inaccuracy of the laboratories. Obviously, we are more interested in the inaccuracy of single laboratories, or rather, of single determinations. As can be seen from figure 2, this inaccuracy has a practically normal distribution within a very broad range spanning from one-half to twice the average value.

Similar observations can be made on the imprecision and inaccuracy of urea, total protein, and cholesterol assays—the last of these being the most imprecise and inaccurate of all. For the sake of brevity, I shall omit details and only say that we detected no significant correlation between accuracy and precision in any given laboratory. This creates some perplexity as to the absolute precision of the laboratories which did give two identical values for the same assay.

A criterion for overall evaluation of the results is offered in Fig. 3, where for each of the assays we show the percentages of replies between ± 10 %, ± 25 %, ± 50 %, and ± 100 % of the reference value.

As can be seen from what I have said so far, inaccuracy and imprecision weigh differently on the various assays made in different laboratories. The laboratories differ from one another on several counts, some of which were taken into consideration as variables to be correlated with the analytical quality of these laboratories (Table I).

This has made it possible to make multiple regression analysis in an attempt to determine to what extent precision and accuracy depend on one or more of these factors. The results of this analysis were negative (Fig. 4), in that the background variability that remains unaccounted for is far greater than the variability attributable to said factors. This, if confirmed by further investigations, may mean that in order to obtain greater precision and accuracy it is not enough to change methods, analysts, or laboratories: what is needed is for every analyst, in each laboratory, and with any method, to submit his work to systematic scrutiny by the daily use of standards, appropriate replications, and quality control.

Above all, the large socialized medicine institutes, hospitals, and the like should organize full-fledged services for the systematic checking and control of clinical laboratory procedures, whether they carry out this work themselves or have it done by others.

As I said before, statistical analysis must tell the analyst not only the magnitude of error in his measurements, but also give information

Figure 3 - *Percentages of determinations made in the* 404 *laboratories, which fall within* ± 10 %, ± 25 %, ± 50 % *and* ± 100 % *of the true value.*

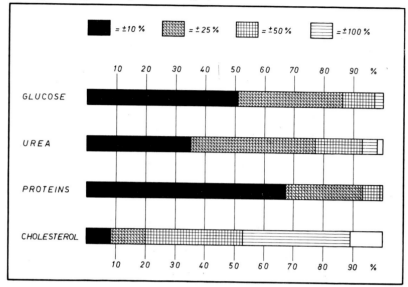

Figure 4 - *The black sector shows the percent of the total variance of inaccuracy and imprecision which can be predicted by the five independent variables listed in table n.* 1 (*SARACCI,* 1968).

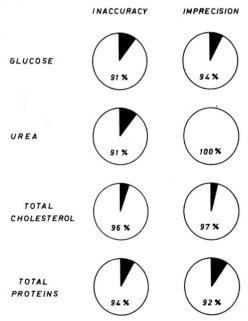

Table I – Variables whose correlation with the accuracy and precision of the 404 laboratories was investigated

Variables	Levels
(1) Laboratory Class	(1) Private (2) Nursing Home (3) Public (4) Hospital (5) University
(2) Laboratory Size	(1) <100 Determinations per Diem (2) 101-300 (3) 301-500 (4) >500
(3) Analyst Qualification	(1) University Degree (2) Technical Degree (3) No Recognized Degree
(4) Analyst Seniority	In Years
(5) Analytical Methods	As Binary Dummy Variables

on the source of error. The magnitude of error may be assessed in terms of accuracy and precision, but also of reproducibility, specificity, and other parameters (Whitby, Mitchell and Moss, 1967).

The sources of error will be identified, apart from the investigative talent of the analyst, by an effective experimental design which will not only reveal their existence but also determine their size.

For the sake of brevity, I shall only illustrate the latest problem of this kind, which Dr. Ettore Marubini of my Department tackled in cooperation with Drs. Sirchia, Ferrone, and Zanella of the Department of Medical Pathology of our University (Sirchia, Ferrone, Marubini and Zanella, 1968). As their paper is being printed, and all technical details will be found there, I shall only mention that the problem was the determination of erythrocyte acetylcholinesterase with dithiobisnitrobenzoic acid by Ellman's method. But what I am going to say applies to any analytical method, including those used in haematology.

Here the purpose of the investigation was to find out how much of the total variability was contributed by sources of error in the object itself, and how much by sources inherent in the analytical technique under discussion.

Table II – Variance analysis of the hierarchic type on the results of an experiment planned as in Fig. 5 (SIRCHIA, FERRONE, MARUBINI, ZANELLA, 1968)

Source of variability	d.f.	Sums of squares	Expected mean square	Mean square	F
B. subjects	4	566622.59	$\sigma^2 + 2\sigma_\rho^2 + 10\sigma_\tau^2 + 50\sigma_\pi^2$	141655.64	6.96*
B. times w. subjects	20	406809.24	$\sigma^2 + 2\sigma_\rho^2 + 10\sigma_\tau^2$	20340.46	14.05*
B. subsamples w. times	100	144762.00	$\sigma^2 + 2\sigma_\rho^2$	1447.62	7.36*
B. replicates w. subsamples	125	24572.50	σ^2	196.58	
Total	249	1142766.33			

* highly significant (P < 0,01)

σ^2 = variance due to random fluctuation = 196.58

σ_ρ^2 = variance due to subsamples = 625.52

σ_τ^2 = variance due to different times of blood collection = 1889.28

σ_π^2 = variance due to subjects = 2426.30

For the former, the following were considered:

1. Variability between subjects (5 healthy adults), and
2. Time variability in the same subjects (five samples, taken on five different and non-coincident days, for the five subjects).

The following technique-bound variables were considered:

3. Variability between 5 sub-specimens taken each time from each subject, and
4. Variability between two assays made on each sub-specimen from each subject at each time.

This is a typical « nested » design as shown in Fig. 5, suitable for variance analysis of the hierarchic type (see Table II), which provides the expected tests of significance, and also affords isolation and measurement of variability, due to the various sources.

This, in turn, allows us to formulate and compare various alternatives for the practical, routine control of the analytical work under discussion, by pre-evaluating the standard error of measurements obtained with each alternative. Some of these alternatives are shown in Table III, from which it is apparent that with 3 samples, 3 sub-specimens, and one single determination the estimate of individual cholinesterase is more precise than with one sample, 3 sub-specimens, and 3 determinations, or with 2 collections, 3 sub-specimens, and 3 determinations. This, I repeat, is an example which I have singled out because it is unpublished: but the basic approach is general and applicable to all cases.

Instead of having five test subjects we can consider five laboratory

Table III – Alternatives for the assay of erythrocyte acetylcholinesterase, and estimate of the corresponding errors

No. of times of blood collection	No. of subsamples	No. of replications	S.E. of AChE values	
			Absolute value	% value
	1	2	51.12	8.87
1	1	3	50.80	8.81
	3	1	47.90	8.31
	1	2	40.85	7.09
2	1	3	40.44	7.02
	3	1	37.28	6.47
	1	2	36.79	6.39
3	1	3	36.34	6.31
	3	1	32.17	5.58

152

Figure 5 - *Experimental design for the analysis of some sources of variability affecting the determination of the RBC-acethylcholinesterase; for more details see in the text.*

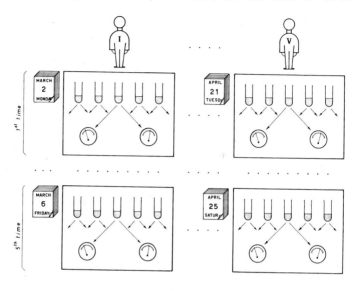

Figure 6 - *A comparison of the variability sources in the hypothetical example described in the text.*

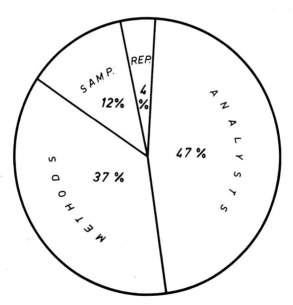

workers, and instead of taking samples at five different times we can consider five different methods for the same assay.

We thus have a situation far from uncommon in the laboratory, as when we are worried by the imprecision of a certain measurement and we wonder how much of this imprecision is due to variability between observers, difference between methods, difference between samples, and variance between replications. To this question we can give an answer like the one formulated in Fig. 6, which also provides some practical recommendations such as informing the analysts of their errors, selecting a method relative to a standard of analysis, and preferring a single determination on two samples rather than two determinations on the same sample.

From considerations such as these, and of course from subtler and more penetrating ones, the analyst acquires, besides his technical knowledge, a methodological knowledge of his procedures. Once he has this added knowledge, he will find it easier to implement the more effective devices for quality control in his laboratory work. Automation encourages the adoption of such devices, or indeed considers them as part and parcel of its procedures. On the other hand, it would be very bad if this were to encourage an automatic, non-critical use of the analytical methods.

I am confident that this will not happen, since I feel that if the analyst is freed from harassing routine, he will have better upportunities for increasing his knowledge and understanding of the underlying methodological problems.

This Symposium is itself a good indication of the interest of the analysts for such a development.

Conclusions

The clinical laboratory, as a mediator of information, is a mixer of signals and noises. A systematic and competent statistical analysis of its outputs may be useful in order to reduce the noise obscuring the signals, to identify the sources of variability and to keep them under control.

Two.examples are given. One deals with a survey of 404 Italian laboratories aiming at studying the factors affecting accuracy and precision in four clinical-chemistry determinations (glucose, urea, total cholesterol, total proteins). Another example deals with the design, the experimental results and the statistical analysis of an assay of RBC-acethylcholinesterase. The error components were evaluated and practical criteria for their reduction have been shown.

The adoption of a systematic quality control procedure for the clinical laboratory is advocated.

154

References

INAM, 1967, *Bilancio Consuntivo dell'Esercizio* 1967, Roma.
Saracci, R., 1968, Accuratezza e precisione nella determinazione di alcune grandezze ematochimiche. *A.b.d.c.e.*, 3, 1968-212.
Sirchia, G., Ferrone, S., Marubini, E. e Zanella, A., Statistical Evaluation of the Determination of Red Cell Acetylcholinesterase Activity by Diagnostic « Kit ». *Clinica Chimica Acta*, in press.
Whitby, L. G., Mitchell, F. I. e Moss, W., 1967, Quality Control in Routine Clinical Chemistry, in Bodansky, O., e Stewart, C. P., *Advances in Clinical Chemistry*, vol. 10, Academic Press, New York.

1.2. *Blood Collection and Preservation for Haematological Analyses*

S. M. Lewis B. Sc., M. D., M. R. C. Path, Department of Haematology, Royal Postgraduate Medical School, Ducane Road, London, W.12, UK

Containers for collecting blood for blood counts and other haematological investigations are used by their thousands each day. There are literally dozens of tubes, bottles and other containers in use, of varying sizes and varying efficiency. It is not my intention to suggest that only one standardized container should be adopted internationally. There are factors to be taken into account which make this impracticable, not least the important factors of personal preference and the requirements for individual specialized work. I shall, however, describe some criteria which are desirable and some which should be avoided in selection of tubes or bottles for blood collection for routine analyses.

Two to three ml of blood are, as a rule, sufficient and the container should have a volume about 30 % greater. The cap should be a screw type, preferably with a liner of a pliable material to ensure that it be leak proof. In Britain we have had considerable experience with plastic containers fitted with push-in caps. These are reported to be convenient to handle, especially by technicians who like to use only one hand for opening them, but their main defect is that they almost invariably leak after they have been once opened and resealed. This is a potentially serious health hazard in the laboratory, as well as being aesthetically objectionable. Moreover pneumatic delivery systems which are becoming more widely used subject the specimen containers to negative pressure which results in leakage if they are not adequately sealed. Plastic containers are not as a rule suitable for tight sealing by means of screw caps, but one type with a close-sealing joint (Fig. 1) has recently been developed and shows promise. It is certainly leak proof when sealed correctly although the seal tends to become less effective after multiple manipulation. In general, however, glass containers are more reliable than plastic with regard to their sealability. They also have the advantage that they can be constructed with a shoulder for easier handling, especially when put into a centrifuge cup. It is necessary to avoid containers which are too bulky or which have top-heavy caps, caps with sharp edges, caps made with hard plastics which are liable to become brittle with age, containers made from certain plastic material which, too, may degenerate with time, leading to brittleness and fracturing especially when the tube is subjected to the stress of centrifuging. The deterioration of certain plastic materials increases rapidly at low temperatures and attention should be paid to the effect on the containers of storage at 4 °C and at − 20 °C or lower. On the other hand, disposable plastics have obvious advantages over the heavier, more fragile and less easily disposable glass. A British Standard is at present being prepared by the British Standards Institution which will include specifications for both materials and will, it is hoped, ensure that the disadvantages of each type will be avoided. It might be necessary to prescribe an expiry date and suitable storage conditions for plastic containers.

Does the material of the container have any effect on blood constituents? Potential sources of contamination of the blood are leaching of soluble materials from the fabric of the container, contamination of the container during preparation and contamination by dust or by material used for packing. This is especially a problem for the clinical chemist but one of which the haematologist must be aware. Of course it would be impractical to have a quality control test for all possible contaminants, and Marks (1967) has recommended sodium and potassium as non-specific indicators. The test procedure is to fill the container with deionized water, shake for one hour and allow to stand for 18 hours and again shake for one hour. The sodium and potassium are then determined by flame photometer. The acceptable tolerance is, of course, a matter for debate; we are proposing that it should not exceed .023 mg/ml sodium and .001 mg/ml potassium, i.e. 1 % of the amount usually present in a blood sample.

Fielding (1968) has shown, however, that even when polystyrene tubes contain negligible contamination with sodium and potassium they may have significant iron contamination unless acid washed. Contamination might also be introduced in the anticoagulant, and this, too, must be tested as part of a quality control.

I shall now turn to the requirements and effects of anticoagulants.

156

Figure 1

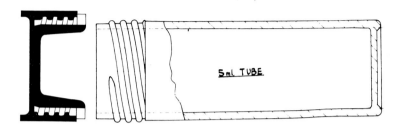

Figure 2

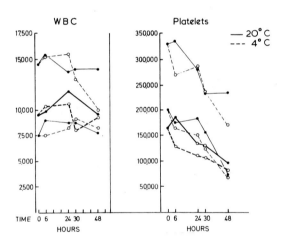

The anticoagulants in common use in haematology are EDTA, ammonium and potassium oxalate mixture, heparin and sodium citrate. The ammonium and potassium oxalate mixture has largely been replaced in clinical haematology by EDTA. Three salts of the latter are generally available — disodium, dipotassium and dilithium. The dipotassium salt is more soluble than the disodium salt and is to be preferred on this account. The dilithium salt appears to be equally effective as an anticoagulant and has the advantage that it can also be used for chemical investigations. On the other hand it is less soluble than the other salts and whether its advantage is sufficient to recommend its use requires further study.

EDTA is by no means a perfect anticoagulant; it has serious limitations. It should be used at a concentration of 1.5 mg/ml blood, and this must be fairly strictly adhered to, as an excess of EDTA results in a significant decrease in the packed cell volume. This has been demonstrated by Lampasso (1965) and by Pennock and Jones (1966) who have shown that more than 2 mg/ml of EDTA results in decreased PCV and increased MCHC. It is, thus, pointless to carry out a PCV measurement if too little blood is added, proportional to the anticoagulant. There is little room for manouvre, as less than 1 mg/ml is ineffective for preventing coagulation.

The main advantage of EDTA over oxalate is that they prevent the clumping of platelets in vitro and thus its use allows an accurate platelet count to be carried out on venous blood samples sent to the laboratory. But here, too, care must be taken to ensure that EDTA is used in correct proportion — a low concentration may cause platelet clumping even if there is no obvious clotting of the sample.

Platelets and leucocytes undergo degenerative changes in anticoagulant; this leads to progressive fall in counts (Fig. 2) and while these effects can be lessened by keeping the blood at 4 °C, the blood count should be carried out within 6 hours of collection.

Anticoagulants affect blood-cell morphology (Dacie and Lewis, 1968). Within three hours the changes are usually well marked. Some of the large mononuclear cells develop extensive changes. Small vacuoles appear in the cytoplasm and the nucleus undergoes irregular lobulation. Some lymphocytes undergo similar changes, with vacuoles in the cytoplasm, budding of the nucleus into two or three lobes and more homogeneous staining of the nuclei. Some of the neutrophils will also be affected — nuclei stain more homogeneously, nuclear lobes become separated, the cytoplasmic margin becomes ragged and vacuoles appear in the cytoplasm. All these changes become progressively more marked until the cells lose all their normal features and cannot be identified. The changes occur irrespective of anticoagulant. They occur more rapidly in oxalated blood than in EDTA blood and appear to be proportional to the concentration of anticoagulant. The changes are not, however, due entirely to the presence of anticoagulant, as they also occur in defibrinated blood, though much more slowly. Red cells alter more slowly than do the leucocytes, and after six hours or longer progressive crenation and sphering occur. I might here mention one other effect of EDTA — basophilic stippling of red cells will not stain in films prepared from venous blood taken into an anticoagulant, especially EDTA, even when clearly demonstrable in fresh films. The reason for this is not clear but the implication in relation to screening tests for lead intoxication is obvious.

EDTA and oxalate also affect enzyme content of blood cells. The effect on neutrophil alkaline phosphatase of storage of blood with EDTA is illustrated in Fig. 3. There is a decrease in score as the blood stands at room temperature, but less so at 4 °C. A similar effect is seen with peroxidase (Fig. 4). The loss of enzyme activity can be overcome by making and fixing films immediately after the blood has been collected.

It is clear that there is need for an improved anticoagulant, which will not affect blood constituents adversely and will enable blood counts and other investigations to be carried out after standing for a considerably longer period than is possible at present. The need to prevent haemolysis should also be taken into account.

Other anticoagulants may be used for specific purposes. Heparin is an effective anticoagulant; it does not alter red cell size and it reduces the chance of haemolysis to a minimum. It is the anticoagulant of choice for osmotic fragility, for enzyme studies, and when a specimen is required for chemical analysis. It does not affect the pH of the blood to the same extent as does EDTA. Heparinised blood is, however, unsuitable for blood films as it gives a blue background staining with Romanowsky dyes. Liquid heparin has a storage life of five years. The storage life of dry heparin should not be different, but whether the condition under which the heparin is stored when in blood containers affects this storage life is not known.

Trisodium citrate is the anticoagulant for coagulation studies and for measurement of sedimentation rate. There has been confusion about the concentration of sodium citrate to be used. Normal human serum has an osmolarity of 289 m-OsM. 3.8 % trisodium citrate is hypotonic; originally trisodium citrate was a salt with 11 parts of water to 2 parts of salt and this was, in fact, iso-osmotic at a concentration of 38 g/l.

159

Figure 3

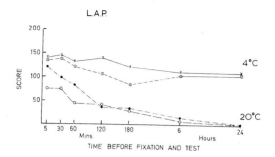

Figure 4

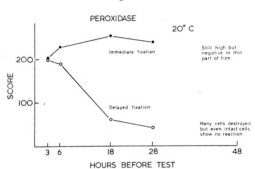

Figure 5

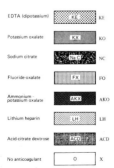

The code letters have since been altered. The recommendations by BSI are indicated alongside Fig. 5.

160

(0.106 mol). The form of trisodium citrate now available contains only 2 parts of water and the equivalent concentration to achieve iso-osmolarity is 31 g/l. Whether this makes any significant difference to the sedimentation rate of blood and other tests is not known but we should at least be consistent and standardize our techniques in this regard. It must also be remembered that this is a liquid anticoagulant which must be used in a precise proportion to avoid irregular dilution of the blood. This demands that prepared containers must contain an accurate volume of the anticoagulant and that evaporation or leakage of the solution will invalidate the container. This is particularly a problem with plastics which are semi-permeable, and as a precaution such containers should be given a relatively early expiry date in the hope that outdated bottles will be discarded and not kept on the stock shelf or in the clinic cupboard for too long. Preferably, such bottles should be kept at 4 °C. It is not known whether plastics have any effect on the citrate which might influence its anticoagulant activity.

It is undesirable to use glass containers for collecting blood for coagulation studies, including routine prothrombin, as glass activation of the clotting mechanism before the tests are carried out results in serious error. Conversely the choice of container for clotted blood is also a problem. As plastics inhibit clotting this results in poor retraction. Nylon is better than most plastics but is an expensive material. Styrene can be rendered wettable by strong gamma radiation but this too is an expensive procedure, and may shorten life of the material. Thus glass has advantages over plastics when serum is required.

Finally, I would like to remark on the labelling of containers. There is urgent need for agreement to overcome the confusion which exists because of the great variation in design, and in colour of the labels which are in current use. We have made recommendations in Britain which will form part of a British Standard, and will, we hope, be acceptable as the basis for an international code (Fig. 5). We would like, also, to see some consistency with regard to the information printed on the labels, and the space available for patient data, having due regard for the needs of automatic sample handling and computer processing. In view of the importance of having a relatively accurate concentration of anticoagulant per ml of blood it is also highly desirable that the label or the container itself should have a precisely placed mark to indicate the level to which the blood must be added.

I have tried to indicate the problems which are still present and the areas in which studies and trials are necessary. It is clear that there is need for an improved anticoagulant, and that there is need for careful consideration to enable us to arrive at a design for the container and a choice of material to overcome the limitations which exist. Without doubt, much can be done to improve the standard of the containers in common use, and the establishment of a rational international specification should be a valuable contribution to the practice of haematology.

References

[1] Dacie, J. V. and Lewis, S. M., *Practical Haematology,* 4th Edition, p. 6, Churchill, London, 1968.
[2] Fielding, J. and Ryall, R., *J. clin. Path., 21,* 415, 1968.
[3] Lampasso, J. A., *Amer. J. clin. Path., 44,* 109, 1965.
[4] Marks, V., Memorandum No. 67/25947; British Standards Institution, 1967.
[5] Pennock, C. A. and Jones, K. W., *J. clin. Path., 19,* 196, 1966.

1.3. *A Study of the Phenomenon of Count Loss in the Coulter Counter*

P.W. Helleman, Dept. of Haematology Univ. State Hospital Utrecht, Nation. Instit. of Public Health, Utrecht

Many of the electronic devices used in counting particles are characterized by the fact that the number of particles counted (N_c) is inferior to the true number of particles present (N_t). This phenomenon occurs when the detection unit of the apparatus is large in relation to the distance between the particles. In this situation, several particles can be present simultaneously in the detection area without being separately discernible (so-called coincidence). The resolving power of the apparatus can be diminished when the impulse produced by a particle is led through an amplifier with an insufficient band width; in that case the amplitude of the pulse decrease appreciably. Count loss can occur also when the discriminator is insufficiently sensitive to distinguish two closely spaced impulses. A third possibility is that the counter used is not sufficiently fast to record all the pulses offered.

When a well-adapted electronic counter is used, the degree of count loss is dependent exclusively on the degree of coincidence.

The detection unit of the Coulter counter consists of a capillary immersed in an electrolyte solution on which an electric tension is generated.

The particles contained in the electrolyte solution pass through the capillary at a certain speed, causing a brief change in resistance within the capillary. This change in resistance gives rise to a brief change in potential, which is translated into an electric impulse. Because the density of the electric field inside and immediately outside the capillary is not homogeneous, the pulse is bell-shaped instead of block-shaped. The rise time, fall time and peak duration of the pulse are determined by the speed at which the particle passes through the capillary; the peak height is determined by the field strength in the midportion of the capillary. The formation of a plateau-like peak depends on the homogeneousness of the field in the midportion of the capillary, on the path of the particle through the capillary and, to some extent, on the velocity of ion displacement in the electrolyte solution as well as, possibly, the particle's own charge. The rate of flow of the fluid which contains the particle, must be so controlled as to ensure that the electronic apparatus can correctly assimilate the resulting pulse; in other words: the rate of flow must be adapted to the band width of the amplifier.

With a view to the occurrence of count loss, a study was made of the band width of the Coulter counter, its effect on the shape of the impulse produced in the detection unit, the shape of this pulse and its assimilation by the discriminator.

Because coincidence depends in part on the distances between particles, a study was made also of the particle contribution in the thread of fluid which passes through the capillary.

Since with increasing particle concentration, the chance of coincidence increases, and therefore also the chance of increased pulse durations and amplitudes, pulse duration- and pulse height graphs were plotted in relation to certain cell concentrations. The changes occurring in the distribution curves as a result of changes in particle concentration, correlate with the occurrence of coincidence. From these changes some insight into the occurrence of coincidence can therefore be gained.

Procedure and discussion of results

1. Block-shaped pulses (with a rise time of < 1 µsec) were offered at the input of the pre-amplifier. From the pulse shapes obtained behind the pre-amplifier and main amplifier, the rise times of the amplifiers were calculated.
   The results showed that the band width of the amplifiers was sufficient and exerted little influence on the pulses offered at the input.

2. The pulses caused by erythrocytes were led from the amplifiers to a memory tube. Some of the pulse shapes obtained with the 70 µm capillary are nearly identical.

3. The pulse shape is determined, not only by the geometry of the electric field, but also by hydrodynamic phenomena in the detection unit.

According to Gutmann [1], the flow of fluid in the capillary behaves in accordance with the law of Poiseuille.

Proceeding from this law it can be calculated, that the mean rate of flow in the capillary should be 8.9 m/sec. This is not consistent with the mean rate of intracapillary flow; the average velocity of that was measured to be about 4.9 m/sec.

According to Bernouilli, the mean rate of flow through an orifice can be calculated from the pressure gradient and the contraction coefficient.

With the aid of the law of Blasius, the contraction coefficient can be calculated, if the length of the capillary and the Reynolds number are known. The Reynolds number can be calculated if the mean velocity, capillary diameter, viscosity and density of the fluid are known. Given these, it could be calculated that the contraction coefficient would be about 0.8. When this factor is used in the calculation according to Bernouilli, a mean rate of flow of 4.8 m/sec is obtained; this is consistent with the measured rate of flow, thus the flow of the fluid in the capillary obeys the law of Bernouilli.

The pulse shapes caused by erythrocytes depend not only on the volume, but also on the path described by the erythrocytes. In view of this, the durations of pulses produced by Celltroll particles passing through 50, 70 and 100 μm capillaries, respectively, were determined.

Taking into account the fluid flow distribution in the capillary, an average pulse shape was calculated from the pulse shapes obtained and the mean pulse durations. On the basis of the rise times calculated, idealized average pulse-shapes were constructed for the 50, 70 and 100 μm capillary, respectively.

With block-shaped pulses offered to the amplifiers, while the pulse frequencies were varied, the speed of the counters was found to range up to 200- to 250- thousand pulses in regular succession per second.

The discriminator and electronic counters used, are thus adequate and are not likely to exert an unfavourable influence on the resolving power of the apparatus. In view of the pressure gradient in the manometer, the *construed averaged and idealized* pulse shapes can therefore be used in determining the occurrence of coincidence in the detection unit.

In principle, count loss due to coincidence can be determined by making counts in several dilutions. The chance of coincidence diminishes by as much as the dilution of a suspension increases. If the dilution is very high, then the chance of coincidence can be assumed to be 0. When the result of the count in the diluted suspension is multiplied by the dilution factor, the true number of cells which has passed through the capillary is obtained. By subtracting from this figure the number of cells counted, the correction required for count loss due to coincidence can be obtained.

The results obtained from counts of *serial dilutions* with the 70 μm capillary indicate that this method of determining count loss is not reliable, and may be influenced by dilution errors, contamination and other disturbances.

Since the above warrants no definite conclusion as to the validity of the correction for count loss due to coincidence, the statistical model from which Mattern proceeded must be considered in order to see whether a different approach to the problem is feasible.

Mattern's statistical model [2] is based on the principle of taking from the thread of fluid in which the count is made, successive samples with the size of the active volume. If the sample contains no particle, then no count is made; if it contains one or several particles, this produces a single count pulse.

On statistical grounds it can be inferred from this conception that, when the particles in the fluid are homogeneously distributed and those in the thread of fluid according to Poisson, the correction factor E (given $N_c = E.N_t$), required for converting the number of cells counted to the true number of cells equals:

$E_M = (1 - e^{-\mu})/\mu$, in which μ indicates the mean number of cells per active volume, which can be calculated according to: μ equals the mean of the number of cells counted divided by the active length of the capillary.

In first approximation this equation becomes: $E_M = 1 - 1/2 \mu$.

Unlike Mattern, Strackee [3] calculates the correction factor on the basis of the assumption that a count pulse occurs only when a particle or series of particles is (are) followed by a volume of fluid the size of the active volume in which no particle is contained. If, proceeding from a Poisson distribution of the particles in the thread of fluid, E_S is derived from this model, then it is found, that $E_S = e^{-\mu}$.

In first approximation this expression becomes $E_S = 1 - \mu$.

If in both equations the same values are used for μ, then the correction factor calculated according to Strackee proves to exceed that calculated according to Mattern.

Because of that, there is a discrepancy between the correction factors calculated from the active volume according to Mattern's and according to Strackee's statistical model. This discrepancy might be explained if the supposition of a Poisson distribution of particles were wrong.

In order to establish this, frequency histograms of the time intervals between consecutive count pulses were obtained using a CAT (Computer of Average Transients). The linear course of the curves (plotting the frequency of occurrence in the class intervals logarithmically along the ordinate and the distances linearly along the abscissa) shows that the count-pulse intervals are characterized by an exponential distribution at various concentrations of the cell suspensions. This is also in evidence at various discriminator settings and various capillary diameters.

This implies that the particles in the thread of fluid obey a γ-distribution. Since pulse intervals the length of the detection unit, could not be measured, it could not be established with certainty that the γ-distribution was of the Ode order, i.e. distributed according to Poisson. What could be established was, that the order had to be quite near 0.

Approximately, therefore, the particles show a Poisson distribution in the thread of fluid up to intervals of the order of the active length. Therefore, the difference between Mattern's correction factor and that of Strackee cannot be explained on the basis of particle distribution.

Coincidence occurs because blood cells pass through the detection unit in such close succession that the pulses caused by the cells overlap in such a manner that count loss occurs, and that possibly two or several cells cause a single pulse, the maximum amplitude of which exceeds that of the pulse caused by the largest particle.

On the basis of this definition, active length can be defined as the distance along which a cell is discerned, projected on the capillary axis.

It is possible to replace the rather static active length concept by a more dynamic concept, to wit: dead length (l_m). This can be defined as the minimum proximity between two particles, which permits of separate detection of these particles. In using this concept, the elevation of a pulse under the influence of another pulse closely proximate in time, is taken into account.

If N_t is the true number of particles in a starting suspension of a serial dilution, and if C equals the reciprocal value of the dilution factor, then the number of particles in the dilution equals: $C.N_t$.

The mean number of particles per dead length (l_m), can then be calculated according to:

$$\lambda = C \cdot N_t \cdot l_m/a,$$

in which « a » is the total length of the thread of fluid.

In accordance with Mattern's model it can then be deduced that:
$N_c/C = N_t \cdot (1 - 1/2\ N_t \cdot C \cdot l_m/a)$ in which $N_c =$ the number of particles counted.

In accordance with Strackee's model it can be deduced that:

$$N_c/C = N_t \cdot (1 - N_t \cdot C \cdot l_m/a).$$

According to Strackee $N_c = (1-k)N_t$, in which $k = N_t \cdot l_m/a$.

Because l_m can be calculated from the pulse duration of the idealised pulse form at discrimination setting d, to be $[\Delta p + (2 - d/D)\tau] \cdot v$, in which D is the discriminator setting at the top of the pulse, and t the rise time of the pulse and « a » can be calculated from the measuring time x v, N_c can be calculated as a function of N_t. From this the count-loss due to coincidence, defined as $(N_t - N_c)\ N_t$, can be calculated as function of N_t.

Zones formed by plotting the counts loss percentages were calculated for $d = o$ and $d = D$ against N_t for the various capillaries, $d = o$ implying that the discriminator position for this limit equals o, and $d = D$ implying that the discriminator position for this limit equals the height of the amplitude of the ideal pulse shape.

The results also indicated the lines calculated on the basis of the corrections supplied by Coulter. These lines coincide reasonably well with the zones calculated.

Another method of determining the count loss percentage makes use of the following procedure.

It follows from $\lambda = l_m \cdot N_t/a$ and $a = t \cdot v$, that λ equals $l_m/v \cdot t/N_t$, in which t/N_t is the mean time interval between two particles, and can be calculated from the mean pulse shape, the mean rate of passage and the mean time interval between two particles.

The last mentioned value can be deduced from the pulse interval diagrams.

The values calculated for λ in this manner are identical to the values calculated for λ as described before.

Another possibility to determine the dead length (l_m) is found in that portion of the pulse interval diagrams in which the time intervals are of the order of the pulse durations.

From the diagrams, the mean dead times of the various capillaries were determined, and the mean dead length can then be calculated with the aid of the mean rate of passage. λ can then be calculated as a function of N_t with the aid of $\lambda = N_t \cdot l_m/a$. Count loss percentages were determined by this method, given a d/D ratio of 1/6.

The results obtained in this way are consistent with those obtained by the two preceding methods.

The correctness of the order of magnitude of count loss percentage calculated according to Strackee's theory can be verified by comparing the frequency distribution curves of the pulse durations, plotted at various cell concentrations.

The count loss percentages calculated according to Strackee's theory in the two suspensions differed by 7%. The difference in area between two curves was 8%. The good agreement between these values is an argument in support of Strackee's theory.

Curves plotted with the aid of a pulse height analyser in combination with a pulse delay, proceeding from suspensions of different cell concentrations.

The fenomena, as observed, are a consequence of coincidence. It is a suspicious feature that the frequency distribution curves at the lower concentrations show only slight differences; from this we may conclude that the skewness, which characterizes frequency distribution curves of erythrocytes at conventional concentrations, results not from coincidence but from a different cause, e.g. the difference in osmotic properties between different cell groups.

As a general conclusion it can be maintained that Mattern's statistical model for calculation of coincidence, errs. Nevertheless, results of calculation for coincidence correction based on this theory are within the correct order of magnitude. This must be attributed to the use of an oversize standard for the active volume in computing coincidence with this formula. This standard was probably deduced from experimental findings, to which the theory has been adapted.

The statistical model introduced by Strackee is correct, but requires some refinements as to the shape of the pulses, as a result of which the count loss due to coincidence becomes dependent on the position of the discriminator.

Results obtained by the above discussed methods of determination of count loss percentage, indicate minimum count loss percentages. The true count loss percentage may be larger because an idealized pulse shape has been used in computations, whereas in reality this pulse shape is bound to show some degree of variation. However, the difference can only be small, and may be within the margins of the constant error of a cell count.

For the time being, there are sound reasons for the continued use of correction tables so far employed.

References

[1] Gutmann J., *Elektronische Verfahren zur Ermittlung statistischer Masszahlen einiger medizinisch wichtiger Daten*, Dissertation, München. 1966.

[2] Mattern C. F. T., Brackett F. C. and Olson B. J., « Determination of Number and Size of Particles by Electrical Gating: Blood Cells », *J. Appl. Physiol.* 10, 56, 1957.

[3] Strackee J., « Coincidence loss in blood counters », *Med. Biol. Engin.* 4, 97, 1966.

2nd Session

Chairmen: P. E. Carson, E. Salvidio, E. Vivaldi

2.1. *On Electronic Methods for Red Blood Cell Sizing*

Dr. A. Ur, Medical Division, Oak Ridge Associated
University, Oak Ridge, Tennessee, USA *

The introduction of electronic methods for particle counting stimulated the development of techniques for sizing the counted particles. In the counting techniques, a suspension of the particles in an electrolyte solution is pumped through a small aperture. The electrical conductivity of the suspension is monitored by a pair of electrodes situated one on either side of the aperture. Because the specific resistivity of the particles is higher than that of the electrolyte solution, the passage of particles through the aperture causes momentary pulse-like decrements in the electrical current. These pulses are counted electronically; and under appropriate conditions, their number represents the number of passing particles. This technique has proved very successful for cell counting and is now popular in haematological laboratories.

The modification of this technique for particle sizing involves the addition of a pulse-height analyser. This not only counts the total number of pulses but also provides a histogram of their distribution according to amplitude. Assuming that the amplitude of a pulse is determined by the volume of solution displaced from the aperture by the passing particle, the histogram also represents the size distribution of the particles. However, such an assumption, even if valid for inert uniform particles like latex spheres, can not automatically be applied to biological particles like Red Blood Cells (RBC) which not only possess a specific shape but may also vary from one to another in characteristics other than size.

---

* Present Address: Physiological Flow Studies Unit, Imperial College, London SW 7.

The amplitude of a pulse is determined by several factors, among which the size of the particle is probably predominant. The accuracy of the sizing method will, therefore, depend on the relative importance of the particle size as compared with that of the other factors. The accuracy will fall, for instance, when the difference between the specific resistivities of the particle and of the solution is small. Moreover, it is possible that biological particles, such as RBC, vary among themselves in their specific resistivity, e.g. in accordance with their lipid content; so that different particles, even if of the same size, would produce pulses of different amplitude. Additional factors are the shape of the particle — whether sphere, disc, rod, etc. — and its orientation in the aperture. For example, a disc, travelling with its flat surface parallel to the axis of the aperture, would give a different pulse amplitude than one which has its flat surface perpendicular to the axis. Other parameters, such as the position of the particle in the aperture, may also affect the amplitude of the pulse. It is therefore wrong to assume that the histogram of pulses amplitude represents the distribution of particle sizes, unless it can be shown that, within the required sizing accuracy, factors other than particle size do not affect the amplitude histogram.

That this assumption is, in fact, erroneous is shown in an experiment in which different pulse amplitude distribution curves are obtained by changing the aperture current (fig. 1). Since all other variables were kept constant, it appears that the intensity of the electrical current affected either the sizing process, or the RBC themselves, or, perhaps, both.

To study the effects of electrical fields on RBC, a suspension of RBC was placed in an electrical field maintained between two platinum wire electrodes mounted on a glass slide. Figs. 2-8 are phase photomicrographs that show the changes in the RBC which occur under the influence of the electrical field. A few seconds after the electrical field was established (by applying about 2 Volts between the electrodes) the cells nearest the cathode underwent crenation, at first slowly and later on more rapidly. With the last stages of crenation the opaque cell content shrank, leaving a clear zone between it and the cell membrane, which had become finely wrinkled and spiculated. Later still, the membrane again became smooth, while the concentrated cell content became round and dark. At this point, the RBC lysed.

While these changes were occurring in cells near the cathode, the cells near the anode became cup shaped, but without crenation. Following this stage, these cells too underwent lysis.

Figure 1

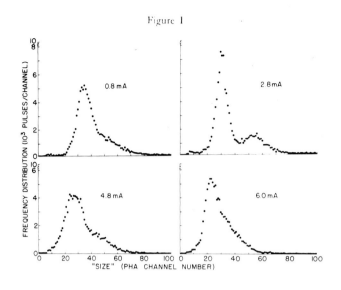

Figure 2

Figure 3

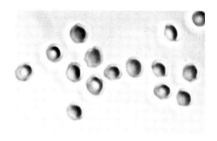

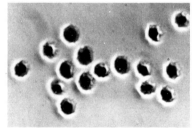

Figure 4

Figure 5

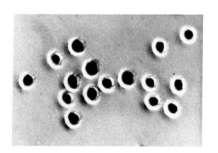

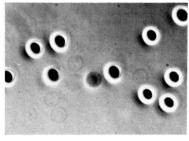

Figure 6   Figure 7

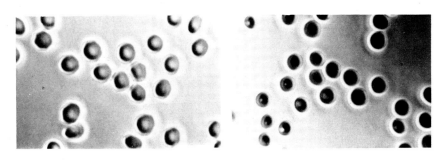

Figure 8

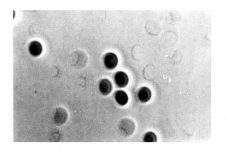

Figure 9

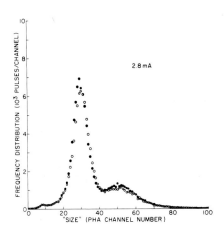

These changes in the RBC are probably caused by the alteration of the pH of the solution near the electrodes (Rand, Burton & Canham, 1965). It takes some time, however, for the change in pH to diffuse from the electrodes to the bulk of the suspension. By selecting an apparatus with certain physical characteristics (volume of the suspension, aperture size, current intensity, etc.) it is possible to avoid the effect of this change for a considerable time. In the conditions under which the 2.8 mA curve (fig. 1) was obtained, significant changes in the RBC were avoided for about 25 minutes (Ur & Lushbaugh, 1968).

It is possible, also, that electrical fields might affect the RBC in other ways which are not manifest morphologically but which would still affect the sizing principle. The high intensity of the electrical field in the aperture subjects each RBC to a potential difference of 2 to 3 volts across its diameter. Such potential differences, when applied to excitable cells, could stimulate the cells and change the permeability of their membranes to ions, i.e. could change the electrical conductivity of these cells. These cells would, therefore, be erroneously counted as of smaller volume. Such membrane changes take place in excitable cells only when the stimulus is of certain duration. While the passage of the cells through the aperture itself is too fast to allow such changes to occur, it is nevertheless possible that some of the cells might be delayed in the space in front of the aperture and so could be subjected to the electrical field long enough to undergo some such changes. In this case, two different cell populations would be sized — those which passed through the aperture with no delay, and, therefore, with no alteration of their membrane permeability; and those which were delayed in front of the aperture and did undergo such changes.

The curve obtained with the 2.8 mA current (fig. 1) in fact displays a bimodal amplitude distribution; so that such membrane alteration seemed possible. To examine this possibility, the speed of flow through the aperture was reduced from 3.7 m/sec to 2.6 m/sec so as to increase the time the RBC spent in the electrical field and hence change the ratio between the two populations. However, as shown in fig. 9, this reduction of flow brought no significant change in the bimodal size distribution.

Another important factor to be considered is the nature of the flow through the aperture and its effect on the pulse amplitude distribution. Gutmann (1966) suggested, for instance, that the bimodal size distribution, observed by Lushbaugh and others, is caused by different orientations of the cells in the aperture. The flow behaviour of particulate suspensions is rather complicated: it involves migration of the particles

174

together with rotation at different angular velocity as well as deformation of certain particles such as RBC (Mason and Goldsmith, 1968). However, it seems that the conditions under which the curves in fig. 9 were obtained, were such that the flow of particles was uniform, with the cells probably parallel with their surface to the axis of the aperture. Otherwise the reduction of flow would have been expected to bring some change in the pattern of the curve.

We believe that, of the sizing systems currently available, the one employing a 100-micron aperture with a current of 2.8 mA is to be preferred for RBC sizing. These are probably still not the optimum conditions, and it is possible that better results could be obtained by designing the apparatus, specifically for sizing, according to carefully planned hydrodynamical and bioelectrical principles.

Even if the bimodal amplitude distribution found for RBC does not truly represent the distribution of cell volume, it still displays some real property of the RBC population. It is difficult to confirm this bimodal distribution by the use of other methods, because the variations in the RBC are too small to be detected in any other way. It seems, however, that the distribution of the RBC's «Sphericity Index» (Canham and Burton, 1968) does show a skewed and perhaps bimodal pattern, though the sensitivity of their method is not sufficient to allow a definite conclusion. (Burton, personal communication).

Meanwhile the bimodal « size » distribution has been found to be a promising diagnostic tool, as the pattern of the curve changes with certain pathological conditions. (Lushbaugh and Lushbaugh, 1965).

References

[1] Canham, P. B., Burton, A. C., « Distribution of Size and Shape in Population of Normal Human Red Cells », *Circ. Res.* 22, 405-422, 1968.

[2] Gutmann, J., « Elektronische Verfahren zur Ermittlung statistischer Masszahlen einiger medizinisch wichtiger Daten », *Elektromedizin*, 11, 62, 1966.

[3] Lushbaugh, C. C. and Lushbaugh, D. B., « Rapid Electronic Red Blood Cell Sizing as an Aid in Clinical Diagnosis », *Sth. med. J.* 58, 1208, 1965.

[4] Mason, S. G., Goldsmith, H. L., « The flow Behaviour of Particulate Suspensions », *Ciba Foundation Symp., London*, July 1968.

[5] Rand, R. P., Burton, A. C. and Canham, P., « Reversible Changes in Shape of Red Cells in Electrical Fields », *Nature (London)*, 205, 977, 1965.

[6] Ur, A., Lushbaugh, C. C., « Some Effects of Electrical Fields on Red Blood Cells with Remarks on Red Blood Cell Sizing », *Brit. J. Haemat.*, 15, 527-537, 1968.

Acknowledgment

I thank Mr. M. Gordon, B. A., M. Sc., for valuable help and consultation.

2.2. Red Cell Suspensions as a Reference in Blood Counting

R. K. Archer, Equine Research Station of the Animal Health Trust, Newmarket, England; S. M. Lewis and B. J. Burgess, Royal Postgraduate Medical School, London W.12, England

A number of commercially prepared products are now available for use as particle standards for electronic and other automatic counting instruments. They are, as a rule prepared from plastic materials, such as latex, from biological materials such as mould spores or pollens and from red blood cells which are treated in one way or another to ensure stability. However, all of these have limited value since the methods of preparation are unpublished and indeed are jealously guarded trade secrets. The absence of information about the method of preparation of these products virtually excludes them from consideration for an international standard, for one of the most important criteria of such a standard must be that it can reliably and reproducibly be manufactured, albeit in small quantities, by reference laboratories using an agreed and published method.

A method for the preparation and use of glutaraldehyde fixed red cells as a stable suspension was published in 1966 by Lewis and Burgess and since then this material has been used with increasing frequency and has proved satisfactory. We have modified the original method. The cell suspensions are prepared by collecting blood into ACD anti-coagulant and immediately washing it three times in iso-osmotic phosphate buffer at pH 7.4. The cells are then fixed by adding a large volume (10-fold) of 0.25 per cent glutaraldehyde in phosphate buffer. After standing for one hour at room temperature the suspension is washed three times in distilled water and then reconstituted with distilled water to a final volume which is adjusted in order to have an appropriate number of cells per cu.mm. One per cent sodium azide in H_2O is added. The suspension is mixed on an ultrasonic disintegrator for thirty seconds and further mixed on a mechanical mixer overnight before being dispensed in aliquot portions in glass containers. Two or three glass beads are added to each container and the containers are then well sealed. The material should be stored at 4 °C. For use a container is brought to room temperature and shaken vigorously by hand to ensure that the material is dislodged from the bottom of the container and there is no obvious clumping. Then the suspension is mixed on a mechanical mixer for at least ten minutes. Thereafter an aliquot portion is taken into diluent for a cell count.

176

Material prepared in this way was used in the first instance for limited trials in Great Britain. When it was found to be a satisfactory preparation it was further tried out by several members of the Expert Panel on Haemocytometry. For this purpose the material was sent by post to these colleagues in various parts of the world. It can be assumed that testing was carried out under especially stringent conditions. The data were recorded as the means of all counts from the particular laboratory, as obtained by electronic counters and, separately, their haemocytometer counts. The results show that even in these laboratories there are discrepancies but from our point of view they indicated that the material was of potential value for its purpose (Fig. 1).

A larger international trial was organised by Dr. A. H. Holtz for the I.C.S.H. from Utrecht which is mentioned on page 232.

The gluteraldehyde-fixed red cells are satisfactory for red cell counting and methods can easily be adapted to count these suspensions accurately. In order that they be most useful, however, it is the suspensions that must be adapted to the automatic counting equipment actually in use, and this necessitates that the cells have a range of size and that most of them, when fixed, have an MCV close to that of unfixed human erythrocytes. For most electronic counters, including the Coulter models other than the « S », fixed red cell suspensions work well, but for the AutoAnalyzer the Erymat and the Coulter « S » only whole, fresh blood can be counted and handled.

Consideration of the use of fixed animal (i.e. non-human) erythrocytes was therefore made. This was particularly influenced by the facts that a range of erythrocyte sizes is readily available, and that to obtain large batches from single donors at one venepuncture is straight forward. Furthermore, at least in Great Britain, no product derived from or including human tissue may be sold or in any way charged for, so that commercial co-operation, for instance in dispensing or distributing material, is impossible.

When erythrocytes are fixed according to the method given above there is a certain shrinkage in size, mostly immediate but continuing slowly for three or four days. Thereafter changes are virtually undetectable, at least for some months. Red cells from a number of animals were examined fresh and also five days after fixation with a Coulter plotter type « J » attached to a Coulter counter model « B ». Some of the results are given in Figs. 2 to 6. In the case of one goat examined, which may have been abnormal since the MCV measured was higher (30.2) than expected (ca. 20), fixed cells were small with an MCV of 24.7 fl. (Fig. 2). In the case of sheep, a very similar MCV for fixed cells

Figure 1

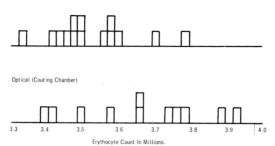

Electronic (Coulter)

Optical (Couting Chamber)

3.3   3.4   3.5   3.6   3.7   3.8   3.9   4.0

Erythocyte Count In Millions.

Figure 2

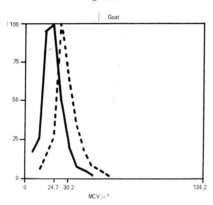

Goat

100

75

50

25

0

0   24.7 30.2   134.2

MCV μ^3

Figure 3

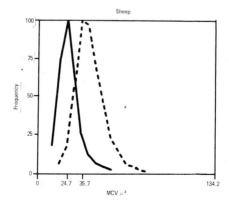

Sheep

100

75

Frequency

50

25

0

0   24.7 35.7   134.2

MCV μ^3

Figure 4

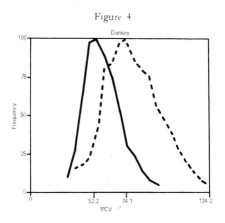

Donkey

Figure 5

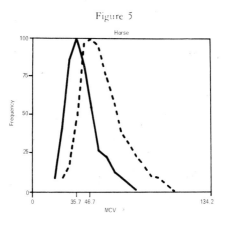

Horse

Figure 6

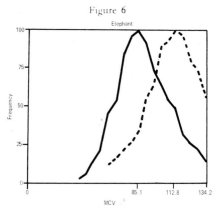

Elephant

Figure 7

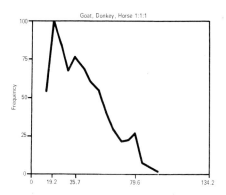

Figure 8

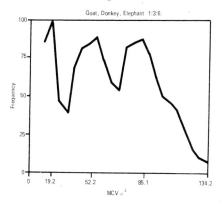

Figure 9

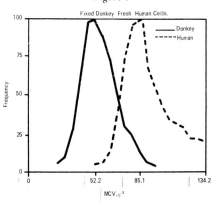

180

was obtained (Fig. 3). In the horse, MCV ranges from 40 to 50 fl. are commonly found; when fixed cells are used this decreases to about 36 fl. (Fig. 4). All these cells are too small for use in a standard intended for human erythrocytes, but the donkey (*Equus assinus*) has red cells with an MCV much nearer that of man (Fig. 5). When fixed, donkey erythrocytes are about 50 to 55 fl., that is towards the lower end of the normal human range. It will be noted, however, that appreciable numbers of fixed donkey red cells have an MCV above 75 fl.

As a general rule, the larger and more deliberate an animal becomes, the larger are its red cells. The elephant is an excellent example of this, having an MCV of about 120 fl. (Fig. 6). When fixed, elephant erythrocytes still show an MCV of about 85, perhaps somewhat above the normal mean figure for man.

In an attempt to provide a cell suspension of fixed material to cover the whole expected range of unfixed human erythrocytes, mixtures of some of these animal red cells were made and examined. Two of these are shown in Figs. 7 and 8. One to one mixtures of goat, horse and donkey are generally too small and have too few cells above 80 fl. When one part of goat cells, three parts of donkey and six parts of elephant are mixed, a smoother pattern showing three peaks is obtained (Fig. 8). In this case, quite large numbers of cells over 100 fl. are present: a distinct disadvantage.

Experiments are now being made with suspensions of fixed donkey cells from several individuals of that species, and it is material of this general kind, which should have an MCV, when fixed, close to 55, and should contain appreciable numbers of cells of 80 fl. or more, which is suggested for consideration (Fig. 9). It should be noted, however, that whilst packed cell volume estimations can be made, the fixed cells do not pack so tightly as fresh ones and abnormally high PCV (and therefore MCV figures calculated from this) will be found.

Acknowledgements

We are obliged to Mrs. Penny M. Close for technical assistance, particularly with the cell size distribution plotting.

Reference

Lewis, S.M. and Burgess, B.J., *Lab. Pract.*, *15*, 305, 1966.

2.3. Stable Standard Suspensions of Particles Suitable for Calibration and Controls of the Electronic Counters

G. Torlontano and A. Tata, Clinica Medica II dell'Università di Roma, Italy

The problem regarding the availability of corpuscles suspensions stable for number, shape and volume, without aggregates and easy to use, is still open to question. Apart from many other numerous possible uses, a type of preparation with these characteristics would be of great value as a standard of reference for the calibration and successive daily control of the electronic counters.

Attempts to provide suitable sized particles suspensions by the use of ragweed pollens, polystyrene latex, various organic materials and tanned cells [1, 2, 3], have not been completely satisfactory [4].

According to de Boroviczény [5], a useful but by no means ideal suspension consists of erythrocytes preserved in Gowers-Kleine solution. Another useful method relies on fixation with formaldehyde [6]. However, according to Lewis and Burgess [4], such a method would give results inferior to those obtained by using glutaraldehyde as a fixative. Even though the preparation of this type of erythrocyte suspension, elaborated by Lewis and Burgess offers several advantages [4], there are a few drawbacks:
1. the packing of the red cells makes resuspension difficult;
2. the red cell volume is reduced.

The erythrocyte standard suspensions now on the market, namely Dade Erythro-trol and Pfizer Celltrol, require repeated shaking to obtain the uniform resuspension of the red cells, and present a reduced mean corpuscular volume. Because of their characteristics, they are more suited to the control than to the initial calibration of only a few of the electronic counters: for example, of the Coulter A and not of the Coulter D and Dl.

In order to obtain a stable standard suspension of particles to be used in the calibration of the electronic counters, we have tested a new fixing solution [7-8].

The fixative has the following composition:

crystallized acetic acid:	42.0 mg
sodium sulphate, anhydrous:	7.0 g
sodium chloride, anhydrous:	7.0 g
distilled water:	1000.0 ml

After preparation, the solution must be carefully filtered.

Whole blood is added to the fixing solution in the proportion of 1 to 200. We thus obtain a stock suspension that should be stored in the freezer.

This stock suspension is suitable for the erythrocyte optical counts, and allows the subsequent preparation of dilutions suitable for every type of electronic counters.

By carrying out our controls with repeated optical counts and electronic counts, using the F and D1 Coulter, the Celloscope 101 and the Biotronics 400/B, we were able to prove the constancy of the numerical counts and the complete absence of stable aggregates for a period of over 2 years.

The red blood cells of the suspension prepared six months ago, showed a mean corpuscular volume of 79 fl. instead of 83 fl. as found during the first weeks after fixation: these volumes were obtained by means of the Coulter F computer, which gives a normal range of 83-85 fl. The morphology of the red cells is well preserved (Fig. 1).

The plateaus obtained after 5 months with our RBC suspension, with the Coulter F Counter (Fig. 2) and the Biotronics 400/B Counter (Fig. 3), are similar to those obtained with normal RBC. Like results have been obtained with the other counters we used: Coulter D1 and Celloscope 101. The volumetric distribution of our suspension by an experimental electronic analyzer,* was found after 5 months, to be similar to that obtained with normal fresh blood cells (Fig. 4).

Therefore, we can state that during several months, the fixed red cells do not undergo relevant changes, and that their behaviour is similar to that of normal fresh blood cell suspensions, no matter what kind of electronic counter is used.

The RBC suspension prepared with our fixing solution had an initial haemolysis rate of more than 3%; we have therefore tried several modified formulas. We could reduce the initial haemolysis to about 1% by increasing the concentration of the sodium chloride to 9 g in the original fixing solution (Fig. 5).

Since the number of white blood cells and of platelets in the fixed whole blood was found to be very stable, in recent months we have studied the possibility of preparing stable suspensions of WBC and of platelets.

1° WBC suspension.

We have utilized plasma rich in leucocytes. This plasma has been diluted by saline solution until a WBC suspension of $10\text{-}20^3/\text{nl}$. This suspension was then diluted 1:20 by the following fixing solution:

crystallized acetic acid: 42.0 mg
sodium sulphate, anhydrous: 7.0 g
sodium chloride, anhydrous: 7.0 g
distilled water: 1000.0 ml

* This experimental analyzer has been constructed by dr. M. Frank, Chief of the electronic laboratories of the « Istituto Superiore di Sanità ».

183

Figure 1

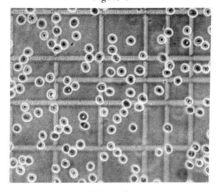

Figure 2

COULTER ˝F˶

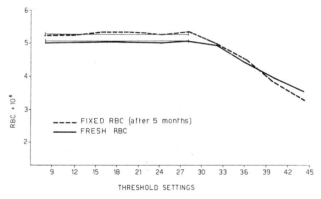

---- FIXED RBC (after 5 months)
——— FRESH RBC

THRESHOLD SETTINGS

Figure 3

BIOTRONICS ˝400 b˶

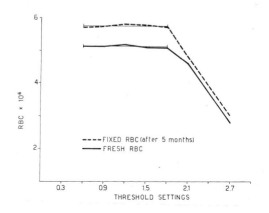

---- FIXED RBC (after 5 months)
——— FRESH RBC

THRESHOLD SETTINGS

184

This stock suspension is suitable for the leucocyte optical count, and allows the subsequent preparation of dilutions suitable for any type of electronic counters.

After the first month of preparation, the WBC pattern is very similar to that of fresh WBC (Figs. 6-7).

Platelet suspension.

We have utilized citrated plasma rich in platelets. This suspension has been diluted 1 : 10 with the following fixing solution:

crystallized acetic acid: 148   mg
sodium sulphate, anhydrous: 12.3   g
potassium sulphate, anhydrous: 12.3   g
sodium chloride, anhydrous: 9.0   g
distilled water: 1000.0   ml

This stock suspension is suitable for optical counts and allows the preparation of dilutions suitable for any type of electronic counters.

After one month, there was no change in the number of platelets and there was no clumping (Fig. 8). Therefore we hope to have a stable suspension of platelets.

This investigation is still in progress. At present, we are not aware of any other stable suspensions of this kind.

Addendum

Subsequent experiments proved that the erythrocytes fixed with our fixing solution did not alter even when resuspended in distilled water (Fig. 9).

References

[1] Gabrieli, E. R., Wertheimer, M., « Standardization of the Electronic Counter of Blood Cells », *Am. J. Clin. Path.*, *36*, 277, 1961.
[2] Hummel, K., « A Standard Suspension for Electronic Cell Counters », *Bibl. Haemat.*, *18*, 21, 1964.
[3] Orthney, G. F., Traynor, J. E., Ingram, M., « Use of Tanned Erythrocytes as Standard Particles in Cell Volume Determinations », *Bibl. Haemat.*, *21*, 14, 1965.
[4] Lewis, S. M., Burges, B. J., « A Stable Suspension for Red-cell Counts », *Lab. Pract.*, *15*, 305, 1966.
[5] De Boroviczény Ch. G., « Standardization in Haematology », *Bibl. Haemat.*, *24*, 1, 1966.
[6] Benedek E., « Experience with a Blood Cell Standard », *Bibl. Haemat.*, *24*, 67, 1966.
[7] Tata A., Torlontano G., « Stabile sospensione standard di eritrociti adatta alla taratura e ai controlli dei contatori elettronici », *Haematologica Latina*, *11*, (Suppl. III), 45, 1967.
[8] Torlontano G., Salvatori L., Tata A., « Sulla standardizzazione dei metodi di conta degli eritrociti. Conteggi ottici, conteggi automatici e problemi di taratura e di controllo dei contatori elettronici », *Haematologica Latina*, *11* (Suppl. III), 25, 1967.

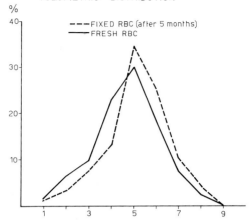

Figure 4
VOLUMETRIC DISTRIBUTION

---FIXED RBC (after 5 months)
——FRESH RBC

Figure 5

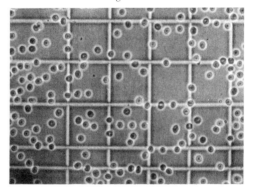

Figure 6

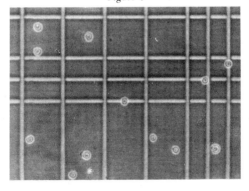

Figure 7

BIOTRONICS ˝400 b„

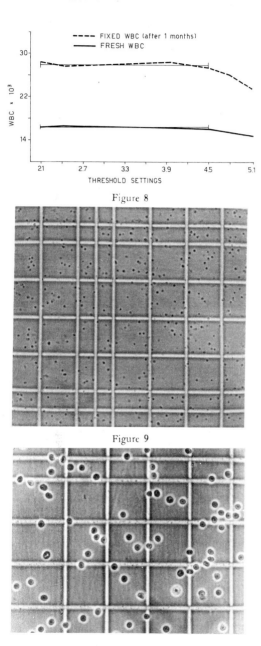

- - - - FIXED WBC (after 1 months)
——— FRESH WBC

WBC × 10³

30

22

14

2.1   2.7   3.3   3.9   4.5   5.1

THRESHOLD SETTINGS

Figure 8

Figure 9

2.4. *A Simple Method for Counting Platelets*

C. Petrini Arisi, F. Giorcelli and G. Vanzetti
Biochemical Laboratories of the Ospedale Maggiore
Ca' Granda and Ospedale Maggiore
San Carlo Borromeo di Milano, Italy

As everybody knows, platelet counting is still a problem for the analyst: many procedures have been recommended but only a few are really satisfactory.

Highly sophisticated electronic cell counters are available, but they are not within the reach of all analysts; hence the need for simple visual methods that can be used in all laboratories.

One basic problem is interference from erythrocytes, normally present in the blood in far higher numbers than the platelets.

Several workers have suggested counting the platelets in the *plasma* after sedimentation of the erythrocytes [1, 4], but the red blood cell sedimentation takes rather a long time and there is the risk of a slight sedimentation of the platelets in the supernatant. In addition, the packed cell volume must be measured in order to compute the ratio plasma volume/blood volume, and to calculate the number of platelets per cu.mm blood.

Another possibility is to dilute the blood with special reagents that induce hemolysis of the erythrocytes without damaging the platelets, and take a direct count of the platelets with a phase contrast microscope. Several methods of this type have been described: Feissly and Lüdin's cocaine method [5], Brecher's ammonium oxalate method [6, 7], Piette and Piette's procain method [8], etc. By means of these methods it is possible to count a large number of platelets and to reduce the statistical error, owing to the limited dilution of the blood.

Already in 1950, a simple method for counting platelets was described by one of us [9]. This method is based on blood dilution (1 to 20) followed by removal of the erythrocytes by brief centrifugation (at 1500 rpm); the platelets are counted in the supernatant, and an empirical factor is used to compensate for their sedimentation. Similar methods based on erythrocyte removal by low speed centrifugation were used by others (Eastham 1963 [10]; Lancastre et al. 1965 [12]; Eastham and Morgan 1967 [4]).

The method that we are presenting now is a modification of the method of Foss et al. (1960) [13]; it is based on the dilution of blood 1 to 20 (0,2 to 4,0 ml) with a 3,0 % solution of Na_2EDTA containing

1 ml concentrated formalin in 100 ml, followed by sedimentation of the erythrocytes, transfer of the platelet-rich supernatant to another test tube and counting of the platelets.

Good results are obtained if attention is given to the following points:

1. Plastic test tubes are used for the sedimentation of the erythrocytes, and plastic pipettes with a large tip are used for the transfer of the platelet-rich supernatant.
2. A small amount of formalin is added to the diluting reagent, in order to reduce platelet stickiness.
3. The test tubes are inclined at an angle of 30° to the horizontal; the time required for the sedimentation is thus reduced to about one hour.
4. In order to get reliable results a large portion of the supernatant must be transferred to another test tube and shaken: direct sampling from the supernatant of the first test tube is not recommended, owing to the large scatter of the results.

The equipment required for our method is illustrated in fig. 1. The reproducibility of our method was appraised repeatedly on 20 samples from the same blood specimen. For each count the platelets contained in 40 rectangles of a Bürker chamber were counted: the resulting figure was divided by 2 and multiplied by 100. The results are shown in table 1. A variation coefficient of ± 5,4 % was recorded; variation coefficients of ± 4,1 % and ± 7,4 % were obtained in two other similar tests. This is satisfactory, if allowance is made for the statistical error of visual counts.

In table 2 we report the results of the platelet counts on 20 samples of another blood specimen, using the cocaine method of Feissly and Lüdin: the variation coefficient was ± 5,4 %. A variation coefficient of ± 5,6 % was found in a similar test carried out with the same method.

A series of 30 parallel determinations were then performed with our method and with Feissly and Lüdin's method. The results are reported in fig. 2.

As shown in the diagram, there are differences in either direction between the two methods, but they are within acceptable limits if allowance is made for the statistical error. The average difference was of ± 10.600, the maximum difference was 43.500.

A slightly lower overall average value was obtained with our method compared with Feissly and Lüdin's method. Two source of error acting in opposite directions can account for this difference: platelet sedimentation, which may result in a lower number of platelets being counted, and erythrocyte sedimentation, which may lead to a concentration of platelets in the supernatant. Compared with the statistical error the

Tab. 1 – Reproducibility of Platelet counts by our method.
20 Samples of the same blood No. of Platelest/CU.MM.

1	223.500	11	205.500
2	196.000	12	195.500
3	202.500	13	184.500
4	192.000	14	197.500
5	204.500	15	193.000
6	190.500	16	194.500
7	182.500	17	193.000
8	195.500	18	175.000
9	188.000	19	189.000
10	184.000	20	203.500

av. $\pm$ st.d. $= 194.500 \pm 10.450$
Confidence limits $= \pm 20.900$
C.V. $= \pm 5.40\%$

Counting technique: introduce a drop of platelet suspension in a Burker's chamber. After 10 min. count the cells contained in 20 rectangles: repeat on a second drop. Divide the total number of platelets by 2, and add two zeroes to the resulting figure.

Tab. 2 – Reproducibility of Platelet counts by Feissly and Ludin's method
20 Samples of the Same Blood
N^O of Platelets / CU.MM.

1	175 500	11	218 000
2	186 500	12	192 000
3	193 000	13	181 000
4	198 000	14	190 500
5	192 000	15	185 500
6	186 000	16	190 000
7	181 000	17	204 500
8	199 000	18	202 500
9	197 500	19	192 000
10	200 000	20	195 000

av. $\pm$ st.d. $= 192\,900 \pm 10\,100$
Confidence limits $= \pm 20\,200$
C.V. $= \pm 5,75$

Figure 1

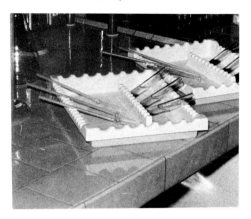

Figure 2

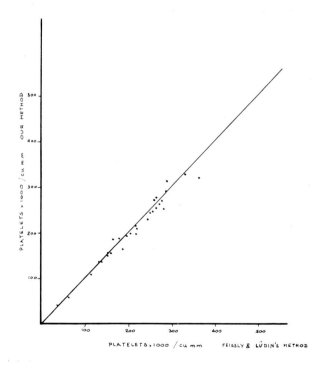

difference between the two averages is small (about 2 %): a correction was therefore not applied.

Comparative determinations are now under way in our laboratories with visual and electronic counts, using a platelet suspension prepared with our method: at present, we are not yet able to report conclusive results.

In conclusion visual counting of the platelets by means of our method is nearly as simple as visual counting of the red and white blood cells; the main advantages are the following:

1. the platelet-rich supernatant is easily prepared;
2. a normal microscope without phase contrast equipment can be used;
3. there is no danger of thrombolysis, that can be a source of error when the red blood cells are hemolysed;
4. there are very few erythrocytes, and the platelets can be easily identified since their refringency is increased by the action of formalin;
5. a large number of platelets can be counted quickly, owing to the limited dilution.

References

[1] Sipe, C. R. and Cronkite, E. P., Ann. N.Y. Acad. Sci., 99, 262, 1962.
[2] Girling, J. H., J. Med. Lab. Techn., 19, 168, 1962.
[3] Eggleton, M. J. and Sharp, A. A., J. Clin. Path., 16, 164, 1963.
[4] Eastham, R. D. and Morgan E. H., J. Med. Lab. Techn., 24, 315, 1967.
[5] Feissly, R. and Ludin, M., Rev. Hémat., 4, 481, 1949.
[6] Brecher, G. and Cronkite, E. P., J. Appl. Physiol., 3, 365, 1950.
[7] Brecher, G., Schneiderman, M. and Cronkite, E. P., Am. J. Clin. Path., 23, 15, 1953.
[8] Piette, M. and Piette, C., Sang, 30, 144, 1959.
[9] Vanzetti, G., Haematologica, 34, fasc. 4°, 1950.
[10] Eastham, R. D., J. Clin. Path., 16, 168, 1963
[11] Eastham, R. D., J. Clin. Path., 18, 248, 1965.
[12] Lancastre, F., Gineste, J. and Maupin, B., Nouv. Rev. Française d'Hématologie, 5, 521, 1965.
[13] Foss, O. P., Rosenlund, B. and Vik, O., Nord. Med., 64, 1350, 1960.

Chairmen: C. G. de Boroviczény, E. G. Torlontano, G. Vanzetti

3.1. *Multiple Haematological Analysis by Means of the S.M.A.-4*
M. G. Nelson, Clinical Pathologist, Royal Victoria Hospital,
Belfast, UK

The work of the hospital laboratory throughout Great Britain has
been rising exponentially and this rise has affected all laboratory discipli-
nes. In haematology a very high proportion of tests are of a routine,
repetitive nature and readily capable of automation. In our own
laboratory more than 50 per cent of the total workload consists of four
tests which could be performed on currently available multi-channel
equipment such as the S.M.A.-4.

By a process of *S*equential *M*ultiple *A*nalysis, this continuous flow
equipment can determine the haematocrit, the haemoglobin, the red
cell count and the white cell count. If a calculator is attached then the
M.C.V., M.C.H.C. and M.C.H. can be derived which converts the
equipment into a SMA-7.

The SMA-4 consists of the following modules: a sampler, a proportioning pump, plastic tubing manifolds and glass helical mixing and
phasing coils, a conductivity flow cell, a tubular flow cell colorimeter,
a dual channel cell counter, a programmer and a single pen recorder.
The anticoagulated whole blood in the sample cup is mixed by twin
paddles and an aliquot taken up by the sampler crook. This is then
split by the « sample splitter » into four streams. These pass along the
plastic tubing manifolds and helical mixing and phasing coils to individual detecting devices for the haematocrit, haemoglobin and cell
count determinations. The output from each detector is monitored by
the programmer and fed sequentially to a single pen recorder. The

instrument operates at a rate of 60 samples per hour and the results are graphically recorded and immediately readable. Variations from the « normal » may be visualised against the range for each sex, which is indicated on the precalibrated graph paper by a shaded zone.

I wish to present our experience with the S.M.A.-4 which we have subjected to technical evaluation in order to determine its precision and accuracy. Subsequently the equipment was put into routine service use in order to find out its reliability, its simplicity of operation in less skilled hands and its operational cost.

During the early scientific assessment of the S.M.A.-4 the results obtained on the haematocrit and red cell count channels, were frequently found to be inaccurate.

The cause of inaccuracy in the haematocrit channel was first investigated. It was found to be necessary, when setting up the equipment, to adjust this channel with two Potassium Chloride solutions of 2.66 and 5.07 grams. per litre which correspond to haematocrit readings of 50 and 19 per cent respectively. However, even when the haematocrit channel was correctly set, occasional vicarious results occurred. In the S.M.A.-4 the haematocrit is derived from the electrical conductivity of the blood sample passing through the conductance chamber. This conductivity is a function of the concentration of ions present in the sample which is altered by a number of factors apart from the relative volume of red cells in the suspending medium. In the first place excess anticoagulant in the specimen container is responsible for a proportion of erratic results. This can be eliminated by ensuring that all specimen bottles are adequately filled with blood. Discrepancies caused by minor variations in the filling of specimen bottles can be made less significant by reducing the concentration of E.D.T.A. anticoagulant from 2 mg to 1.6 mg per ml. This latter concentration is adequate for anticoagulant purposes and does not result in any measurable increase in the number of clotted specimens (see fig. 1).

Other causes of discrepancy when the haematocrit is determined by conductance have been investigated by Davis, Bresland and Green (1966) who showed that electrolyte concentration, protein content and the presence of leucocytosis all had a significant effect. These workers reported that « variation in plasma electrolytes up to 150 mEq/litre, leucocyte counts up to 30,000 per mm^3 and protein concentration up to 9 grams per cent did not influence the results ». Davis et al also reported that 86 per cent of 500 samples gave results which were within ± 2 per cent of the microhaematocrit centrifugation method, and our studies would confirm these findings.

The results obtained in the red cell count channel, using the original manifold, were unsatisfactory and gave coefficients of variation from 3.6 to 5.3 per cent. These unsatisfactory results were considered to be due, in large measure, to irregular pumping along large diameter tubes in the manifold which tended to wear out quickly and to lose their elasticity. Consequently the manifold was re-designed and large diameter tubes were replaced by a number of tubes of narrower bore. This necessitated the introduction of a second pump and the extra capacity of this pump permitted the elimination of wide diameter tubing throughout the rest of the manifold. The modified manifold had no tubing of a diameter greater than 0.073 in. internal diameter.

The S.M.A.-4 with this modified manifold was then subjected to a scientific assessment. Basic to the scientific evaluation of an instrument which operates on the continuous flow analytical system is the need to determine the presence and degree of cross contamination. In the S.M.A.-4 the most likely place for such interaction is at the point where carry-over from one sample cup to the next can occur. This was investigated using a radioisotope dilution method with ^{131}I-albumin according to a technique by Skentelbery and Neill (1968) which involves the measurement of the effect of samples of abnormally high values upon the result of a blank immediately following. The amount of carry-over from this cause was found to be less than 1.5 per cent which is within an acceptable range.

The precision of a measurement is the agreement between a series of determinations of the same quantity. In an instrument it can be regarded as a reflection of its mechanical consistency. It is usually determined by the repeated analysis of the same sample and then by calculating the standard deviation and the coefficient of variation. Using the modified flow system, a study of the precision of each of the four channels of the S.M.A.-4 was made by twenty or more replicate determinations of the same sample, and the results are summarized in Table 1.

The accuracy of an analytical procedure is a measure of how close the observed value is to be « true » value. Thus accuracy in the biochemical sense is more related to the design of the chemistry than to the mechanics of the measurement. In haematology the « true » value is not absolute but can be derived by mathematical computation. To this end 100 blood samples were divided into two aliquots and submitted to analysis on the S.M.A.-4 and by acceptable standard methods. The methods chosen for comparison were as follows: the haemoglobin content was determined as cyanmethaemoglobin at 540 nm in an Optica CF4 spectrophotometer which had been calibrated against the I.C.S.H.

Tab. 1 – Precision of S.M.A. 4.

	Coefficient of Variation (Per Cent.)	
	Range	Mean
Haemoglobin	0.38 – 0.92	0.54
Packed Cell Volume	0.0 – 2.08	0.83
Red Cell Count	1.52 – 3.62	2.37
White Cell Count	1.65 – 3.23	2.43

Tab. 2 – Accuracy of S.M.A. -4.

	Correlation Coefficient.	Regression Equation.
Haemoglobin	*0.9942*	$y = 1.003 \ x - 0.04$
Packed Cell Volume	0.9668	$y = 0.9205 \ x + 3.41$
Red Cell Count	0.9583	$y = 0.9902 \ x + 0.034$
White Cell Count	0.9905	$y = 1.003 \ x + 0.150$

International Reference Standard. A Coulter electronic cell counter Model « A » was used for white cell counts by the method of Richar and Breakall (1959) and for red cell counts by the method of Brecher, Schneiderman and Williams (1956). The packed cell volume was determined by the microhaematocrit centrifugation method (Hawksley) and the results read on the standard reader. Each pair of results was then subjected to statistical analysis by calculating the regression equation and the correlation coefficient. The haemoglobin and red cell count values are presented on a scattergraph and all the results summarized on Table 2. In figs. 2 to 5, I report the results of parallel determinations of Ht, WBC, Hb and RBC performed by the SMA 4 and by reference methods and instruments.

Once the scientific assessment had been completed, and we were satisfied that the S.M.A.-4 was producing precise and accurate results, the equipment was transferred to the routine laboratory to see if it was capable of being handled by less skilled workers, that it was free from troublesome breakdowns and that it could be operated at an economic cost.

Before each batch of tests approximately one hour is needed to start up the equipment, to run through the reagents and the blood primers for zeroing and the standards for calibration. During the run we have found it advantageous to carry out concurrent recording of the results directly on to a worksheet.

196

Figure 1 - *Effect of concentration of EDTA anticoagulant on the PCV determination.*

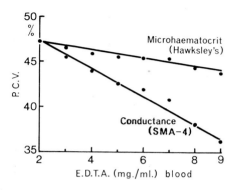

Figure 2 - *Comparison of duplicate haematocrit determinations.*

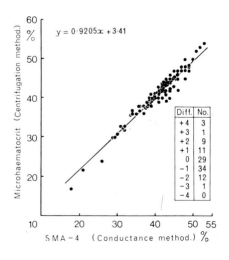

197

Figure 3 - *Comparison of duplicate leucocyte determinations.*

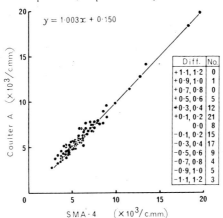

Figure 4 - *Comparison of duplicate haemoglobin determinations.*

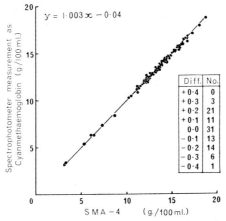

Figure 5 - *Comparison of duplicate erythrocyte determinations.*

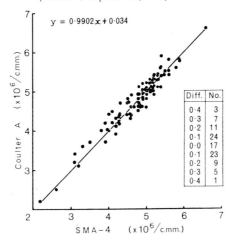

Because of this the part-time services of a second but less experienced operator has proved to be necessary in order to mix the samples, fill the sampler plate and carry out less skilled tasks.

It has been our experience that a fault will occur in the equipment at least once every day and it need hardly be stated that all such stoppages should be quickly corrected. The main cause of stoppage is mechanical blockage of the flowlines at certain critical points mainly at the sample splitter. The number of stoppages due to this cause can be reduced but not eliminated by attention to the regular washing of the flowlines at the end of each run.

We have found the equipment to be particularly vulnerable to dust in the laboratory atmosphere and protection of the reagent containers from contamination by dust is necessary. Dust is also deleterious to the electrical components of the programmer particularly the printed circuits and the micro switches. Preventive maintenance of the electronic components of the programmer at least once every two weeks is needed.

Two quality control systems are routinely employed. We prepare our own red cell suspension as a working reference standard. For this purpose fresh whole blood is collected in Alsever's solution, adenine and inosine are added as erythrocyte preservatives and the suspension is stored at 4 °C for four weeks. This suspension is used to set the haemoglobin, red cell count and haematocrit channels. The same red cell suspension is used to detect instrumental drift by introducing it into the sample plate in every twentieth slot. We also maintain a statistical method of quality control, using the cusum technique. The results of the haemoglobin and P.C.V. determinations are collected each day, the mean is determined and the difference from the « grand mean » is algebraically calculated and cumulatively plotted on a graph.

The results obtained on the S.M.A.-4 are graphically recorded on the chart and an individual set of results for one patient can be torn off for transfer to the ward or delivery to the physician. However, the large sheet of graph paper is not always record compatible and translation into digital form with subsequent transcription onto currently used record documents may be desirable. Concurrent recording, directly from the chart onto a worksheet or report document, is most satisfactory but this requires the technician to observe the chart continually, and to record the results. The introduction of an electronic analogue-digital converter and some form of automatic recorder would free the technician from this responsibility. It is for this reason that we are trying to develop a system which involves the interfacing of an A/D converter, together with a lineariser and scaler linked to an automatic punch. Digitized results could then be punched onto an 80-column card for subsequent automatic typing on to a report document. The laboratory data can then be stored either on the punch card or transferred to the memory store of a computer.

A cost analysis of the S.M.A.-4 for one year was carried out. This included the salary of the personnel, the cost of materials and reagents, the maintenance of the apparatus and amortization of the equipment over a ten year period. This showed that salaries and wages constituted about 50 per cent of the total and that amongst materials the most expensive by far was the chart paper. The operational cost worked out at £65 per 1,000 specimens or 1.3 shillings per specimen.

The basic requirements of an automated analytical system are that the results should be precise, accurate and free from carry-over, that the equipment should function at as high a speed as possible compatible with accuracy, and that the data should be automatically produced with the minimum of clerical work. At the same time the equipment should be mechanically and electronically reliable, and operate at an economic cost. The S.M.A.-4 certainly meets most of these requirements. The ultimate test of any scientific equipment is how it behaves when subjected to a large daily workload in a service laboratory. The fact that this equipment is in daily use in our hospital department of haematology is a measure of its acceptability.

References

Brecher, G., Schneiderman, M. and Williams, G. Z., *Amer. J. Clin. Path.*, 26, 1439, 1955.
Davis, R. E., Bresland, R. and Green, R., *Laboratory Practice*, 15, 1376, 1966.
Richar, W. J. and Breakall, E. S., *Amer. J. Clin. Path.*, 31, 384, 1959.
Skentelbery, R. G. and Neill, D. W., Personal Communication, 1968.

3.2. *SMA-4 A and SMA-7 A: New Developments in Automated Cell Counting Techniques and Systems Operation*
Claude Studievic, Technicon, Domont, France

Introduction

It became apparent during the latter half of 1967 that, while SMA-4 and SMA-7 systems were capable of providing accurate and useful data to the hematology laboratory, it was necessary for technologist who operated the system to constantly monitor its performance and perform numerous checks and adjustments to maintain optimum working characteristics.

This required an experienced technologist and an upgraded training class at Technicon to maintain optimum function. Visits were made to check installations during the Fall of 1967 and an improved training course was instituted by the end of 1967. In January, it was realized that operation of the equipment still gave rise to serious problems in many laboratories. In view of this, the continuing program of technical improvement of these systems was upgraded to a major research effort. The decision was made to delay fulfilment of outstanding orders until the full range of advances could be incorporated. A further decision was taken to incorporate the same advances into all existing systems without charge to the user.

The details and the results obtained by the SMA-4 A and SMA-7 A modifications are presented in this report.

The following facts provided the basic starting point for the research effort that has resulted in the SMA-4 A and SMA-7 A systems.

A. *Calibration curves of RBC/WBC*

To control conformity to calibration (accuracy) 3 independent criteria were necessary:

1) Initial manifold dilution must conform.
2) Dilution must not deteriorate significantly with age of manifold (hours of running time).
3) Stable and accurate standards should be available to maintain constancy of calibration and confidence that conformity check results are valid.

B. *Downtime due to adjustments of system other than conformity checks* for example:

1) PT-6 fitting was often a cause of blockage;
2) Some counter valves tended to leak;
3) Plastic flowcell collected debris;
4) Lack of positivity of flowcell focussing.

C. *Reproducibility*

The reproducibility of the SMA-4 and SMA-7 counting systems was not as good as the original single channel cell counter Autoanalyzer technique, although it was much better than manual and about equal to semi-automatic techniques.

Specific aims

The aims of the research program with respect to these facts were:
1) To produce an instrument with linear calibration (no coincidence);

2) To design an appropriate manifold for a linear counter having improved dilution characteristics in regard to initial dilutions and constancy of dilution over a realistic manifold life-time;
3) To improve component parts by redesign, to reduce downtime and necessity for frequent system monitoring;
4) To investigate and improve reproducibility thereby upgrading instrument performance and decreasing the frequency of quality control.

These four aims have been achieved with the SMA-4 A and SMA-7 A by a combination of modifications, many of which contributed to more than just one of the aims above.

Modifications

The modifications incorporated into the current SMA-4 and SMA 7 systems to produce 4 A and 7 A systems can best be described by considering the following:

1) Manifold and reagent changes;
2) Changes in Counter mechanics and optics;
3) Changes in Counter electronics;
4) Programmer changes.

Manifold

Here are, in short, the main features of the new manifold:
1) The first point to note is that no pump tube is larger than .073 inches (nominal delivery 2.0 ml/min.). It was found that the larger tube used in the original manifold decreased in delivery with age up to 20 %, thus causing a similar change in manifold dilution as the sample tubes are (relatively) constant in delivery. The diluent tubes selected for this manifold have shown consistently to decrease in flow rate only by 5 % over a 125 hour pumping time (about 4-5 week normal usage) without stretching the end-block position. The constancy of flow rate, together with linear calibration (non coincidence), eliminates the necessity of checking conformity to calibration that is required once a week on the present system. Additionally, phasing requires virtually no attention with this new manifold after initial adjustment.
2) Calibrated pump tubes are used for the RBC sample and resample lines. They ensure that the manifold starts and maintains a dilution compatible for linear calibration without the need for conformity checks. They are not necessary for WBC since normal tolerances

are sufficient to maintain correct dilution ranges for linearity. The dilution attained and maintained by an average manifold are 1 : 10,000 for RBC and 1 : 40 for WBC. (The new Counter allows considerable departure from this figure before linearity is affected.)

3) The A 12 fittings on the RBC resample line·was designed to ensure that a portion of every air bubble is drawn into the resample line. This ensures consistent second stage dilution and provides necessary wash.

4) The new stream splitter (PT-16) replacing the PT-7 is stainless steel with a surrounding plastic holder. During laboratory tests this has never become occluded by a normal (clot-free) sample. Simple as it is, it should be a major factor in ease of system operation.

5) The RBC and hemoglobin sample line is a common one. This assists in reduction of sample volume, reduction of blockage at the stream splitter and elimination of unnecessary pump tubes. The hemoglobin system is fundamentally unchanged except that lysis before addition of the Drabkins reagent is now performed by Triton X-100 instead of water. Due to the RBC count requirement, the initial dilution is made in saline. A typical correlation of this technique with the SMA-4 and 7 hemoglobin technique shows the method to be identical.

6) The pull-through tubes on the flowcell have been reduced (4.0 ml/min nominal instead of 6.8 ml/min). However, due to Counter flowcell design changes, this does not mean a reduced count (see later).

7) Reagent filters and air line filters have been added to the manifold to eliminate background count errors and flowcell obstruction by small particles. They have been shown to be an effective and important addition to operation of the system.

8) The introduction of a new white cell diluting fluid incorporating certrimide together with a great reduction in acetic acid concentration is a major contribution towards improved reproducibility and smooth operation. The reason for this is the virtual elimination of any protein precipitate that in the present system requires monitoring and rigorous periodic cleaning. Non-reproducibility can occur in the present system if theflowcell collects protein particles. This could produce irregular flow patterns in the flowcell both for red and white cell counts. An apparent unexpected bonus was the diluent's ability to destroy nucleated red cells, so giving an accurate white count. This does, however, require substantiation, since only one sample of this type was encountered in the initial evaluation.

9) The sample consumption is reduced by 28 %. Reagent consumption is reduced by 40 %.

Counter - mechanical and optical changes

1) To enable adjustment should any seepage occur at the valve situated immediately prior to the flowcell, a simple mechanical modification has been made.
2) Firm precise flowcell positioning is built into the optical bench. A two-way micrometer adjustment positions and holds the flowcell in an exact position for focus. Once selected this position is rigidly held. Flowcell focusing is important to maintain linear calibration.
3) A glass flowcell is now substituted for the original plastic unit. This is important for a number of very practical reasons:
    a) It is easier to handle — plastic flowcells can scratch easily giving excessive background noise as a result;
    b) The characteristics of glass are such that it has greatly reduced tendency for collecting debris. (This coupled with the new white cell diluent has made particulate matter in the flowcell a thing of the past!)
    c) Production of glass flowcells results in a more precise product. Flowcells can be freely interchanged without recourse to realignment of optics.
4) The flowcell dimensions have been considerably modified together with modifications to the optical apertures. The new view volume is less than 1/10 of the old view volume and this is the primary reason for linearity of calibration, not the fact of increased sample dilution although it does play a supporting role. (See also the comments on electronic modifications.)

The reduced view volume does not mean a reduction of cells counted which statistically would lower reproducibility. The opposite is the case, we now count twice as many cells as we did previously. This is due to the flowcell dimensional modifications.

Counter - electronic changes

1) In order to measure the new linear (non-coincident) optical system, photomultiplier bandwidth resolution has been greatly improved. (The smaller the view volume in the flowcell, the shorter the pulse generated, hence the more sophisticated are the electronics required.)
2) The electronic improvement has not been obtained at the expense of component reliability. The opposite is the case. This is due to

the extensive redesign of the electronics with substitution of solid state circuitry.

3) The gain setting has also been improved and simplified. The user no longer has to adjust the gain of the instrument (and more important perhaps, is no longer able to misadjust it!). Furthermore, a two-position gain switch is provided to facilitate the precise flowcell alignment mentioned earlier. The background can be amplified on the oscilloscope display so that the flowcell position for minimum background be found easily.

Programmer

1) For obvious reasons the SMA-7 A programmer will have a different signal conditioner card due to the change in the RBC calibration curve.

2) An apparently minor but very important change is a simple modification that is being made to the recorder damping for the counter circuits when the recorder is in the « non-read » position immediately prior to read time. Slightly increasing the amount of damping has made a significant improvement in the appearance and reproducibility of the recordings both for RBC and WBC.

Recorder

No substantial changes have been made to the recorder. WBC and RBC scales are linear except for a very small percentage at full scale. Another change to improve readability as made by printing smaller subdivisions for WBC and Hgb. The final chart paper change is the addition of a blue colored area for each scale indicating the correct reading position.

Standards

We consider that the introduction of the new automated SMA-4 A and 7 A hematology systems is incomplete without introduction of « primary » standards for the system. We have long been aware that the accuracy of a user's SMA-4 or 7 was only as accurate as the method to calibrate the whole blood used as the instrument standard. Manual and semi-automated counting techniques are subject to a variety of inherent errors. Among them: high irreproducible dilution in both techniques; subjective counting by manual means; and electronic and diluent background errors of semi-automated systems. These shortcomings cause serious doubt as to the advisability of employing these methods for routine standardization as insufficient time is available to statistically eliminate the errors by multiple tedious determinations. The « Stabicel » standards soon available represent an important step in consistent, accurate cell counting. As described in a separate bulletin, they are fully compatible with the Autoanalyzer system when used as directed and have excellent stability characteristics.

Figure 5 shows the typical threshold curves of RBC, WBC, and the fixed horse cells (microcytic with respect to human cells) used for both RBC and WBC standards. It should be noted that good agreement is obtained over a wide threshold range setting making this another non-critical adjustment that is critical in semi-automatic counting systems currently available.

This then completes the list of modifications that result in an SMA-4 A or SMA-7 A system. However, a brief review of the results of these changes is worthwhile.

Three major advances have been made in SMA-4 and 7 operation with respect to cell counting. They insure accuracy, reproducibility and ease of system operation.

Accuracy

The basic cell counter system resulting from optical and electrical improvements is fundamentally the most accurate system available. This is based on the fact that the detection point particle concentration is 5 to 6 times higher than any other instrumental system while still maintaining linear calibration (no coincidence effects). At full scale (RBC) cell concentration in the flowcell is approximately 700 cells/cu. mm compared to 112 and 140 cells/cu. mm for systems using dilutions of 62,500 and 50,000 respectively. Errors of dilution are therefore greatly reduced as also are errors in background count. This would be the case even if diluent background count was not eliminated by the zero baseline setting and continuous reagent and air filtration in the SMA-4 A and 7 A. These facts are, of course, only pertinent to the subject of accuracy if calibration standard is accurate. The SMA-4 A and 7 A systems can realize the potential of this fundamentally superior counting system now that:
1) Stable standards are available;
2) These standards are thoroughly, statistically counted.

Reproducibility

A typical reproducibility date is that on hospital bloods for RBC on SMA-4 A using 2 separate samples of the same blood (in effect 2 different dilutions) and SMA-4 A versus 7 A using 2 separate samples of the same blood (2 different dilutions, 2 different systems). The same standard was used in each case for calibration. The same picture could be repeated on a semi-automatic counter only if the same dilutions were used. If two different dilutions were made the scattergram was noticeably worse.

Coefficients of variation of $\pm$ 2.0 % are attainable in SMA-4 A and 7 A systems on up to 40 samples randomly loaded without re-calibration in the run. We now recommend no more than one check standard every 20 samples in routine operation. This reproducibility is representative of the original single cell counter reproducibility where the entire curve is visible. The major reasons for improvement apart from the linear calibration, are the counting of twice as many cells, modified programmer damping, and the realization that the proper place to read the curve is *at the end of the flat* shown on the blue area on the recorder paper. The system is always more reproducible at that point due to the longer time interval which enables the recorder pen to achieve the true mean count value. Other contributing factors are: 1) Stable manifold pumping and dilution; 2) Better white cell diluent, etc.

Ease of system operation

A thorough study of this report will enable the present SMA 4 or 7 user to understand that this new system is relatively easy to operate. All the modifications made, without exception, result in elimination of many checks and changes necessary for optimum performance of the existing SMA-4 and 7 systems. This has introduced a new feeling of confidence in the operation and has enabled production of fast, yet consistently reliable and accurate results.

3.3. *Multiple Hematologic Analyses by Means of a Coulter Counter Model S* *
Arthur W. Gottmann, St. Joseph Hospital, Denver, Colorado, USA

The new Coulter· Model S has been in our laboratory for almost four months and during this time seven parameters on more than

* Manufactured by Coulter Electronics, 590 W. 20th St., Hialeah, Florida.

20,000 blood samples have been studied. Duplicate determinations were done on the hematology samples passing through our laboratory and up to 50 multiple determinations on single selected samples during the same day. Results have been evaluated on a computer using standard statistical techniques and an algorithmic interpretation of histograms.

The Coulter Model S simultaneously determines values for seven blood parameters. Red counts (RBC), white counts (WBC), hemoglobin (Hgb) and mean corpuscular volume (MCV) are directly determined whereas the other three results are calculated. The hematocrit (Hct) represents the product of the MCV x RBC, the mean corpuscular hemoglobin concentration (MCHC) is the product of Hct x Hgb, and the mean corpuscular hemoglobin (MCH) is the product of the MCV x MCHC.

The principles of cell counting are the same as those used in earlier models of the « Coulter Counters » although each sample is now counted three times instead of once. Hattersley and Ragusa [1] showed the error for this red cell counting technique is 1.3%. The hemoglobin is done by the routine cyanmethemoglobin method with a blank. The MCV is determined as the red count is being done by measuring the size of the voltage drop as the red cells pass through the aperture. Studies of this technique for MCV determinations by Copeland [2] showed a coefficient of variation of 1.0%. Hattersley and Ragusa's work also showed the calculated hematocrit as the product of MCV x RBC when compared with the Wintrobe macro-hematocrits had a coefficient of variation of 1.0%.

Briefly, the Model S is a combination of electronic, hydraulic and pneumatic systems. It is a combination of five separate components including the power supply unit, the printer unit, the vacuum-compressor unit and the electronic-computer unit together with the dilutor unit. The design provides us with distinct advantages. First, the results are printed out by the unit and/or the instrument may be interfaced directly to a computer. These approaches help in decreasing the paper work load present in any laboratory today and enhances the quality control capabilities. Second, a unique diluting system provides for a level of reproducibility not previously attainable. This is possible on both whole blood and capillary blood. Third, because of the design the unit may be tested and balanced electronically. Finally, the instrument may be easily calibrated against known standards.

In counting, the three RBCs and WBCs are done separately but simultaneously and are averaged. If for some reason, one of the counts is greater than three standard deviations from the mean it is not included in the average. In the rare event that two of the three counts are greater than three standard deviations, no numbers at all will be produced for that count and the related calculated parameters. Two determinations for the MCV are averaged for the final printed result. Of utmost importance is the fact that the user of this instrument may separately calibrate each of the seven parameters measured. By introducing a blood standard with known values into the Model S one may, by means of a potentiometer in each of the seven circuits, adjust the instrument so that it will print these known values. Table I shows a comparison of our initial calibrations in relation to the same standard run 33 times during a three week period. We deliberately left the hemoglobin value 0.3 gm % less than the standard because we had been using this level in our laboratory on our previous instrument. The standard we used is one produced by Coulter Diagnostics.

From a practical standpoint the instrument is easy to operate and can process large numbers of specimens in far less time than was previously possible. The cycle time is 40 seconds for all seven parameters. We have not used the instrument long enough to evaluate its durability but electronic components are on modular circuit boards that are easily replaced.

The other parts are readily accessible and the preliminary instruction manual contains an easily understandable and well illustrated trouble shooting section.

In our testing of the precision or reproducibility of the instrument we began by doing 30-50 determinations of the seven parameters on six to ten tubes of blood drawn in sequence from a single patient. As expected, we found a progressive decrease of up to 500 white cells and 100,000 red cells with related declines in the hemoglobin and hematocrit which we have related solely to the removal of a rather large volume of blood from a single vein. Without modifying the results related to this decline, Tables II and III illustrate the standard deviation and coefficient of variation for each of the seven parameters measured. These tables also show the comparison of these values with those calculated for the Standard which we originally used to calibrate the Model S.

Simultaneously, we did duplicate studies on all the blood work routinely passing through our laboratory. Duplicates were run to analyze the effect of carry-over within the system. On the WBC the difference between the first and second determination averaged approximately 150 cells, the RBC difference averaged 40,000 cells, the hemoglobin difference averaged approximately 0.1 gm. and the MCV difference averaged less than one cubic micron. These findings suggest that carry-over

Table I

	Standard (Coulter)		Hospital Mean
WBC	5.9	(Thousands)	5.8
RBC	5.2	(Millions)	5.1
HGB	17.3	(gms %)	17.0
HCT	47.7	(%)	47.7
MCV	91	($\mu3$)	91
MCH	32.8	($\mu\mu g$)	33.0
MCHC	36.5	(%)	36.3

Table II

	Donors (200) Standard Deviation	Standards (33) Standard Deviation
WBC	.170	.211
RBC	.057	.073
HGB	.166	.145
HCT	.602	.776
MCV	.719	1.064
MCH	.263	.408
MCHC	.314	.475

Table III

	Donors (200) Coefficient of Variation	Standards (33) Coefficient of Variation
WBC	3.363	3.649
RBC	1.197	1.427
HGB	1.063	.850
HCT	1.313	1.627
MCV	.766	1.175
MCH	.806	1.233
MCHC	.904	1.301

is a factor in the reproducibility of the instrument and that its magnitude is in the range of 3%. Minor design changes, such as changes in the caliber of tubing, are being made by the manufacturers to reduce this carry-over even more. In the future, when we have a computer interface installed we shall examine this facet again.

We have felt that the classical statistical approaches which have been used in the past for quality control fail to be of much value in day to day performance evaluation. According to Mainland [3] and others, application of laboratory standard deviation and coefficients of variation to non-gaussian curves and discrete data not only yield misleading but also occasional frankly erroneous information. As a result, Mr. Joseph Robbins, our Chief Medical Programmer, and I have evolved a tentative approach to quality control which uses daily histograms of replicate blood samples to test the stability of the process under scrutiny. The algorithm which we utilize to evaluate the results incorporates the following:

$$\frac{\text{Number of values in major mode}}{\text{Total number of values}} + \text{Major modal tendency} - \text{Gaps in Array} = \text{Process Stability}$$

This provides a gross quantification of the events leading to the results and to the production of the histogram pattern. Subsequent variations in the pattern and index point to variations or a breakdown somewhere in the overall process.

Tables IV, V, VI and VII show histograms of the WBC, RBC, Hgb and MCV over 50 sequential determinations on the same blood sample. The WBC histogram shows a process which fails to produce a distinct major mode but does not have any gaps from outliers and so suggests moderate process stability. The RBC histogram shows less precision and stability with evident outlier development. The Hgb and MCV histograms show other variations which are unique for each measurement. It is suggested that any variation affecting the process at any level will cause a degeneration of the reproducibility of the system. Some distinct pattern aberrations emerged from the data we have collected to date. We believe that in the future we shall be able to diagnose specific problems within the system by our methods of computer monitoring utilizing these deviations in established patterns. We intend to also extend these techniques to all the tests done in the laboratory.

I feel at this point that this Coulter Model S has proven to be an important improvement in our laboratory instrumentation. The instrument does have some minor imperfections such as the carry-over problem. It also does not reproduce white counts as well in the

Table IV

6,6	X X X X X
6,7	X X
6,8	X X X X X X X X X
6,9	X X X X
7,0	X X X X X X X
7,1	X X X X X X X
7,2	X X X X X X X
7,3	X X X X X
7,4	X X X X

Table V

4.56	X	4.66	X X X X X X X X
4.57	X	4.67	
4.58	X X	4.68	X X X X
4.59		4.69	X
4.60	X X	4.70	X
4.61	X X	4.71	X
4.62	X X X X X X X X X X X	4.72	
4.63	X X X X	4.73	
4.64	X X X X X X X X	4.74	X X X
4.65	X	4.75	

Table VI

15.8	X X X X X X X X X X X X X X X X X X X
15.9	X X X X X X X X X X
16.0	X X X X X X X X X X X X X X X X X X
16.1	
16.2	X X X X X X
16.3	X

Table VII

90	X X X X X X X X X X X X
91	X X X X X X X X X X X X X X X
92	X X X X X X X X X X X X X X X X X X X X X X X X X X X X

lower ranges as it does in the higher ranges. We concur with Brittin [4] when he suggests that this is the result of small bubbles produced in the system which raise the background count when the lysing agent is added. The problem of the lysing agent destroying more fragile white cells in diseases such as chronic leukemia persists as it did in the old model Coulter Counters.

Philosophically, one must expect problems to develop with any new instrument. In the solving of problems we frequently get greater insight into the value of the result and the overall quality and usefulness of the data relative to the patient's well-being and ultimate benefit. This is evolution!

In summary, we have an instrument which is capable of a high degree of precision and accuracy. It has been thoughtfully designed and significantly incorporates complete calibration capabilities. Because of its improved function, more reliable standards are necessary than have been needed in the past both to match the capabilities of the instrument and so that each hospital, no matter where located, can produce equivalent results.

References

[1] Hattersley, P. G. and Ragusa, D., « An Electronic Mean Cell Volume Computer and Hematocrit Accessory », *Amer. J. Clin. Path.*, 47, 229, 1967.
[2] Copeland, B. E., « Standard Deviation », *Amer. J. Clin. Path.*, 27, 551, 1957.
[3] Mainland, D., « Notes on Biometry in Medical Research », *VA Monograph* 10-1, supplement 4, August 1968.
[4] Brittin, G. M. and Brecher, G., « Evaluation of Coulter Counter Model S », Read at the Amer. Soc. of Clin. Path. Program, Oct. 1968, to be published.

3.4. *Automated Hematology (Red Cell Counts, White Cell Counts, and Hemoglobin Determinations) Using the Hem-alyzer TM*
Robert J. Frost, Michigan City, Indiana, USA

Introduction

The Fisher Hem-Alyzer automatically determines and records the white cell count, the hemoglobin content and the red cell count of a whole blood specimen—all without operator intervention, and all within 96 seconds.

A programmed diluter samples each specimen in sequence and prepares the proper dilutions. These in turn are processed through an optical counting system composed of two separate optical assemblies, one is for the photometric determination of hemoglobin in blood, the other is for the determination for red and white blood cells. The specimens are fed into the system by means of a turntable which can handle up to 48 specimens requiring only 500 ml of diluent and 2 ml of lysing agent.

Upon completion of all measuring functions, the values are printed in succession on paper tape, being numerically identified.

Hemoglobin determinations are made using a null balance filter photometer. In the photometer, light from a common source is split into two beams by a fiber-optic conductor. One beam is directed to fall upon a reference photo cell; the other is directed to pass through a cuvet containing a prepared hemoglobin sample and into the sample photocell. Since the electronical output of the sample photocell varies with the absorbance of the solution in the cuvet, and the output of the reference photo cell remains unchanged, a voltage difference develops. When the output of the reference and sample photocells are compared, the difference between them — related to hemoglobin concentration — is measured into electrical pulses, proportional to the concentration.

Blood cell counts are made by electronically counting the flashes of light refracted from the cells in a dark field optical system. During operation, a 0.5 ml. aliquot of diluted blood sample is drawn through the channel of the micro counting chamber. As blood cells pass through the sensing zone of the dark field they produce flashes of light which are directed onto the face of the photomultiplier tube where they are converted into corresponding electrical pulses, which are then counted. Since the red and white cells are different in size, they reflect different intensities of light. Therefore, the sensitivity of the instrument must be adjusted to operate at two different sensitivity levels. This is accomplished by setting the red and white threshold adjustments for optimum response to red and white blood cells (fig. 1).

Operation

In operation, the apparatus is turned on at the beginning of the day and left on throughout the day since there is an initial warm-up period of some 20 minutes. The dilutor is primed and checked to see that the lines are free of bubbles. The counting chamber, which is cleaned once a day, is checked through the view eye piece using the view control Figs. 2.1. The shutter adjustment and focus of the counting chamber are then checked. The hemolyte reservoir is filled and hemolyte is added to the white cell cuvet.

214

Figure 1 - *Front view of instrument.*

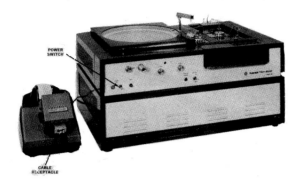

Figure 2.1 - *Top front panel controls and indicators.*

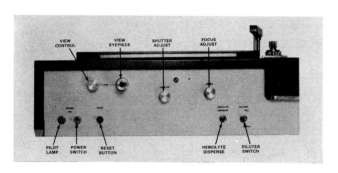

Figure 2.2 - *Bottom front panel controls and indicators.*

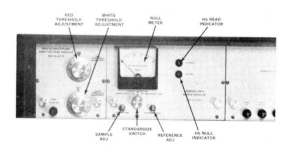

The hemoglobin servo module calibration is checked after the warm up period just prior to use (Fig. 2.2). The standardize switch is set in the sample cell position, and the sample adjustment switch is adjusted until the needle indicates the closest reading to 0 that is possible. The standardize switch is then set to the reference cell position and the reference adjustment is turned to bring the reading on the null meter to the same position as for the sample adjustment. The standardize switch is then placed in the normal position and the hemoglobin calibration is then complete. The RBC and WBC threshold adjustments are then checked for their proper settings: for our instrument, 85 for RBC's, 71 for WBC's. Checks are made for background counts of the diluent. This is accomplished by and letting the machine cycle through positions # 1 and # 2 without any specimens in the cups. The readings then printed out are the background counts and should be less than 200 for WBC's, less than 0.3 grams for hemoglobin, and less than 300,000 RBC's.

Blood is then added to the disposable cups to just cover the radial fins and placed in the turntable, and their sample positions noted.

At the end of any run, regardless of the number of specimens that have been previously processed, the instrument can be placed in the stand-by position (i.e. ready for immediate use).

If a Stat count is received while the instrument is counting, the instrument may be stopped and the Stat specimen placed in the turntable at position 5 from the sampling position. (If necessary a well mixed specimen could be placed in the location prior to the sampling station. We, however, have utilized position 5 to be certain that the specimen is well mixed prior to counting).

In our laboratories we use EDTA vacutainers for the collection of anticoagulated blood. There are however, no special requirements and any anticoagulated blood may be used. Only 1 ml. of blood is required. The results of a white cell count, hemoglobin determination and red cell count—in that order are recorded automatically on the printer tape.

In the Hem-Alyzer blood samples are diluted with and measured in normal saline solution. During an analysis, samples are transported to and from the measuring system by synchronized pumps and valves that make up the fluid handling system.

The sample probe initially descends into a blood specimen on the turn table, then the sample syringe dilutor draws 20 microliters (lambda) of blood into the probe (Fig. 3). Simultaneously 5 ml. of saline solution is drawn into the diluent syringe from the diluent reservoir. The sample probe then moves over and into the WBC/Hb cuvet and discharges the

Figure 3 - *Top deck of instrument.*

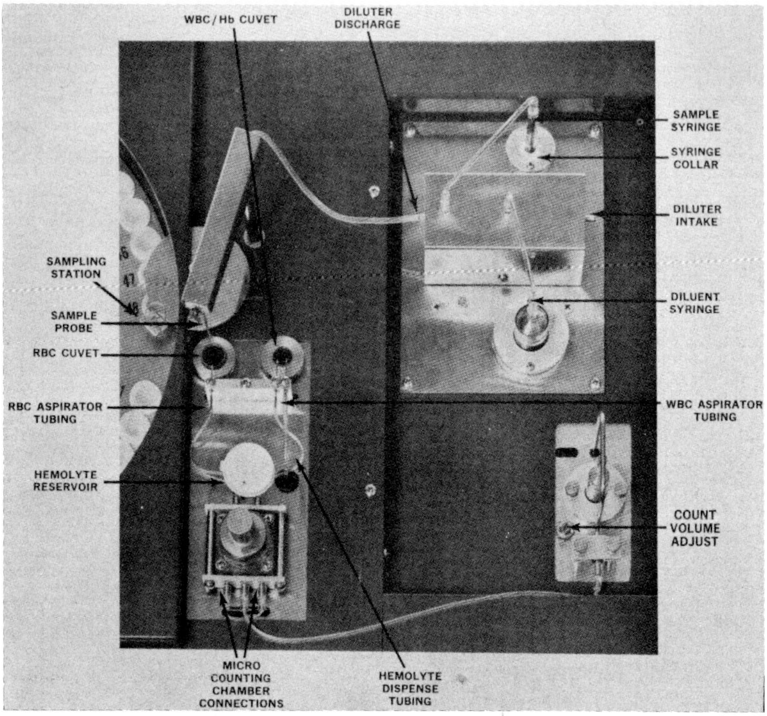

metered blood and saline. Part of the 1 : 250 dilution then remains in the cuvet for WBC and hemoglobin measurment.

With the sample probe still in the WBC/Hb cuvet, the sample syringe draws 20 microliters (lambda) of the 1 to 250 dilution into the probe, and 5 ml. of saline solution are drawn again into the diluent syringe from the diluent reservoir. This latter will provide 1 : 62,500 dilution for RBC counts. After the tip of the probe clears the top of the WBC/Hb cuvet 40 microliters of hemolyte from the hemolyte reservoir are injected into the cuvet by the hemolyte pump through the hemolyte injector needle. The hemolyte lysis the red blood cells in the cuvet to prepare the sample for WBC and Hemoglobin measurements. In addition to destroying red blood cells to prevent interference with the white cell counts, the hemolyte also releases and reacts with the hemoglobin in the red cells to form oxyhemoglobin. Approximately 1 milliliter of diluted sample from the WBC cuvet and the RBC cuvet are drawn through the micro counting chamber.

The white cells are counted over the 0 to 99.99 thousand cells per cubic millimeter range. The hemoglobin content, reported in grams of hemoglobin per 100 ml. of whole blood is measured over the 0 to 20.0 grams percent hemoglobin range.

The red cells are counted over the 0 to 9.99 million cells per cubic millimeter range.

Standardization

Initial standardization of the instrument in our laboratory was carried out as follows. Using whole bloods, threshold curves were made by taking counts at various threshold levels, first for the red counts and then for the white counts. By processing numerous blood specimens which had previous manual counts performed to compare with the threshold curves, the optimum threshold for our instrument was found to be 85 for RBC's and 71 for WBC's.

The hemoglobin servo was then standardized against a known hemolysate standard which we have used in our laboratory for years as well as against a College of American Pathologists Certified cyanmethemoglobin standard using a Fisher hemophotometer as the reference instrument, since the Hem-alyzer measures oxyhemoglobin and not cyanmethemoglobin.

Fresh whole blood was drawn from normal male donors and the following was done:

Five replicate RBC's, Microhematocrits, WBC's and hemoglobin determinations were done by each of four technologists to obtain the

Table 1

0 7 W 0 7 3 3	0 3 W 0 6 8 4		
0 7 H 0 1 1 5	0 3 H 0 1 0 9		
0 7 R 0 4 5 3	0 3 R 0 4 2 8		
0 8 W 0 7 2 4	0 4 W 0 6 9 0		
0 8 H 0 1 1 5	0 4 H 0 1 1 3		
0 8 R 0 4 7 5	0 4 R 0 4 5 4		
0 9 W 0 7 1 6	0 5 W 0 7 0 8		
0 9 H 0 1 1 5	0 5 H 0 1 1 5		
0 9 R 0 4 6 4	0 5 R 0 4 5 6		
1 0 W 0 7 1 6	0 6 W 0 7 1 4		
1 0 H 0 1 1 1	0 6 H 0 1 1 3		
1 0 R 0 4 7 9	0 6 R 0 4 6 4 Diff.		
W 7220	6990	360	
Mean H 11.4	11.25	0.15	
R 4.68	4.51	170,00	

Table 1 - *Quadruplicate count on two successive days. It shows that on one day the white count varied from 7,160 to 7,330 for a mean value of 7,220. On the following day the values varied from 6,840 to 7,140 for a mean value of 6,990. The difference between the two mean values is 360 cells. The hemoglobin values on the first day varied from 11.1 to 11.5 and on the second day varied from 10.9 to 11.5, with a mean value on the first day of 11.4 and on the second day of 11.25, and a difference of 0.5 grams. The red cells on the first day varied from 4,530,000 to 4,790,000 and on the second day the values varied from 4,280,000 to 4,664,000. This gave a mean on the first day of 4,680,000 and a mean on the second day of 4,510,000 and a difference 170,000. The differences between the mean values are well within the Quality Control limit, the hemoglobin and red cell being less than one standard deviation and the white cells being just slightly more than one standard deviation.*

mean values in each specimen. The Microhematocrits were used as a check on the manual red count and as will be shown, is still a part of our daily standardization.

Utilizing this method, we were able to adjust the instrument to obtain values within plus or minus 300 cells for the mean WBC, within plus or minus 100,000 cells for the RBC, and the hemoglobin within plus or minus 0.1 gram of those determined manually.

We continue to use a modification of the original standardization procedure for the daily standardization of the apparatus to be sure of day to day duplication of our results (tables 1-2).

1. 15 ml. of EDTA anticoagulated blood is collected from a patient with a presumed normal count. Duplicate microhematocrits and duplicate hemoglobins on a hemophotometer are done on this specimen. In addition the technologist estimates the WBC's as follows: If the WBC's are less than 5,000, to the nearest 1,000. If between 5,000 and 10,000 to the nearest 2,000, and if more than 10,000, within a range of 3,000 to 5,000. She also estimates whether the MCHC is normal or below. These examinations then serve as a check in the evaluation of the count of this blood specimen.

Table 2

0 0 W 0 0 0 7	0 9 W 0 7 2 6	1 7 W 1 2 2 0
0 0 H 0 0 0 0	0 9 H 0 1 3 2	1 7 H 0 1 1 5
0 0 R 0 0 2 9	0 9 R 0 4 2 4	1 7 R 0 4 6 3
0 1 W 0 0 0 5	1 0 W 0 7 1 5	1 8 W 1 2 8 8
0 1 H 0 0 0 0	1 0 H 0 1 3 5	1 8 H 0 1 1 0
0 1 R 0 0 2 8	1 0 R 0 4 4 6	1 8 R 0 4 4 1
0 2 W 0 0 0 7	1 1 W 0 7 0 9	1 9 W 1 3 4 6
0 2 H 0 0 0 0	1 1 H 0 1 3 3	1 9 H 0 0 9 2
0 2 R 0 0 2 6	1 1 R 0 4 5 1	1 9 R 0 2 9 8
0 3 W 0 0 0 8	1 2 W 0 7 3 6	2 0 W 1 3 5 6
0 3 H 0 0 0 0	1 2 H 0 1 3 6	2 0 H 0 0 9 4
0 3 R 0 0 2 5	1 2 R 0 4 6 4	2 0 R 0 2 9 6
0 4 W 0 0 0 5	1 3 W 2 0 2 0	2 1 W 1 1 3 2
0 4 H 0 0 0 0	1 3 H 0 1 4 4	2 1 H 0 1 2 6
0 4 R 0 0 2 5	1 3 R 0 4 6 6	2 1 R 0 4 0 9
0 5 W 1 4 2 1	1 4 W 2 1 2 1	2 2 W 1 1 7 3
0 5 H 0 1 3 7	1 4 H 0 1 4 6	2 2 H 0 1 3 0
0 5 R 0 4 6 6	1 4 R 0 4 7 6	2 2 R 0 4 0 6
0 6 W 1 5 4 1	1 5 W 0 6 2 3	2 3 W 0 5 7 0
0 6 H 0 1 4 4	1 5 H 0 1 5 9	2 3 H 0 1 5 8
0 6 R 0 4 9 6	1 5 R 0 5 2 1	2 3 R 0 5 1 8
0 7 W 1 4 7 7	1 6 W 0 6 5 1	2 4 W 0 5 8 3
0 7 H 0 1 4 2	1 6 H 0 1 6 5	2 4 H 0 1 5 6
0 7 R 0 4 6 5	1 6 R 0 5 2 3	2 4 R 0 5 2 2
0 8 W 1 5 1 7		2 5 W 1 0 5 5
0 8 H 0 1 3 7		2 5 H 0 1 2 6
0 8 R 0 4 7 4		2 5 R 0 4 9 9

(handwritten annotations in margins: "Henry QC", "Kalenda", "Staurat", "D'leiper", "Barnes", "Freukout", "Roukay", "Zenny")

Two segments of a single day's tape showing the background counts of the diluent, 0 trough 4.

Two duplicate counts, 5 through 8 and 9 through 11, and then six additional counts all done in duplicate.

Note that for hemoglobin there is a zero background count. The quadruplicate counts rapresent the two quadruplicate counts that we have to do each day, one for the current day to be compared with the previous day and then the current day to be compared with the succeding day.

In the early stages of the use of the machine, until we were satisfied that we were getting adequate results, all of our counts were done in duplicate. However, we now have confidence that this is not necessary.

2. The specimen is run in quadruplicate (4 cups) on the Hem-alyzer. The remainder of the specimen is kept in the refrigerator at 4 °C.
3. The mean WBC, hemoglobin, and RBC of this specimen are determined and this is reported as the patient's results for the day.
4. The following day, this same specimen is rerun in quadruplicate (4 cups) and the mean WBC, hemoglobin and RBC determined.
5. If the second days results are within plus or minus two standard deviations of the mean for the preceding day, the Hem-alyzer is performing within the required limits and may be used.
6. If the means are not within plus or minus two standard deviations, adjustment of the apparatus must be made before the machine can be put into use.
7. Utilizing this procedure, we continue to calculate standard deviations for WBC, Hb, and RBC on a monthly basis utilizing the high and low counts of the quadruplicate specimens. Our records indicate that we continued to have standard deviations in the range as outlined below.

	± 1 S.D.	± 2 S.D.
WBC	425/cmm	850/cmm
Hb	0.27 Gms	0.54 Gms
RBC	230,000/cmm	460,000/cmm
WBC	755/cmm	1510/cmm
Hb	0.30 Gms	0.60 Gms
RBC	140,000/cmm	280,000/cmm
WBC	372/cmm	744/cmm
Hb	0.29 Gms	0.58 Gms
RBC	120,000/cmm	240,000/cmm

Since putting this apparatus into use in our laboratory, we have been able to reduce our standard deviations for red counts, white counts, and hemoglobin determinations by one-third to one-half of what had been our experience with manual methods previously in use.

In our laboratories we have been using a standard hemolysate preparations which we prepare yearly as a standard, and check monthly against a College of American Pathologists Certified cyanmethemoglobin standard. Utilizing this as a control, we have obtained a one standard deviation of ± 0.1 Gms between the Hem-alyzer and a hemophotometer using our quadruplicate specimen.

Our hospital participates in a professional activities survey in which the admission hemoglobin on all admission in recorded, analyzed by computer with other information that is submitted, and an average monthly admission hemoglobin for our hospital is calculated. For years the admission hemoglobin to our hospital has been 13.4 ± 0.4 grams.

Since putting this instrument into use, our monthly hemoglobin has continued to remain in this same range, indicating that our current hemoglobin procedure is comparable to that previously in use.

At the time of introduction of this apparatus into our laboratories, we undertook a one month familiarization program in that we permitted only two of our best qualified Hematology technologists to use the equipment, doing duplicate counts on the Hem-alyzer in duplicate with those done by the other laboratory personnel manually. During this time minor problems were encountered in the nature of discrepancies between duplicate counts and random counts giving ridiculous results. However, as the familiarization process continued, these discrepancies decreased in frequency and eventually completely disappeared, indicating to us that these problems were of human origin rather than machine origin.

Orientation and familiarization with any new apparatus is essential and will lead to less problems with the eventual operation of any automated apparatus, since it will reveal problems that originate with the operator and the specimens as well as with the instrument.

Subsequent to the familiarization program, an indoctrination training program of the other laboratory personnel was undertaken with the instruction being given by one of the two original technologists who worked with the machine. We now have essentially all of our laboratory personnel at all levels of training and competance able to satisfactorily operate the Hem-alyzer.

The Hem-alyzer gives only red cell counts, white cell counts, and hemoglobin determinations. In the average general hospital we do not feel there is a need to calculate the indices, thus I do not feel that the lack of a hematocrit determination is of any consequence. Where the indices are indicated, we do a microhematocrit and calculate the indices using the Fisher Hematology Calculator.

The Hem-alyzer has been in daily use in our laboratories for approximately 7 months, during which time, we have had two minor mechanical difficulties, one of which, a line voltage problem required the services of an outside service man, the other a plugging of the hemolyte line which was readily corrected by replacing tubing which can be done by our own personnel.

Conclusion

This instrument has performed unusually well in our laboratories and in addition to markedly reducing the number of personnel required to do our hematology work load, has given us, as shown by our Quality Control Statistics, significant increased reliability in our hematology determinations.

References

[1] Copeland, B. E., « Standard Deviation, A Practical Means of Measurement and Control of the Precision of Clinical Laboratory Determination », *American Journal of Clinical Pathology, 27*, 551-558, May 1957.
[2] Dorsey, D., *Manual of Quality Control in Hematology,* ASCP, 1964.
[3] Fisher Hem-alyzer, *Modell 400 Instruction Manual,* 1968.

3.5. Measurement of Mean Corpuscular and Packed Cell Volume with the Coulter Counter

A. Carter, P. J. Crosland-Taylor and J. W. Stewart, Bland-Sutton Institute, Middlesex Hospital, London, W.1, UK

There are now two small computers which can be attached to a Coulter Model B or F which will calculate and display a mean corpuscular volume and a packed cell volume whilst the machine is doing a red cell count. These machines are incorporated in the Coulter Model S. This communication is concerned with the performance of these attachments used in conjunction with a Coulter Model F. The apparatus was loaned by Coulter Electronics Ltd, Dunstable, Bedfordshire, England.

As used by ourselves, we had to prepare the 1 : 50,000 dilution of blood by the usual two dilution process. It is important to use a buffered saline solution. 0.85 sodium chloride solution alone is not suitable as changes in red cell size occur in this solution and this invalidates the results. The solution we used was:

NaCl	- 8	grams
KH_2PO_4	- 0.2	grams
KCl	- 0.2	grams
$Na_2HPO_4 \cdot 12 H_2O$	- 1.15	grams
Disodium versene	- 0.2	grams
Distilled water to 1 litre		

Before we describe the results it is important to appreciate how the apparatus works. The M.C.V. is calculated by one computer attachment which measures the height of the pulses over a period during the actual count, summates the results and divides by the number of pulses recorded in the same period. This gives the average volume of the particles counted after suitable calibration of the apparatus. We calibrated the apparatus, with the aid of a technician from the manufacturers, using blood cells whose M.C.V. was calculated from the red cell count and the packed cell volume obtained by centrifuging for 10 minutes at 6,400 g. in an M.S.E. microhaematocrit centrifuge. The apparatus is equipped with a lower threshold which eliminates very small particles such as platelets from the calculation. There is no top or upper threshold so that the results of the M.C.V. of erythrocytes would not be correct in such conditions as leukaemia in which the leucocytes are markedly raised. The packed cell volume is calculated from the red cell count as determined by the counting apparatus. The computer used for this determination must work in conjunction with that used for the M.C.V. It automatically accepts the reading from this first computer and the red cell count from the counting machine, calculates the coincidence correction and then the P.C.V. from the total cell count and the M.C.V. The results are available within 1 second of completion of the count. It is evident that the P.C.V. so determined is a total P.C.V. of all the particles counted and their mean volume. Whereas the M.C.V. as determined by the apparatus is independent of the count the P.C.V. calculation is dependent on it. Thus if the 1 : 50,000 dilution is incorrectly made, the M.C.V. displayed will be correct but the P.C.V., although correct for that dilution, will be erroneous for the original blood sample.

In our first experiment ten dilutions from the same blood sample were prepared so as to give red cell counts varying between 10,000 and 100,000 on the machine after coincidence correction. This is equivalent to counts of between 1 and 10 million per cu. cmm in blood before dilution. The results are shown in Fig. 1. It can be seen that the P.C.V. displayed by the machine is exactly proportional to the dilution of the blood sample. The M.C.V. displayed by the apparatus varied between 91.5 and 94 μ^3 in this experiment.

We then recorded the M.C.V. and P.C.V. on 100 blood samples received in the laboratory. On the same blood samples the P.C.V. was obtained on the M.S.E. microhaematocrit centrifuge and the M.C.V. calculated from this value and the red cell count obtained from the counter after correction for coincidence using the Coulter correction chart. The results of the P.C.V. as displayed by the computer and obtained from the microhaematocrit are shown in Fig. 2. It can be seen that all the results are closely grouped around the diagonal. The

Figure 1

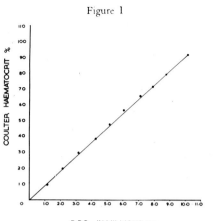

R.B.C.   IN MILLIONS /c.mm.

Figure 2

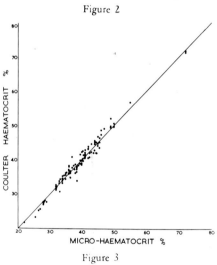

Figure 3

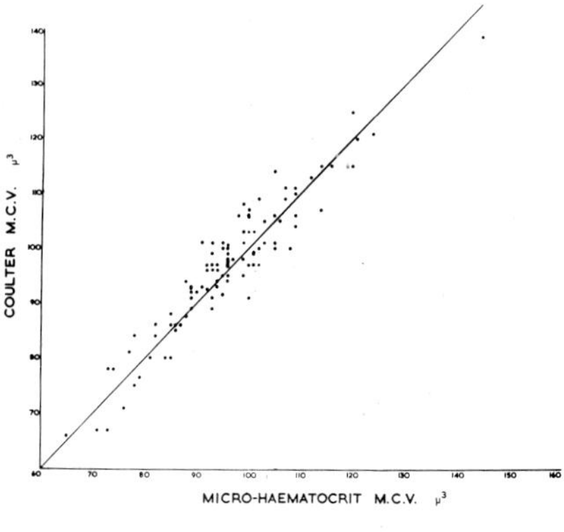

standard deviation of the difference was 1.7 divisions. 74 of the 100 samples agreed within 2 divisions and all but four agreed within 3 divisions. Of these 4, it was possible to repeat the observations on 3 samples in duplicate. In two, the microhaematocrit reading of the centrifuged specimen changed and was now in agreement with the Coulter measurements and the original readings were therefore incorrect. In the third specimen, the red cell count and the P.C.V. as displayed by the Coulter apparatus changed and were now in agreement with the value obtained by centrifuging. In this instance, the dilution of the blood sample presented to the machine must have been inaccurate.

Fig. 3 shows the Coulter M.C.V. plotted against the M.C.V.'s calculated from the red cell count and the centrifuged P.C.V. The standard deviation of the differences was 4.1 μ^3 72 of the hundred observations agreed within these limits. In four instances the difference exceeded 8 μ^3. It was possible to repeat the observations on two of the four samples. As already stated, the centrifuged P.C.V. was wrong.

During the time of use we found the performance of the apparatus was comparable in every way with the usual method using the microhaematocrit provided the very occasional patient with a high white count was excluded. There was no consistent difference between then values obtained by the machine and those obtained from the microhaematocrit and any significant differences were due either to errors in reading the P.C.V. obtained by centrifuging or lack of uniformity of the bore of the tubes used in this determination. Even the best tubes used in the microhaematocrit are allowed a variation of up to $\pm 2.0\%$ in bore. Another source of difference was errors in preparing the dilution of the samples for the Coulter counter but this occurred in only 1 of the 100 observations. We found that the most valuable feature was the saving of time required to obtain the results. It was also evident that calibration would be vastly simplified if a suitable standard of known size and count was available.

This paper is reproduced from the publication of the same title in the *Journal of Clinical Pathology* (*21*, 222, 1968) by kind permission of the Editor.

Chairmen: J. F. Coster, T. De Sanctis Monaldi, S. Eridani

4.1. *A Program for the Collection of Normal Hematological Values in Italy*
L. Tentori, Istituto Superiore di Sanità, Rome, Italy

Within the framework of recent initiatives taken in order to implement its statute, the CISMEL organization has established a panel for the study of normal values in hematology. This is regarded as one of the fundamental tasks of the organization, along with standardization of analytical methods and of clinical nomenclature. In my capacity as moderator of the panel, and also on behalf of my associates, I wish to thank the organizing Committee of this Symposium for including our subject matter in the agenda.

It is quite obvious, but it bears pointing out, that knowledge of the normal values of hematological variables in healthy subjects is of prime importance both as a technicality and because of its practical reflections.

The phrase « normal values » naturally applies to the concept of good health, this being regarded as a normal condition. Obviously, therefore, our first task is to define good health and normality.

A classical medico-legal definition states that health is the absence of disease: in other words, a subject is said to be healthy when there are no objective impediments to the implementation of his physiological functions and to his survival. However, I believe that a more serviceable and realistic definition is that incorporated in the charter of the World Health Organization (WHO), according to which health is a state of complete physical, mental, and social well-being, and not only the absence of disease or infirmity. This definition is currently accepted as an expression of an ideal situation to which modern men and nations are entitled. In a later WHO report we find it further explained that health is the state of the human organism that reveals a perfect functional adjustment to genetic and environmental situations. Thus we may say that a subject is in good health when all his functions operate within the limits of normal variability, and when he meets all the standard criteria of normal health relative to his age, sex, ethnological group, and geographical location.

At this point, we shift from an ideal and theoretical definition of normalcy to the concept of experimentally determined normal values constituting an index of normality in the population under discussion.

The value of statistical normality based on relative frequencies defines the upper and lower limits of variation; the central values within this band are accepted as normal averages for a given homogeneous population.

These premises are important on two counts. For one thing, the practicing physician must have suitable tables of normal values to help him solve diagnostic, prognostic, and therapeutic problems. And on the other hand, health authorities are interested in normal values because a rigorous survey of the amplitude of normal deviation provides essential information on the general state of health of the population; this, in turn, is indispensable for correcting social and economic disparities and for a rational planning of preventive medicine.

There are essentially two methods for gathering this type of information. One is mass survey of relatively simple parameters, and the other is the specialized investigation of a single item in a more complex problem.

Mass survey is obviously easier to carry out; it is also cheaper, does not call for highly specialized personnel, and yields a large number of information items. The data thus gathered are extremely useful because their elaboration provides the grounds for finer investigations to be carried out by experts at a higher technical level.

Specialized surveys, on the other hand, must be planned with due consideration for the principles of probability.

In the field of hematology, the first data on normal values for men and women were based on observations made over a century ago in a total of four clinically healthy subjects, and it was not until 1933 that a list of data gathered somewhat systematically became available. At that time a number of investigators became preoccupied with the lack of precise standards; but the average practicing physician was still unconcerned. After World War II, fairly rigorous studies were made, particularly in Anglosaxon and Scandinavian countries, and numerous papers were published with data on average normal values for hemoglobin, hematocrit, RBC, and WBC counts in adult males and females, and in children. More specialized papers dealt with the variations of these parameters according to age, sex, race, environment, and work or athletic activities, as well as with variations connected with the day-and-night rhythm and with the seasons.

In addition, the WHO recommended and sponsored large-scale, national or international surveys concerning the state of health and nutrition of various populations. And more recently, two important Symposia on the subject of normal hematological values were organized by ICSH: one in Stockholm in August 1964, and one in New York in September 1968; both were part of the programs of the International Society of Hematology, and both stressed the value of investigations of this kind, carried out with absolute scientific rigor.

Now if we want to plan this type of work in Italy, we must first decide (a) how many, and which, variables should be investigated; (b) what analytical methods should be used; and (c) how the normal population should be sampled. Making these decisions is far from easy, as we must always bear in mind the characteristics of the Italian mentality and general situation. In other words, we must take into consideration the degree of maturity and responsiveness of the general population called upon to cooperate in such an investigation and supply the blood samples, and then we must look into the existing or potential structures available for the job.

Thus we feel that for the time being we should confine our observations to the hemoglobin value, and that the method of assay should be the assay of cyanmethemoglobin, according to the recommendations and standards set forth by ICSH. These two suggestions are based on several considerations. In order to eliminate all possible variations caused by the use of different methods both in sample collection and in assay, standard methods are obviously needed; and today we do have a standard method for hemoglobinometry that is fairly simple and universally accepted. And we do have standard preparations of CNHb readily available, being produced under the supervision of CISMEL in accordance with the international standard. CISMEL also guarantees the perfect calibration of photometers to be used in mass survey. Further, the stability of CNHb solutions from the time of collection to the time of photometric reading is quite adequate.

The per cent concentration of hemoglobin in normal subjects is influenced by a number of individual factors such as sex, age, body weight, race, diet, partial oxygen pressure in the inspired air, physiological day and night variations, pregnancy, physical activity, and others. All these factors must obviously be taken into account in figuring out a normal value.

Concerning the sampling of population, it would be easier to investigate certain preconstituted groups such as students, Army draftees, firemen, the personnel of large industrial Companies, and the like; but the results of a survey so biased could certainly not be taken as representative of the whole population. Thus we find it desirable to use a population sample that includes subjects of all age groups, both sexes, and diversified work activities: this can easily be done with the population receiving medical assistance from the two main organizations of socialized medicine in Italy, namely INAM and ENPAS. These two institutions have in their care 60 per cent of the Italian population, with practically all work activities being represented (INAM takes care of manual workers and farmers, ENPAS of white-collar workers; both organizations also care for the workers' dependents).

What is requested of the clinics or institutes taking part in the experiment is as follows. Firstly, they must select INAM and/or ENPAS territories so that they are near enough to the clinic or institute, and so that their populations of workers, office workers, and farmers are representative. Secondly, they must effect a random selection without replacement of individuals in the lists of the INAM and/or ENPAS territories under discussion. This, in turn, requires access to the INAM and/or ENPAS files, and more particularly, knowledge of the number of primary sample units (eg classifiers) and of secondary sample units (eg drawers in each classifier) with the average number of file cards contained in each secondary unit.

Sampling is done by random selection of primary and secondary units. The selection of subjects is done by a random number of n + 1 digits, of which the first n digits identify the holder of the file card (by its position in the drawer) and the last digit identifies the dependent relative. Sampling is continued thus until the number required for each punched hole of the sample is filled. It is anticipated that twice as many subjects should be selected as are needed for the test.

Next, the participating institute must transcribe the data relative to each selected subject, and instruct the subject to report to the institute in a fasting state on a certain day.

Statistical considerations

Statistical elaboration will apply only to subjects pronounced clinically normal according to suitable criteria. The sample is organized according to a fixed module of 3 factors, namely *age* (14 classes), *sex*, and *occupation of the holder* (3 classes). Any combination of factors, totaling 84 punched holes, represents a case. If n is the number of subjects per case (this being a constant number), and if we assume a normal distribution of hemoglobin values and a standard deviation not exceeding 1.25 [6], for each case we expect that:

1. The error in estimate of the average, expressed as confidence interval, will not exceed the values:

$$\pm \frac{2.09 \times 1.25}{\sqrt{20}} = \pm 0.58 \text{ for } n - 20,$$

$$\pm \frac{2.02 \times 1.25}{\sqrt{40}} = \pm 0.40 \text{ for } n = 40, \text{ and}$$

$$\pm \frac{1.99 \times 1.25}{\sqrt{80}} = \pm 0.28 \text{ for } n = 80.$$

2. In order to cover 95 % of the normal values with a 90 % confidence, tolerances in excess or in defect of the average must not exceed:

$$\pm 2.56 \times 1.25 = \pm 3.20 \text{ for } n = 20,$$
$$\pm 2.33 \times 1.25 = \pm 2.91 \text{ for } n = 40, \text{ and}$$
$$\pm 2.20 \times 1.25 = \pm 2.75 \text{ for } n = 80.$$

Should the standard deviations relative to type of occupation not differ significantly, the intervals of confidence would be reduced to:

$$\pm 0.32 \text{ for } n = 20,$$
$$\pm 0.22 \text{ for } n = 40, \text{ and}$$
$$\pm 0.16 \text{ for } n = 80$$

and the intervals of tolerance would go down to:

$$\pm 2.81 \text{ for } n = 20,$$
$$\pm 2.69 \text{ for } n = 40, \text{ and}$$
$$\pm 2.60 \text{ for } n = 80.$$

It emerges from these considerations that each participating clinic or institute must examine a number of subjects between 1680 and 6720, equally spread among the 84 punched holes (Table 1).

For each of the subjects, the clinic must fill out a special form containing, in addition to complete identification of the subject, all pertinent facts in the clinical history of the subjects and in his (or her) physical examination, the latter being carried out and recorded in care of the participating institute or clinic.

Table 1

Schema di organizzazione del campione

Classi di età

Occupazione del Capofamiglia	1	2	3	4	5	6 10	11 13	14 24	25 34	35 44	45 54	55 64	65 74	75 85	Per maschi e per femmine
Impiegati															
Operai															
Agricoltori															1680 6720 individui

1) Ogni casella comprende 20 – 80 individui
2) Su ogni individuo si esegue 1 osservazione, *in doppio*, al mattino.

232

We believe that this way of planning the sample is both rigorous and realistic, and would be serviceable for the intended purpose. Accordingly, we hope that the concerned authorities, being convinced of the need for a survey of normal hematological values in the Italian population, will issue directions and appropriate the funds needed for our panel to carry out the task.

References

[1] Wintrobe, M. M., *Clinical Hematology*, Fifth Edition, 1968.
[2] World Health Organization, *Technical Report Series* No. 137, 1957.
[3] « Standardization, Documentation, and Normal Values in Hematology », *Biblioteca Hematologica, 21*, 125-168, 1965 (S. Karger, Basel).
[4] *Hematology of Normal Man: Hemoglobin Concentration*, Symposium organized by ICSH - New York, 1968. Reference in this publication.
[5] « Recommendations and Requisites of ICSH for Human Blood Hemoglobinometry (in Italian) », *Biochimica e Biologia Sperimentale, 4*, 1-2, 79, 1965.
[6] Milan, D. F., Meunch H., *J. Lab. Clin. Med., 31*, 878, 1946.

4.2. An International Comparative Trial on Cell Counting
Dr. A. H. Holtz, Rijks Instituut voor de Volksgezondheid (National Institute of Public Health), Utrecht, the Netherlands

In March-May 1968 an international haematological trial was organized by the Rijks Instituut voor de Volksgezondheid (National Institute of Public Health), Utrecht, the Netherlands. One of the aims was to obtain information on the reproducibility of and the methods used for the red-cell count in laboratories in different countries. The testing material consisted of two fresh blood samples and a stabilized red-cell suspension.

A report on the trial has already been given elsewhere (Holtz, 1970). There also a general survey of the cell-counting results has been presented. Figures 1-3, which give the values found for the three testing materials, are taken from that publication.

In Figures 4-6 the results of the electronic counters are classified as to type of counter. The most widely used instruments were the Coulter Counter and the Ljungberg Celloscope. The group « other machines » contained:

4 Fisher Autocytometers,
3 Hellige Erymats,
2 Eel Blood Cell Counters,

2 Marius Cyt-o-Counters (Dutch instrument),
2 Mascia and Brunelli Biotronics (Italian instrument),
2 Toa Microcellcounters,
1 ZG 1 Elmed (East-German instrument),
1 Hellige Elektrohaemoskop,
1 Klett Summerson Photo-electric Colorimeter,
1 Sanborn/Frommer Cell Counter,
1 Technicon AutoAnalyzer SMA-4.

No particular type of instrument seemed to perform better than the others.

The variation of the counting chamber results around the reference values (plus and minus about $0.7 \times 10^6/\mu l$) is only slightly larger than that which can be expected on theoretical grounds (Poisson distribution). The variation of the counter results is not much smaller; here, however, the theoretical limits are far exceeded. For the suspension some completely wild results were even found:

$1.64 \times 10^6/\mu l$ Celloscope *
$1.91 \times 10^6/\mu l$ Celloscope *
$2.3 \ \times 10^6/\mu l$ Cyt-o-Counter *
$2.84 \times 10^6/\mu l$ Biotronics
$2.9 \ \times 10^6/\mu l$ Celloscope
$2.98 \times 10^6/\mu l$ Biotronics
$5.35 \times 10^6/\mu l$ Coulter

It seemed worthwhile to investigate whether the large variation in the counter results could be attributed to systematic errors in the various techniques as applied in the laboratories and whether correction of the values found for the blood samples on the basis of the value found for the suspension in the same laboratory, would bring improvement.

When applied to the over-all results as presented in Figures 1-2, no effect of such a correction could be noted. When, however, the procedure was applied after grouping the results as to type of counter, a distinct improvement was observed for the Coulter Counters (Figures 7-8).

The results of the Celloscopes and those of the « other machines » did not improve. As regards this latter group, there is no need to wonder in view of its heterogeneity. That the correction had no or even an adverse effect on the Celloscope results, was rather surprising, however. It could be that certain characteristics of the stabilized cell suspension make this preparation less suited for use in the Celloscope, at least when

* Not included in the graphs.

234

Figure 1

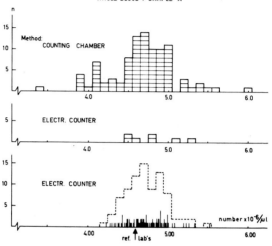

Figure 2

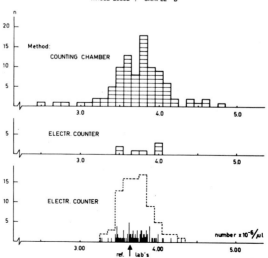

Figure 3

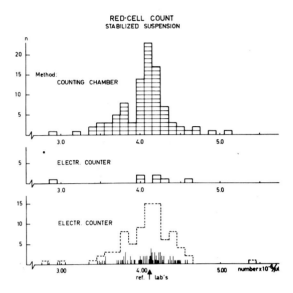

RED-CELL COUNT
STABILIZED SUSPENSION

Figure 4

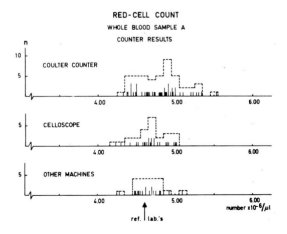

RED-CELL COUNT
WHOLE BLOOD SAMPLE A
COUNTER RESULTS

236

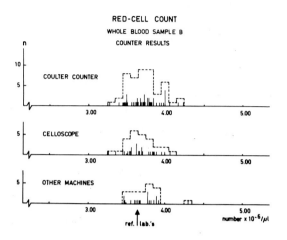

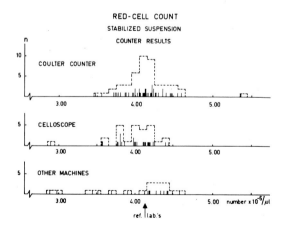

Figure 7

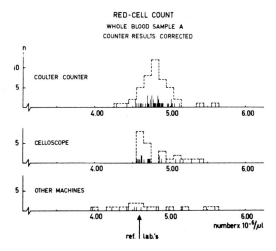

RED-CELL COUNT
WHOLE BLOOD SAMPLE A
COUNTER RESULTS CORRECTED

Figure 8

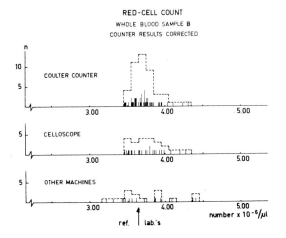

RED-CELL COUNT
WHOLE BLOOD SAMPLE B
COUNTER RESULTS CORRECTED

238

operating with its normal setting for fresh blood. The fact that 3 out of the 7 outlying results came from Celloscopes (and even 6 if one includes the Celloscope-related instruments Cyt-o-Counter and Biotronics) is a strong indication in that direction. Investigations on this point are being continued.

Summary

The results of an international trial on red-cell counting are reported. Counting chambers and electronical counters were used in about the same proportion. Particularly as regards the results obtained with the latter instruments, the uniformity leaves still much to be desired.

Evidence was obtained that at least part of the variation in the counter results was due to systematic errors in the technique, since re-calculation of the results on the basis of a simultaneously analyzed reference sample brought about improvement. This procedure, however, only had effect in the case of Coulter Counters, not in the case of Celloscopes. This may be due to the type of the reference used (a stabilized red-cell suspension).

Reference

Holtz, A. H., in: Standardization in Hematology, Franco Angeli Publ., Milano, 1970, p. 113.

4.3. *The Value of Standardized and Controlled Erythrocytometric Parameters in Differential Diagnosis*

C. G. de Boroviczény and E. Coordes, Institut für Standardisierung und Dokumentation im Med. Laboratorium E. V., Freiburg, Germany

Analysis of the measured and calculated erythrocytometric parameters is of considerable assistance in the differential diagnosis of hematological disorders. The more commonly used erythrocytometric parameters that can be measured directly are the RBC count, the hemoglobin content of whole blood, the packed cell volume of erythrocytes, and the mean diameter of the erythrocytes. From these four values we can calculate the values for mean cell hemoglobin, mean cell hemoglobin content, mean cell volume, and mean cell thickness. The mutual relationships of these parameters are shown in Table I.

Since it is very difficult to scan eight values at a time, each being of two or three digits, we have constructed a nomogram showing the various measured values; from these, the calculated values can be read with the help of a ruler. The nomogram is so constructed that the values on the various limbs form a straight or curved line when joined together: more precisely, normal values lie approximately on a straight line, whereas pathological values form fairly typical curves. Fig. 1 shows the form currently used in our Institute, with the results of erythrocytometric analysis expressed numerically and inscribed in the nomogram.

Obviously the usefulness of a diagnostic system based on four measurements and four calculated parameters is primarily determined by the degree of accuracy with which the measured parameters are assessed; accordingly, special efforts were made toward standardization and effective quality control in hemoglobinometry, RBC counts, and packed cell volume and mean cell diameter determinations. So far, an international standard is available only for hemoglobinometry; however, there are some good published methods for the preparation of stable erythrocyte suspensions that would be suitable for international standardization of RBC counts and packed cell volume determinations. For hemoglobinometry we have both a good reference and several excellent routine methods. For packed cell volume, a microhematocrit method is currently used all over the world with very good comparability of results. An International Expert Panel is working toward standardization of this method. For RBC counts we are still wanting an acceptable reference method, but a serviceable principle has already been published. Here, too, an International Expert Panel is at work. For all three determinations, national standard descriptions are available in England and Germany. For the determination of mean cell diameter, however, the situation is quite different and not nearly so satisfactory. Two unrelated methods are used, namely the halometric method and direct microscopical measurement of the erythrocytes. Further, we know that there are significant differences between the diameter of red blood cells suspended in their own plasma or serum and the diameter of dry, fixed erythrocytes in a blood smear. Unfortunately, no efforts were made so far to standardize the measurement of mean cell diameters. On the other hand, calculations relative to mean cell hemoglobin, mean cell hemoglobin content, mean cell volume, and mean cell thickness are made in the same way anywhere in the world; thus, acceptance of adequate definitions is all that is needed concerning these four parameters.

In the matter of measurements, however, it is not enough to use standardized methods; to obtain precise, reproducible, accurate, and comparable results, one must implement a systematic quality control on such work. This can be done essentially in two ways. Repeat measure-

Figure 1

NAME AND ADRESS OF THE LABORATORY   Sealevel

in m

PARTICULARS OF

THE   DIAGNOSISES

PATIENT

measures	ERYTHROCYTOMETRIC VALUES		computed
c-vB Ery	(±) $10^{12} . 1^{-1}$	M. C. H.	(±) pg
c-vB Hb	(±) g . 1^{-1}	M. C. H. C.	(±) %
c-vB P. C. V.	(±) . 10^{-2}	M. C. V.	(±) fl
c-vB M. C. D.	(±) . μ m	M. C. T.	(±) μ m

MICROSCOPIC OBSERVATIONS: inconspicuous
Pro-normo/megalo-cytes   %; Normo/megalo-blasts   ; Heinz/Howell-Jolly/semilunar-bodies
Round   %, not round   %, elliptic   %, narrowelliptic   %; Elliptocytosis - Drepanocytosis
Aniso - Macro - Micro - Megalo - Poikilo -cytosis; Polychromasia; Erythrocytes en rouleaux;
Ring - Spheric - Target - Burr - Thornapple -cells; Basophilic stippling; Cabot's rings; Schistocytes
Schüffner's granules; Parasites:

PRICE-JONES / VOLUMETRIC -CURVE (cells were measured):
1. population: mean at μ m =   %;   99% of the cells are between   and μ m
2. population: mean at μ m =   %;   99% of the cells are between   and μ m

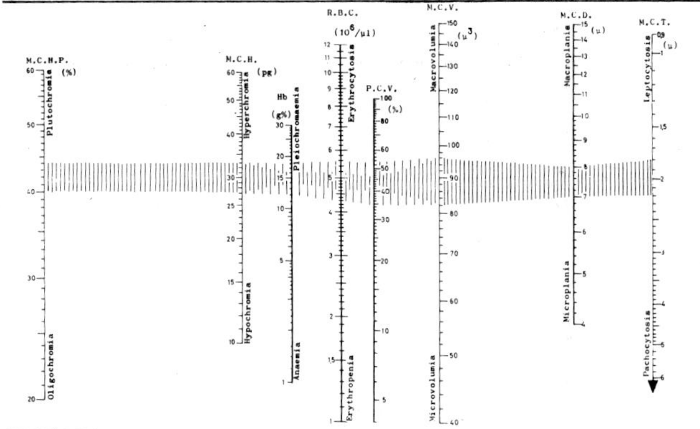

REMARKS:

DATE   SIGNATURE

241

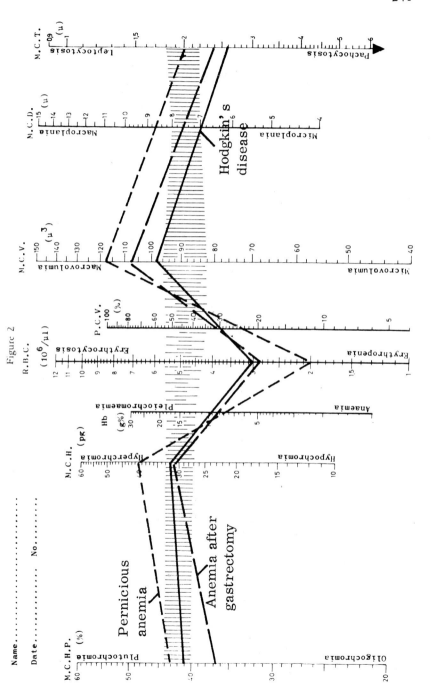

Figure 2

242

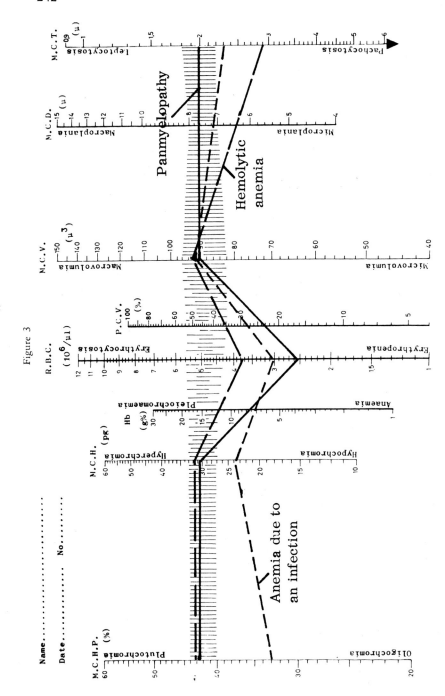

Figure 3

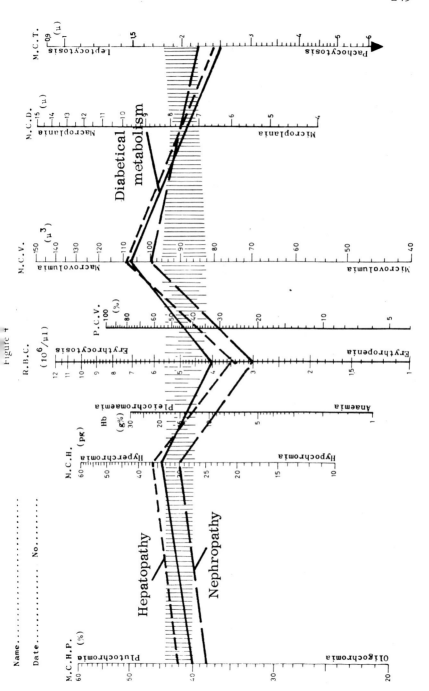

Figure 4

244

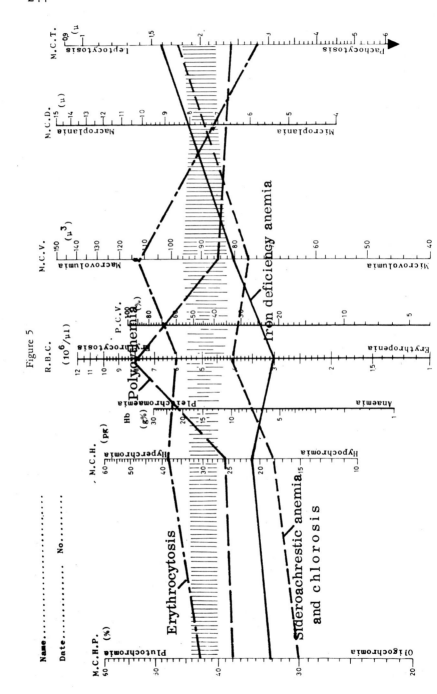

Figure 5

Figure 6 - *RBC value distribution in pathological conditions.*

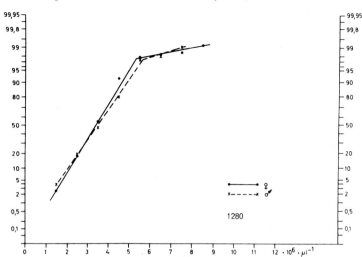

Figure 7 - *Hb value distribution in pathological conditions.*

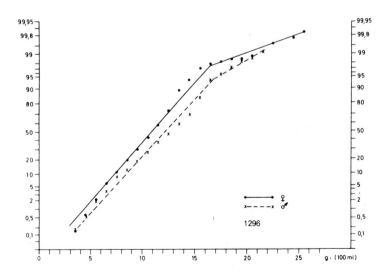

246

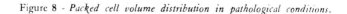

Figure 8 - *Packed cell volume distribution in pathological conditions.*

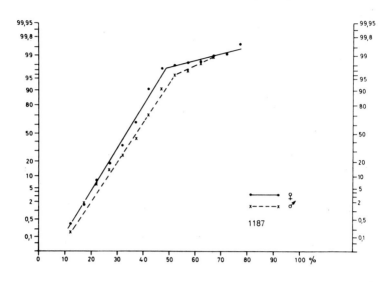

Figure 9 - *Mean cell hemoglobin concentration, and quantity, and mean cell volume distributions in pathological conditions.*

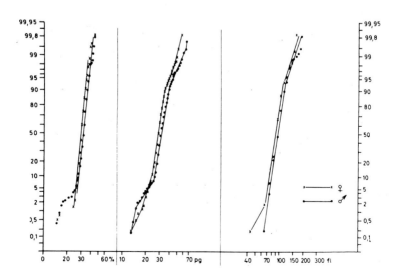

Figure 10 - *Mean cell thickness and mean cell diameter distributions in pathological conditions.*

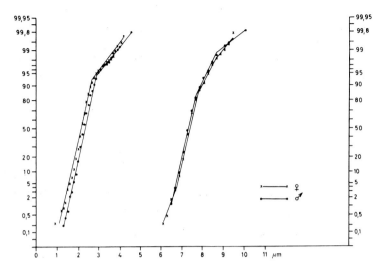

248

Table I. The Mutual Relationship of Erythrocytometric Parameters

Measured Parameters	Computed Parameters	Dimensions, Formulas
Blood Hemoglobin Concentration (Hb)		g/l, or mmol/l, or g/100 ml;
	Mean Cell Hemoglobin	pg/Ery; Hb (g/l)/Ery $(x10^{12}/l)$;
Red Bloodcell Count (Ery)		part.$x10^{12}/l$, or part.$x10^{6}/\mu l$;
	Mean Cell Hemoglobin Concentration	% (v/v); Hb (g/l)/10xKrit (l/l);
	Mean Cell Volume (M.C.V.)	fl; 10^{3}xKrit (l/l)/Ery $(x10^{12}/l)$;
Packed Cell Volume (Krit)		liter/liter, or %;
	Mean Cell Thickness	μm; 4..M.C.V.(fl)/πx(Diam, $\mu m)^{2}$
Mean Cell Diameter (Diam)		μm;

Tab. II.a. Correlation between the Packed Cell Volume and the Hemoglobin concentration

Hemoglobin	0-9	10-19	20-29	30-39	40-49	50-59	60-69	70-79	80-89	Σ
24,0 – 26,9							2		2	4
21,0 – 23,9					1	2	7	10		20
18,0 – 20,9					18	80	13	1		112
15,0 – 17,9			1	30	688	139	6			864
12,0 – 14,9		1	8	450	824	7	2			1292
9,0 – 11,9			227	636	56	2				921
6,0 – 8,9	4	29	284	48	1					387
3,0 – 5,9	3	41	6							50
0,0 – 2,9	1									1
Σ	7	71	526	1164	1588	230	30	11	2	3630
Hematocrit										

Table II.b. Correlation between the P.V.C. and the R.B.C.

R.B.C.										Σ
10,00 – 10,99									2	2
9,00 – 9,99							1	1		2
8,00 – 8,99						3	8	4		15
7,00 – 7,99					1	20	13	2		26
6,00 – 6,99					71	83	5	1		160
5,00 – 5,99				72	594	105	6	2		789
4,00 – 4,99			13	475	798	40	2			1328
3,00 – 3,99		1	216	513	109	10				849
2,00 – 2,99		22	267	93	7	1				390
1,00 – 1,99	3	46	24	2	1					76
0,00 – 0,99		1								1
Σ	3	70	520	1155	1581	252	35	10	2	3628
Hematocrit	0-9	10-19	20-29	30-39	40-49	50-59	60-69	70-79	80-89	

Table II.c. Correlation between the Hemoglobin content and the R.B.C. in patients of a medical department

R.B.C.										Σ
10,00 – 10,99									2	2
9,00 – 9,99								2		2
8,00 – 8,99						3	6	6	1	16
7,00 – 7,99						6	12	8		26
6,00 – 6,99					12	98	48	2		160
5,00 – 5,99			3	27	281	544	50	1	2	908
4,00 – 4,99			11	213	815	198	5	1		1243
3,00 – 3,99		2	99	568	192	23	1			885
2,00 – 2,99		8	236	151	22	1				418
1,00 – 1,99	1	39	35	5	1					81
0,00 – 0,99		1								1
Σ	1	50	384	964	1323	873	182	20	5	3722
Hemoglobin	0,0-2,9	3,0-5,9	6,0-8,9	9,0-11,9	12,0-14,9	15,0-17,9	18,0-20,9	21,0-23,9	24,0-26,9	

ments may be taken by the same investigator working with the same method, or parallel measurements may be taken by two different investigators working with the same method or with different methods. While parallel estimations are generally more useful than double estimations by the same worker, the policy in our Laboratory is to use parallel estimations for RBC counts, and double estimations for the other parameters. In double estimations it is important that the second run should be unbiased by the first. We feel that it is important to have parallel or double estimations for all tests done in our laboratories because we are interested not only in quality control of our average work, but also in the control of each single value. With this policy, the precision of our measurements is between $\pm 1\%$ and $\pm 3\%$ (c.v.).

Concerning pathological findings, we have so far been able to determine the typical erythrocytometric curves for a number of diseases, as shown figs. 2-5. These curves clearly show the degree of diagnostic discrimination afforded bv erythrocytometric analysis. They also confirm the well-known fact that the greater differences are usually found in the middle part of the nomogram, i.e. in the part showing the values for mean cell hemoglobin, hemoglobin content of the blood, RBC count, packed cell volume, and mean cell volume, whereas variability is much less in the nomogram limbs showing mean cell diameter and mean cell thickness, and least of all in the limb showing mean cell hemoglobin concentration. The distribution of values in pathological cases is shown in figs. 6-9, where one can easily see the ranges that can be used for statistical quality control, as introduced by Hoffmann.

The values for RBC count, hemoglobin, and packed cell volume usually increase or decrease together, but not to the same extent. We have found that certain levels of probability obtain in the relationships between each of these values and the others. The results of this analytical work (Table II) are also useful for quality control of individual findings.

4.5. *An Automated System for the Preparation of Blood Smears*

M. Ingram, Department of Radiation Biology and Biophysics, University of Rochester School of Medicine and Dentistry, Rochester, N.Y. 14620, USA

The system which I will describe for automatic preparation of blood films is a direct outgrowth of another, more extensive research effort to develop an automatic pattern recognition system for blood cells. The latter program has been in progress for several years, in collaboration with Mr. K. Preston, Jr., Mr. P. E. Norgren, and others at the Perkin-Elmer Corp., Norwalk, Conn. [1, 2].

The method described in this report is based upon a procedure used commercially for coating small optical parts with « photoresist ». It was initially suggested to me by Mr. Preston and Mr. Norgren who were familiar with the commercial process. Briefly, the method consists of completely flooding a coverglass, edge to edge, with a layer of blood and then centrifuging it rapidly in a plane parallel to the plane of rotation of the centrifuge. The excess blood spins off to leave a monolayer of well-spread blood cells on the coverglass. The preparations are referred to as « spinner smears ».

The machine used for these studies is a Plat Model 102 M blood film centrifuge. The instrument may be adjusted to centrifuge the coverglasses at speeds ranging from 1,000 rpm to 10,000 rpm. A clutch mechanism allows the operator to select two rates of acceleration, reaching full speed in either 30 milliseconds or in one second. A timer is set to the desired time of centrifugation so that the spinner stops automatically (and quickly) after the appropriate interval. Ten to fifteen seconds of centrifugation at speeds of 5,000 rpm (or greater) produces good smears that are completely dry when the spinner stops.

Blood smears have been evaluated by counting and classifying leukocytes in various concentric areas of the smears. Details of the evaluation of spinner blood smears are presented in a report which is in press [3]. The present report is intended simply to describe the technique and the apparatus and to emphasize some of the characteristics of spinner smears.

Using the centrifugal device, it is possible to spread blood in an even monolayer of well-flattened cells over virtually an entire coverglass. The differential leukocyte count is uniform over the entire smear.

Spinner smears are particularly remarkable for the exceptionally low incidence of broken and disrupted cells. Grossly disrupted, distorted or torn cells make up more than 15 % of all leukocytes encountered on conventionally prepared smears, in contrast to approximately 2 % on spinner smears. The human observer is likely to be unaware of the high incidence of disrupted cells on conventional smears unless a deliberate, careful effort is made to determine this. Man's own image-processing system functions so extraordinarily well that he quickly learns to eliminate visual « noise » of this type. A high incidence of distorted or damaged cells is important, however, because the differential leukocyte count is altered if the preparation of smears disrupts predominantly one or two types of cells, leaving other types unaffected.

In normal blood, the granulocytes and monocytes appear to be particularly susceptible to disruption by the shearing force applied when smears are pulled. The effect is exaggerated if coverglasses are not scrupulously clean, if smears are too thin, or if blood is diluted excessively with saline solution, or if the cell suspension is dilute to begin with as in severe anemia. Small lymphocytes appear to be relatively resistant to disruption during preparation of conventional smears, but larger lymphocytes, with more abundant cytoplasm and less compact nuclei, are more vulnerable. Very few « smudge cells » are found on spinner smears of blood from patients with chronic lymphocytic leukemia in contrast to the high incidence of such cells on corresponding conventional smears. The differential classification of various types of lymphocytes is quite different on conventional and spinner smears of chronic lymphocytic leukemia blood.

Since spinner smears have both uniform distributions of cells over an entire coverglass and a very low incidence of disrupted cells, such preparations have distinct advantages for both routine differential leukocyte counting and for studies of cytological detail. The uniform thickness of spinner smears makes them well suited to automatic scanning techniques [3, 4]. The greater spreading (flatness) of leukocytes on spinner smears should be especially advantageous in high resolution autoradiography of cells, especially when tritium is the isotopic label and the preparations are used for grain counting [4, 5, 6].

For instrumental analysis, it is best to work with blood in which the leukocyte count is not greater than approximately 20,000 cells/mm³ in order to minimize the number of contiguous leukocytes. Blood in which leukocyte counts are very high may be diluted with either an isosmotic solution of bovine serum albumin or with autologous plasma or serum.

It appears that those leukocytes and platelets that are in contact with the glass surface before the spinner is started adhere firmly to the glass and are not dislodged or distorted by centrifugation. Nuclei and cytoplasmic contents are not displaced within cells and leukocytes are not distorted by cells that flow over them or strike them while being spun off. On the contrary, erythrocytes conform to the outline of leukocytes and platelets where they abut against them.

Red cells are not uniformly round in contour on spinner smears as on conventional smears but they are intact. When something looks different from what one is accustomed to seeing, it is, perhaps, instinctive to suspect that there is something wrong. In the case of the red cells on spinner smears, however, I believe this assumption is not necessarily justified. The red cells tend to be somewhat elongated and the area of « central palor » is often displaced to one side or appears in the « tail » of an elongated cell. I suspect that the spinner may, in fact, represent an interesting approach to the study of normal and abnormal red cell deformability. One gets the impression that the shapes of red cells on spinner smears may correspond to the shapes of these cells when circulating.

Although most of the studies evaluating the blood film centrifuge have been carried out using normal human blood, preliminary studies using blood from patients with hematological disorders, normal blood from species other than man, bone marrow (mouse, rat and dog), suspensions of isolated nuclei and tissue cultures of PHA-stimulated lymphocytes indicate that the technique gives equally good preparations from such samples. Spinner smears of cell suspensions other than blood and marrow have not been studied in our laboratory, but it seems reasonable to predict that good quality smears of many types of cell suspensions could also be prepared using the spinner technique.

References

[1] Ingram, M. and Preston, Jr., K. « Importance of Automatic Pattern Recognition Techniques in the Early Detection of Altered Blood cell Production », Ann. N. Y. Acad. Sci., 113 (Art. 2), 1066-1072, 1964.
[2] Ingram, M., Norgren, P. E. and Preston, Jr., K., « Advantages of Topology as a Basis for Automatic Analysis of Blood Cell Images », Ann. N.Y. Acad. Sci., in press.
[3] Ingram, M., Minter, N. « Semi-Automatic Preparation of Coverglass Blood Smears Using a Centrifugal Device », Am. J. Clin. Pathol., in press.
[4] Falk, G. and King., R. C., « Radioautographic Efficiency for Tritium as a Function of Section Thickness », Rad. Res., 20, 466-470, 1963.
[5] Feinendegen, L. E., Tritium Labeled Molecules in Biology and Medicine, Monograph of Am. Inst. of Biol. Sci., Academic Press, 1967.
[6] Kisieleski, W. E., Baserga, R. and Vaupotic, J., « The Correlation of Autoradiographic Grain Counts and Tritium Concentration in Tissue Sections Containing Tritiated Thymidine », Rad. Res., 15, 341-348, 1961.

Acknowledgement

It is a pleasure to acknowledge the collaboration of Miss F. M. Minter and the highly skilled technical assistance of Miss B. Morehouse and Mrs. G. Yettewich in the research described.

This work was supported under National Institutes of Health contract # PH 43-66-1159 with the Perkin-Elmer Corp., Norwalk, Connecticut, and, in part under contract with the U. S. Atomic Energy Commission at the University of Rochester Atomic Energy Project and has been assigned Publication No. UR-49-

Note added in proof:

Since this paper was written, the manufacturer has introduced improvements in the Blood Film Centrifuge so that it is now possible to prepare blood films on slides as well as on coverglasses and to prepare them so that erythrocytes retain a circular outline if the operator so wishes.

5th Session

Chairmen: G. Izak, E. Polli, L. Tentori

5.1. *Progress in Haemoglobinometry*
E.J. van Kampen, Clinical Chemical Laboratory,
Diakonessenhuis, Groningen, the Netherlands;
O. W. van Assendelft and W. G. Zijlstra, Laboratory
of Chemical Physiology, University of Groningen,
the Netherlands

Standardization

A reference point must be chosen before standardization is possible.
Establishing the reference point in haemoglobinometry primarily involved a double decision. The first decision concerned the selection of
a physical or chemical property of haemoglobin which could be measured
both easily and accurately. The second decision involved the adoption
of one or more methods to exactly correlate the results of the physico-
chemical measurement with a certain amount of haemoglobin.

Of the few physico-chemical properties of haemoglobin which can
be measured easily and accurately, the absorption of visible light has
been the one most widely used. Using modern spectrophotometers, the
optical density of a clear haemoglobin solution can be measured to within
0.5 %. All haemoglobin must, of course, be converted into one and the
same derivative, or at least into derivatives which are photometrically
indistinguishable at the wavelength of measurement. There is little or
no difference of opinion that the haemoglobin derivative most suitable
in this respect is haemiglobincyanide (HiCN). HiCN is the most stable
of all known haemoglobin derivatives, has a favourable absorption spectrum with a flat maximum around $\lambda = 540$ nm and follows Lambert-

Beer's law over a wide concentration range. Finally all haemoglobin derivatives commonly present in human blood can be completely converted into HiCN by simple means. Thus the first decision could be made without evoking much controversy: the quantity to be measured will be the optical density of HiCN solutions at $\lambda = 540$ nm (D_{HiCN}^{540}).

The second decision involved a choice of either a method based on some functional property of haemoglobin, e.g. O_2 or CO binding capacity, or an analytical method based on the chemical composition of the haemoglobin molecule. The technical difficulties and uncertainties in blood gas analysis and the existence of temporarily inactive haemoglobin in normal blood both favoured the use of an analytical method aimed at the chemical composition of haemoglobin. A strong argument was added when the composition of the haemoglobin molecule was completely elucidated [1, 3].

Having decided on chemical analysis, the most suitable atomic species within the haemoglobin molecule had to be considered. Although N has been proven suitable [13], the atom of choice appeared to be iron, bringing about the last, perhaps the most crucial, certainly the most debated choice to be made. Which method(s) to be selected to determine haemoglobin iron.

It should be noted in this connection that the determination of « absolute » chemical values must always be ultimately based upon a direct method of analysis, i.e. a gravimetric or a volumetric one. Indirect methods are only suitable for the determination of chemical quantities when properly prepared standard solutions based on weight analysis, are used and when all possible interfering factors have been thoroughly studied, preferably by repeated comparison with a direct method of analysis. These safeguards having been taken, the spectrophotometric iron determination using α,α-'dipyridyl [20] and the haemoglobin iron determination by X-ray emission spectrography [8] have been developed into reliable technics, next to the titrimetric method with titanous chloride [20]. Atomic absorption spectrophotometry, on the other hand, has been shown to be inadequate for the « absolute » determination of haemoglobin iron, mainly because of the influence of the method of sample preparation upon the results [15].

Thus, after measuring D_{HiCN}^{540} of a clear solution of exactly known millimolar haemoglobin concentration in a calibrated 1.000 cm glass cuvette with a spectrophotometer checked as to wavelength using mercury emission lines and checked as to optical density scale using a NBS carbon yellow or similar reference filter, the millimolar extinction coefficient of HiCN at $\lambda = 540$ nm could be calculated.

Table I – ϵ^{540}_{HiCN} as reported by different authors, based on iron or nitrogen determination.

author	material	ϵ^{540}_{HiCN}	$s/\sqrt{n}$	n	method
Meyer-Wilmes and Remmer (6)	horse Hb	11.0	0.04	12	Fe; o-Phenantrolin
	horse Hb	11.0	0.04	12	Fe; TiCl$_3$
Remmer (9)	human whole blood	11.09	0.03	11	Fe; TiCl$_3$
	human whole blood	11.19	0.065	4	Fe; complexon
Minkowski and Swierczewski (7)	foetal whole blood	11.15	–	5	Fe; o-Phenantrolin
Zijlstra and Van Kampen (20)	human Hb, toluene haemolysis	10.99	0.01	123	Fe; α, α' – dipyridyl
		10.94	0.03	35	Fe; α, α' – dipyridyl
		11.05	0.02	101	Fe; TiCl$_3$
Wootton and Blevin (19)	human Hb, toluene haemolysis	10.68	0.04	14	Fe; ferric perchlorate
Van Oudheusden et al. (17)	human whole blood	10.99	0.05	10	Fe; α, α' – dipyridyl
	human whole blood	11.06	0.08	8	Fe; α, α' – dipyridyl
Salvati et al. (10)	human Hb purified on CMC column	10.95	0.03	46	Fe; α, α' – dipyridyl
Tentori et al. (13)	human Hb purified on CMC column	10.90	0.05	55	N analysis
Morningstar et al. (8)	human whole blood	11.02	0.03	10	Fe; X ray emission spectrography
	human washed cells	10.97	0.07	6	
Stigbrand (11)	human Hb purified on CMC or Sephadex column or by dialysis against Na$_2$ –EDTA	11.00	0.02	55	Fe; sulfosalicylic acid

s/√n = standard error of the mean; n = number of determinations

The results of 16 series of determinations of the quarter millimolar extinction coefficient (ε_{HiCN}^{540}) by 10 research groups in 7 countries is shown in table I. In all but 2 series adult human blood was used, in most, haemoglobin solutions more or less purified by various methods, in a few, whole blood. One group used horse blood, another human foetal blood. All but one series were based on iron analysis, only Tentori et al. [13] resorting to N analysis.

From the data of table I a total mean value and corresponding standard error of the mean have been calculated using the equations

$$x_g = \frac{1}{n_{tot}} \cdot \Sigma_i \, n_i \cdot x_i$$

and

$$\frac{s^2}{n_{tot}} = \frac{1}{n_{tot} \cdot (n_{tot} - 1)} \cdot \Sigma_i \, (n_i - 1) \cdot s^2_i + n_i \cdot (x_i - x_g)^2$$

where x_g = mean value of all determinations
x_i = mean value of the i-th series of determinations
n_{tot} = total number of determinations
n_i = number of determinations in the i-th series
s_i = standard deviation of the i-th series of determinations
s = standard deviation of all determinations

Excluding the work of Minkowski and Swierczewski [7] who did not publish their standard deviation, a mean value of 10.98 is obtained for ε_{HiCN}^{540}, n = 502, s/√n = 0.009. Exclusion of the series of Wootton and Blevin [19], which differs more than 3 times the standard error of the mean from the total mean value, brings ε_{HiCN}^{540} to 10.99, n = 488, s/√n = 0.009. The quarter millimolar extinction coefficient thus having been determined, standardized haemoglobinometry may be performed by any spectrophotometer adequately checked as to wavelength and optical density scale. To allow the use of a filter photometer a HiCN standard solution of exactly known concentration is necessary for calibration. As clear HiCN solutions follow Lambert-Beer's law, a single concentration of the standard suffices to establish a reliable calibration line. An international reference solution is prepared on behalf of the International Committee for Standardization in Haematology (I.C.S.H.) by the Dutch Institute of Public Health (R.I.V., Utrecht, the Netherlands) to enable manufacturers of HiCN standard solutions to check their products as to conformity with the requirements put forward by I.C.S.H. [4]. The wide range given for $D_{HiCN}^{504}/D_{HiCN}^{540}$ in these requirements should be regarded as a concession to the manufacturers of commercial standards and may well be restricted in the future as proposed by Matsubara and Shibata [5]. Each batch of the international reference standard is tested at regular intervals by laboratories in Germany, the Netherlands, Sweden, the U.K. and the U.S.A. Recently, the control data collected from November 1964 to March 1967 have been published [14].

Although some technical points, primarily concerning clinical haemoglobinometry (methods of obtaining blood samples, calibration of pipettes, stability of reagent solutions etc.) are still under discussion, the fundamentals of standardized haemoglobinometry have now been firmly established. The extinction coefficient of HiCN, the molecular weight of haemoglobin and the international reference solution are, in our opinion, the solid basis upon which haemoglobinometry should rest.

It needs no saying, that once having an internationally accepted, accurate and reliable standardized method, one has to be reluctant to bring about alterations.

In connection with this I plan to say a few words on the haemoglobin-azide method, in which field excellent work has been done by Vanzetti.

As the next speaker will cover this in detail, I only want to say that there are — without doubt — differences already on the grounds of spectral characteristics — and we are happy that, in the near future, we shall be able to work together with Prof. Vanzetti on the azide-method.

At this very moment we can, however not see any clear advantage of this method over the HiCN-method, and thus we would like to wait before contemplating the HiN_3 method as a real alternative to the HiCN method.

Using the HiCN method

That spectrophotometry of clear HiCN solutions by various average operators is non-problematical, is clearly demonstrated in table II. The spectrophotometric procedure adhered to by the I.C.S.H.-nominated control laboratories was used. This procedure is as follows. After adjusting zero and sensitivity controls, the instrument is balanced with the sample in the light path. Sensitivity and zero are then checked and only if no shift has occurred is the absorption scale read. If a shift has occurred, the entire procedure is repeated.

The application of the standardized method in routine clinical haemo-

Table II – D^{540} and D^{504} measurement of International HiCN Reference Solution 60400. Beckman Du spectrophotometer. 20 Operators, slit width fixed.

operator	D^{540}	D^{504}	D^{540}/D^{504}	operator	D^{540}	D^{504}	D^{540}/D^{504}
1	0.385	0.240	1.60	11	0.384	0.239	1.61
2	0.385	0.240	1.60	12	0.385	0.240	1.60
3	0.385	0.240	1.60	13	0.385	0.239	1.61
4	0.385	0.240	1.60	14	0.384	0.239	1.61
5	0.385	0.240	1.60	15	0.386	0.241	1.60
6	0.384	0.239	1.61	16	0.384	0.239	1.61
7	0.385	0.240	1.60	17	0.385	0.240	1.60
8	0.385	0.239	1.61	18	0.385	0.239	1.61
9	0.385	0.239	1.61	19	0.385	0.240	1.60
10	0.385	0.240	1.60	20	0.384	0.240	1.60

mean value $D^{540} = 0.385$, s = 0.0005
mean value $D^{504} = 0.240$, s = 0.0006

$$s = \sqrt{\frac{\Sigma' (x - \bar{x})^2}{n - 1}}$$

Table III – The influence of centrifugation and detergents on the measurement of HiCN solutions using both large exit aperture, LKB multichannel, and small exit aperture, Zeiss PMQ II, instruments. For centrifugation an International centrifuge Pr2 was used for 30 min at 19300 rpm.

| | c_{Hb} stated | | LKB Multichannel | | | | Zeiss PMQ II | | | |
| | | | not centrifuged | | centrifuged | | not centrifuged | | centrifuged | |
	by manu-facturer	detergent	D^{540}	c_{Hb} (g%)	D^{540}	c_{Hb} (g%)	D^{540}	c_{Hb} (g%)	D^{540}	c_{Hb} (g%)
1	15.7	none	.446	16.4	.426	15.7	.478	17.6	.427	15.7
		Sterox SE	.436	16.0	.432	15.9	.450	16.5	.431	15.8
2	14.8	none	.414	15.2	.399	14.7	.436	16.0	.392	14.4
		Sterox Se	.405	14.9	.401	14.7	.409	15.0	.395	14.5
3	16.3	none	.460	16.9	.440	16.2	.514	18.9	.443	16.3
		Sterox Se	.449	16.5	.443	16.3	.469	17.3	.443	16.3

260

globinometry, however, still affords some problems. Errors up to 10 %
relative have been encountered due to the following. Differences in
pipettes, many of which do not deliver the stated volume within 2 %.
Differences in haemoglobin content found by various technicians due
to individual differences in the sampling technic, e.g. squeezing the
sample out of the finger tip. These may be circumvented by calibration
of each pipette and by careful training of personnel. Of a more fundamental character, however, are errors due to turbidity.

When a blood sample and the reagent solution are mixed, a crude
HiCN solution, containing, among others, precipitated proteins, lipid
particles and erythrocyte ghosts, is obtained. If, in a photometer, the
incidental light strikes such a particle, part of the light will be dispersed
and less light will reach the photocell (tube). The photometer will
thus indicate a higher density reading of the solution. The degree to
which a given turbid solution in the cuvette disperses the light depends
primarily on the size of the particles with respect to the wavelength of
the incidental light. The magnitude of the error thus obtained is
greatly influenced by the optical geometry of the instrument used. A
given photocell will only measure the light having passed through the
sample cuvette within a certain angle. The larger is the angle, the smaller
the distance between photocell and cuvette. Thus a photometer with a
short cuvette to photocell distance, i.e. a large exit aperture, is to be
preferred. Errors due to turbidity may be largely eliminated by centrifugation or filtration of the samples or diminished by the addition of
detergents to the reagent solution. To achieve optimal results with
the HiCN method, the reagent solution should thus contain an adequate
detergent and measurement should be carried out with instruments
having a large exit aperture. The resulting error in haemoglobin concentration, primarily due to erythrocyte ghosts not influenced by the
detergent, will be kept to within 2 % relative. Table III, summarized
from the work by Haglund [2], illustrates clearly the effect of centrifugation or detergents on the measurement of turbid HiCN solutions
using both a large exit aperture instrument, LKB multichannel, and a
small exit aperture instrument, Zeiss PMQ II.

Thus it is not yet quite possible to strictly come up to the requirement
of I.C.S.H. that the reagent « must be of such a quality that after dilution of the blood there is no turbidity » [4].

That turbidity errors are prevalent even among commercial standards
is amply illustrated by table IV. Standards were obtained and studied
in the Netherlands in 1964 and in Sweden in 1966. The Swedish results
have been summarized from the work by Haglund [2]. The haemo-

Tabel IV – Haemoglobin determination of commercially available HiCN and diluted whole blood standards with and without centrifugation using a Beckman DU (N. '64) and a Zeiss PMQ II (S. '66). International centrifuge PR2, 30 min, 19300 r.p.m.

standard	material	c_{Hb} stated (g%)		c_{Hb} measured (g%) not centrifuged	centrifuged
Walter Reed Hospital	HiCN	14.9	N. '64	15.2	
Dade Reagents	HiCN	20.0	N. '64	25.8	
Acuglobin	HiCN	14.9	N. '64	15.2	
Diagnostic reagents Ltd.	HiCN	high 22.5	N. '64	22.8	
		low 3.7	N. '64	4.0	
Hycel	HiCN	20.0	S. '66	21.7	20.7
Schweizerhall	HiCN	18.0	N. '64	18.9	
		18.0	S. '66	17.7	17.7
Haury	HiCN	20.0	S. '66	21.0	17.7
Hyland	whole blood	14.1	N. '64	13.1 (1)	
		13.7	S. '66	15.3	13.5
Hemotrol	whole blood	15.0	N. '64	13.8 (1)	
		16.3	S. '66	19.9	15.8

(1) diluted with reagent containing Sterox SE.

Table V – Haemoglobin values in different age groups, both male and female. Samples diluted 251 times with the reagent according to Van Kampen and Zijlstra (16). Measurement using filter photometers (HbF 100, Vitatron, the Netherlands) calibrated with HiCN reference solutions (R.I.V., Utrecht, the Netherlands).

group	sex	n	c_{Hb} (g%)	s (g%)
blood donors (12)	male	100	15.8	1.8
blood donors (12)	female	100	14.5	1.6
healthy volunteers	male	644	14.9	1.5
over 65 years	female	593	14.1	1.3
$\leqslant$ 15 years	female	38	13.7	0.8
16 – 18 years	female	260	13.9	1.1
19 – 21 years	female	309	14.0	1.2
22 – 40 years	female	190	13.9	1.3

globin content when given in mg/100 ml, was recalculated to comparable haemoglobin content of blood in g/100 ml.

Normal values

Although many references to the determination of haemoglobin in normal subjects may be found in the literature, the authors know of no systematic study incorporating the use of the HiCN method, aimed to arrive at normal haemoglobin values. That such a study is filled with pitfalls is, of course, common knowledge. To name but one, daily variations in one and the same individual, due to greater or smaller fluid loss, have been encountered. Much work needs to be done as regards e.g. defining conditions to obtain a normal value and standardization of sample collection.

A few pilot investigations have, however, been held, all using the standardized HiCN method. Some results of these investigations are given in table V. Much work, however, remains to be done to establish the range of normal haemoglobin values in man.

References

[1] Braunitzer, G., Gehring-Müller, R., Hilschmann, N., Hilse, K., Hobom, G., Rudloff, V. and Wittmann-Liebold, B., Hoppe-Seylers Z. physiol. Chem., 325, 283, 1961.
[2] Haglund, H., personal communication.
[3] Hill, R. J., Konigsberg, W., Guidotti, G. and Craig, L. C., J. biol. Chem., 237, 1549, 1962.
[4] International Committee for Standardization in Haematology, Brit. J. Haemat., 13 (Suppl.), 71, 1967.
[5] Matsubara, T. and Shibata, S., to be published.
[6] Meyer-Wilmes, J. and Remmer, H., Arch. exp. Path. Pharmakol., 229, 441, 1956.
[7] Minkowski, A. and Swierczewski, E., in Oxygen Supply to the Human Foetus (Editors: J. Walker and A. Turnbull), Blackwell, Oxford 1959 (pp. 237-253).
[8] Morningstar, D. A., Williams, G. Z. and Suutarinen, P., Amer. J. clin. Path., 46, 603, 1966.
[9] Remmer, H., Arch. exp. Path. Pharmakol., 229, 450, 1956.
[10] Salvati, A. M., Tentori, L. and Vivaldi, G., Clin. chim. Acta, 11, 477, 1965.
[11] Stigbrand, T., Scand. J. clin. Lab. Invest., 20, 252, 1967.
[12] Strengers, Th., personal communication.
[13] Tentori, L., Vivaldi, G. and Salvati, A. M., Clin. chim. Acta, 14, 276, 1966.
[14] Van Assendelft, O. W., Holtz, A. H., Van Kampen, E. J. and Zijlstra, W. G., Clin. chim. Acta, 18, 78, 1967.
[15] Van Assendelft, O. W., Zijlstra, W. G., Buursma, A., Van Kampen, E. J. and Hoek, W., Clin. chim. Acta, 22, 281, 1968.
[16] Van Kampen, E. J. and Zijlstra, W. G., Clin. chim. Acta, 6, 538, 1961.
[17] Van Oudheusden, A. P. M., Van de Heuvel, J. M., Van Stekelenburg, G. J., Siertsema, L. H. and Wadman, S. K., Ned. T. Geneesk., 108, 265, 1964.
[18] Vanzetti, G., J. Lab. clin. Med. 67, 116, 1966.

[19] Wootton, I.D.P. and Blevin, W.R., *Lancet*, 434, 1964, II.
[20] Zijlstra, W. G. and Van Kampen, E. J., *Clin. chim. Acta*, 5, 719, 1960.

5.2. Similarities and Differences between the Azide-methemoglo-bin- and the Cyanmethemoglobin Methods

A. von Klein-Wisenberg, Institut für Standardisierung und Dokumentation im Medizinischen Laboratorium, Freiburg i. Breisgau, Germany

A certain reluctance towards the routine use of a reagent solution for the determination of hemoglobin (Hb) containing poisonous cyanide set the impulse to looking into the analytical application of other Hb compounds of sufficient stability comparable to the well known cyan-methemoglobin (HiCN). Each of the possible Hb species occurring normally or under pathological conditions in human blood should be convertible to this single compound. Next to HiCN, having a stability constant of $10^{+5,5}$ according to Lemberg and Legge (1949), azide-methe-moglobin (HiN$_3$) of Smith and Wolf (1904) with $K \sim 10^{+5,1} \ldots 10^{+5,2}$ (Kellin 1936, Kiese and Kaeske 1942) would serve for this purpose and has consequently been proposed as analytical alternative to HiCN (Vanzetti 1966).

Both methods have in common the use of hexacyanoferrate [III] as electron acceptor (0,606 mMol), the maintainance of a rather low pH (7,2...7,4) at a low osmolality through moderate amounts of buffer (1,03 mMol dihydrogenphosphate resp. 8,25 mMol THAM/ 2,38 mMol citric acid) and 0,05 % v/v of detergent. The former solution (recipe Van Kampen-Zijlstra) contains 0,77 mMol cyanide, the latter (recipe Vanzetti) 0,46 mMol azide as potassium, respectively sodium salt.

The keeping qualities of both reagents are quite different: the de-composition scheme of the cyanid-/hexacyanoferrate [III] system can tentatively be assumed as

$$CN^- + 2\,Fe\,(CN)_6{}^{3-} + H_2O = CNO^- + 2\,Fe\,(CN)_6{}^{4-} + 2\,H^+$$

with lg K > 7, followed by irreversible hydrolysis of cyanate to am-monia and carbon dioxide (von Klein-Wisenberg 1966, Winkelmann et al. 1968). Considering the above equation, the reaction from left to right of this inherently metastable system sets in, and enhances its rate due to the Le Chatelier-Braun principle by concentration; therefore the solution decolorizes upon freezing.

The azide-hexacyanoferrate (III)-system remains unchanged after freezing and thawing. This becomes clear considering the mechanism of decomposition of azide. The heat of formation of the azide ion is fairly high (65,5 Cal · Mol^{-1}, aqueous solution, infinite dilution, 25 °C *). Photolysis experiments with hydrazoic acid make evidence of the intermediate formation of the imide radical (NH) and also possibly the azide radical (N$_3$) leading to an overall reaction:

$$3 \; HN_3 \rightarrow NH_3 + 4 \; N_2 \quad \text{(Joffe 1966)}$$

Using accessible thermochemical data, Latimer (1952), in his standard compilation of electrode potentials allows for two ways of decomposition of hydrazoic acid: oxidative decay to the elements and reductive formation of ammonia and nitrogen. Table I lists these three possible modes of decomposition of azide ion in aqueous solution: by oxidation, by reduction, and by disproportioning. It is interesting to note that the equilibrium concentration of azide in solution, assuming a partial pressure of nitrogen corresponding to air, a 1 % content of hexacyanoferrate (II) in hexacyanoferrate (III), pH 7,2, and ubiquitous concentration of ammonium ion of 1 mMol, can be estimated as $\sim 10^{-53}$ Mol.l^{-1} whichever reaction path is considered. It is also clear from the estimated equilibrium concentration of azide that this system is even more metastable than the cyanide-/hexacyanoferrate(III)-system. The activation energy necessary to start these highly exergonic processes must be very high. Moreover, it can be deduced from table I that neither mode of decay will be favoured by freezing the solution in closed vessels because of the counteraction of increasing solubility at lower temperatures and higher pressure of nitrogen. Following these considerations it would be highly advisable to remove the azide reacting solution from the refrigerator only shortly before use. On the other hand there is a certain probability that inconsiderate personnel will dispense this reagent before its attaining room temperature, thus introducing a positive volumetric error resulting in a negative concentration error.

As would be expected from the similar electronic configuration of cyanide and azide and by the slightly different stability constants of their complexes with methemoglobin, the spectra of HiCN (fig. 1) and HiN$_3$ (fig. 2) are very similar. As already described by Lemberg and Legge and confirmed by Vanzetti (1966) and Van Assendelft (1968) there are bands at 542 and 575 nm with a feeble band at 630 nm. The bandwidth

---

* The main use of inorganic azides, specially of lead, mercury and silver is made as detonating agent in cartridges. Even sodium azide decomposes rapidly upon gentle heating or irradiation with ultraviolet light (253,7 nm). There are restrictions in postal and air mail of this substance in various countries.

Table 1 – Decomposition schemes of azide ion

I. Oxidizing decomposition:

I.a $Fe(CN)_6^{3-} + e^-$ $= Fe(CN)_6^{4-}$ $-\ 6,02$

I.b $N_3^- + H^+$ $= HN_3\,(aq)$ $+\ 4,7$

I.c $HN_3\,(aq)$ $= 3/2\ N_2\,(g) + H^+ + e^-$ $+\ 52,3$

I.d $N_3^- + Fe(CN)_6^{3-}$ $= 3/2\ N_2\,(g) + Fe(CN)_6^{4-}$ $+\ 51$

Equilibrium concentration assuming $p_{N_2} = 0,782$ atm, $/Fe(CN)_6^{3-}/ : /Fe(CN)_6^{4-}/ = 100 : /N_3^-/ = 10^{-53,2}$

II. Reducing decomposition:

II.a $2\ Fe(CN)_6^{4-}$ $= 2\ Fe(CN)_6^{3-} + 2\ e^-$ $+\ 2.6,02$

II.b $N_3^- + H^+$ $= HN_3\,(aq)$ $+\ 4,7$

II.c $HN_3\,(aq) + 3\ H^+ + 2\ e^-$ $= N_2\,(g) + NH_4^+$ $+\ 66,2$

II.d $2\ Fe(CN)_6^{4-} + N_3^- + 4\ H^+$ $= 2\ Fe(CN)_6^{3-} + NH_4^+ + N_2\,(g)$ $+\ 83$

Equilibrium concentration assuming $p_{N_2} = 0,782$ atm, $/Fe(CN)_6^{3-}/ : /Fe(CN)_6^{4-}/ = 100,\ pH = 7,2 : /N_3^-/ = 10^{-53,3}$

III. Disproportioning decomposition:

$3\ (I.b) + 2\ (I.c) + (II.c) : 3\ N_3^- + 4\ H^+ = 4\ N_2\,(g) + NH_4^+$ $+\ 185$

Equilibrium concentration assuming $p_{N_2} = 0,782$ atm, $pH = 7,2,\ /NH_4^+/ = 10^{-3} : /N_3^-/ = 10^{-53}$

(data from Latimer (1952) and Sillen (1964))

266

Figure 1

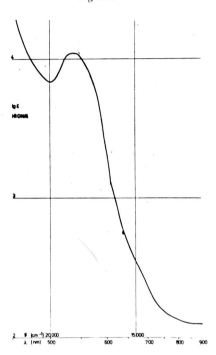

Figure 2

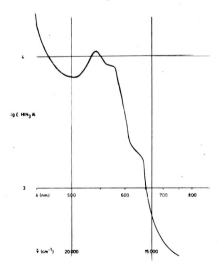

of the Soret band as well as of each of the three overlapping bands in the visible is smaller compared to HiCN, leading to a broader intermediate « saddle » at 505 nm (63,5 ± 0,5 % of absorbance at 542 nm). This could be a disadvantage when using a filter photometer with incandescent lamp, causing a calibration line bent towards the concentration axis. However, the shoulder at 575 nm (77 % of absorbance at 542 nm) could suggest the use of an ad-hoc-hemoglobinometer with mercury discharge lamp and broad-band-width-green-filter, the high intensity allowing to choose a much simpler detector-amplifier-meter combination, because of the fortuitous circumstances of a mercury triplet at 578 nm being roughly of the same magnitude of intensity as the resonance line at 546 nm.

There seems not to be much difference in the speed of hemolysis between both reagents. If not immediatly mixed after the addition of blood, in both reagents the formation of Hb-containing clots indestructible over 6 hours could occasionally be observed. As stated by Vanzetti (1966) no significant difference in the molar absorbance at 540 nm could be ascertained, however, absorbance at 750 nm is about three times higher with HiN_3 compared with HiCN.

In summary it is up to the user to consider the two methods with their advantages and disadvantages and select the suitable one according to his opinion and judgement. The HiN_3 method is equally suitable for the routine use as the HiCN one.

There are the following

Advantages:

— less toxicity,
— no decomposition when frozen,
— obligation to change reagent in time,
— possibility of differential spectrophotometry through subsequent conversion to HiCN,

Disadvantages:

— lower stability at room temperature,
— more rapid deterioration
— inducement to use insufficient temperature adapted reagent,
— higher background in the NIR.

As the sensitivity is exactly equal, there is no particular argument in favour of either on this important point. In the authors opinion future development of hemoglobinometry should strive for a method sufficient sensitive to determine photometrically plasma-, urin-, and spinal fluid Hb and at the same time to be reliable in higher concentration. This would involve the alternative measurement in the Soret band and the visible region, implying the use of an electron acceptor practically colourless with defined redox potential, i.e. a redox buffer. On this subject work is in progress and I hope to report on it in due time.

References

Van Assendelft, O. W., *Rept. XII Int. Congr. Haemat.*, New York, 1968.
Joffe, A. D., Chapter II, « The Inorganic Azides », pp. 72-146 in C.B. Colburn (Ed.), *Developments in Inorganic Nitrogen Chemistry*, Vol. I, Amsterdam, London, New York, Elsevier Publ. Inc., 1966.
Van Kampen, E. J., Zijlstra, W. G., *Clin. Chim. Acta*, 6, 538, 1961.
Keilin, D., *Proc. Roy. Soc.*, 121 B, 165, 1936.
Kiese, M., Kaeske, H., *Biochem. Z.*, 312, 121, 1942.
Von Klein-Wisenberg, A., pp. 150-5 in C.G. de Boroviczény (Ed.), « Standardization in Haematology III », *Bibl. haemat.*, 24, 1966, Basel, S. Karger.
Latimer, W. M., *The Oxidation States of the Elements and their Potentials in Aqueous Solutions*, 2nd. ed. Englewood Cliffs, N. J., Prentice Hall, 1952.
Lemberg, R., Legge, J. W., *Hematin Compounds and Bile Pigments*, New York-London, Interscience Publ. Inc, 1949.
Sillén, L. G., *Stability Constants of Metal Ion Complexes, Sect. I: Inorganic Ligands*, 2nd ed. London, The Chemical Society, Special Publ. 17, 1964.
Smith, L., Wolf, G. G. L., *J. Med. Res.*, 12, 451, 1904.
Vanzetti, G., *J. Lab. & Clin. Med.*, 47, 116, 1966.
Vanzetti, G., *Rept. XII Int. Congr. Haemat.*, New York, 1968.
Winkelmann, M., Mantei, E., von Klein-Wisenberg, A., *Rept. XII Int. Congr. Haemat.* New York, 1968 (this volume p. 50-52).

5.3. A Comparison between the Azide-methemoglobin and Cyanmethemoglobin Methods on 268 Pathological Blood Specimens

C. Franzini, P. L. Morosini and G. Vanzetti, Biochemical Laboratory, Ospedale Maggiore Ca' Granda di Milano, Italy

We have performed parallel determinations of blood hemoglobin by means of the cyanmethemoglobin and azide-methemoglobin methods on 268 pathological blood specimens. The determinations were carried out in duplicate using diluting reagents prepared according to the formulas of Van Kampen and Zijlstra (1961) and of Vanzetti (1966); the absorbance of the dilute blood specimens was read at 542 nm using a Beckman spectrophotometer mod. DBG. A concentrated standard suspension of red blood cells (Hemoglobin reference control of Hyland) was used as reference for both methods.

Concordant results were recorded in 252 blood samples, and discor-

Figure 1 - *Comparative determination of hemoglobin on* 268 *random blood specimens by means of the HiCN and the HiN₃ methods. Cases giving results differing by more than* 3 % (16 *out of* 268) *are marked by crosses.*

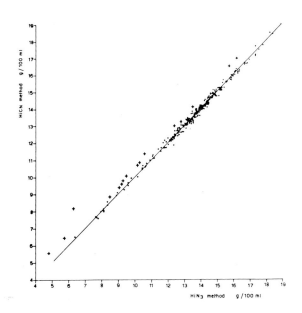

dant results in the other 16: higher values were found in these cases with the cyanmethemoglobin than with the azide-methemoglobin method (see fig. 1 and table 1).

The blood specimens giving discordant results were subjected to careful examination. If the plasma was replaced by a similar amount of isotonic saline, the two methods gave nearly concordant results. This pointed to the plasma proteins as the source of the discrepancies: the presence of turbidity due to flocculation of the less soluble plasma globulins (so called euglobulins) was suspected.

The presence of a slight turbidity in the blood specimens diluted with the cyanide reagent was verified in several instances by visual inspection, observing the dilute blood specimens under strong incident light against a black background, and was confirmed by measuring the absorbance of some of the dilute blood specimens in the near infrared, at 750 nm.

To prevent turbidity we increased the ionic strength of the reagents by dissolving 8 g NaCl per liter. The determination of hemoglobin was repeated in several blood specimens giving either concordant or discordant results: in the former we obtained similar absorbancies and hemoglobin values with the sodium chloride containing reagents, while in the latter the development of turbidity was prevented, and concordant hemoglobin values were obtained with the sodium chloride reagents (table 2): the values were similar to those supplied by the azide reagent, except in specimen N. 14 in which they were lower (-5%).

The results supplied by the sodium chloride containing reagents must be regarded as valid, owing to the absence of turbidity. As shown in the table, turbidity with the cyanide reagent may give rise in some case to large errors, up to 29% of the true hemoglobin value.

The source of the higher turbidity given by the cyanide reagent is not fully understood. The pH of the reagents can play a role: the solubility of the euglobulins is lower at an acidic pH, since this is nearer to their isoelectric point [4]. The pH of our diluting reagents was verified; it was found to be 7,3 for the cyanide reagent and 7,6 for the azide reagent. The lower pH of our cyanide reagent is likely to contribute to its greater flocculating action. The pH of the azide reagent depends on the purity of the THAM preparation used for buffering the solution: this can be critical, since wide differences of pH were found using different commercial preparations of THAM.

Modified reagents with different pH values and similar ionic strength were prepared and tested on blood specimens giving discordant results: a slight turbidity was recorded at an acidic pH with the azide reagent,

Table 1 – Blood specimens giving discordant results with the cyanmethemoglobin and azide – methemoglobin methods. Hemoglobin concentration in g/100 ml

Specimen N.	HiCN Method a	HiN₃ Method b	Difference a − b	Difference % $100 \cdot \frac{a-b}{b}$
1	17.02	16.32	0.70	4.3
2	16.51	15.78	0.73	4.7
3	14.00	13.44	0.56	4.2
4	13.21	12.76	0.45	3.5
5	12.78	12.40	0.38	3.1
6	11.25	10.43	0.82	7.9
7	11.11	10.68	0.43	4.0
8	10.69	10.17	0.52	5.1
9	10.07	9.50	0.57	6.0
10	9.80	9.28	0.52	5.6
11	9.58	9.23	0.35	3.8
12	9.40	9.06	0.34	3.8
13	8.84	8.50	0.34	4.0
14	8.19	6.32	1.87	29.2
15	6.48	5.77	0.71	12.3
16	5.57	4.81	0.76	15.8

Table 2 – Influence of the addition of NaCl to the diluting solutions of the cyanmethemoglobin and azide–methemoglobin methods. Hemoglobin concentration g/100 ml.

Specimen No.	Without NaCl		With NaCl	
	KCN	NaN₃	KCN	NaN₃
1	17.02	16.32	16.32	16.20
3	14.00	13.44	13.57	13.51
5	12.78	12.40	12.58	12.41
6	11.25	10.43	10.15	10.32
7	11.11	10.68	10.64	10.68
8	10.69	10.17	10.26	10.25
9	10.07	9.50	9.36	9.54
14	8.19	6.32	6.05	6.00
16	5.57	4.81	4.81	4.81

but a greater turbidity was found at the same pH with the cyanide reagent. At an alkaline pH (about 7,8) the turbidity disappeared with both reagents.

Our results are in contrast with those reported recently by van Assendelft et al., who performed parallel blood hemoglobin determinations by means of the cyanmethemoglobin and azide-methemoglobin methods on 24 blood specimens, and obtained discordant results in three cases with higher values with the azide reagent: this was attributed to the development of turbidity with this reagent. The divergence between our results and van Assendelft's has to be clarified: we hope that this may be accomplished in the near future through a cooperative effort with Dr. van Assendelft's group.

In summary, according to the preliminary results reported here it appears that the plasma euglobulins can be flocculated in several pathological blood specimens by the cyanide reagent, and possibly in some very rare instance also by the azide reagent: they can thus play a disturbing role in hemoglobinometry, giving rise to turbidity and to significant errors. The turbidity effect is strongly influenced by the pH of the diluting fluid, and can be prevented by using more alkaline reagents, or by adding sodium chloride and thus increasing the ionic strength. This source of error should be carefully evaluated when comparing different methods of hemoglobin determination: a reassessment of the methods in current use for hemoglobinometry will perhaps be required.

References

[1] Van Kampen, E. J. and Zijlstra, W. G., *Clin. Chim. Acta, 6*, 538, 1961.
[2] Van Kampen, E. J. and Zijlstra, W. G., *Bibl. haemat., 18*, 68, 1964
[3] Vanzetti, G., *J. Lab. Clin. Med., 67*, 116, 1966.
[4] Vanzetti, G. and Tarantino, M., *Atti Soc. Lomb. Sc. Medico-Biol., 13*, 366, 373 and 379, 1958.
[5] van Assendelft O.W. et al., this volume, p. 54.

The technical help of Mrs. Adriana Nardeschi and of Miss Carla Campi is gratefully acknowledged.

5.4. *Concentrated Reference Solutions for Hemoglobinometry*
G. Vanzetti and C. Franzini, Biochemical Laboratory, Ospedale Maggiore Ca' Granda di Milano, Italy

To obtain reliable results in carrying out his work load, the analyst should be able to check the analytical procedure as well as the analytical instruments every day. As a minimum, he should perform an overall control by carrying a reference solution of known composition through the entire analytical procedure.

For hemoglobinometry, a concentrated reference standard of known hemoglobin content should be subjected together with the blood samples to the two steps of the procedure: dilution and photometric reading. Analytical errors can arise from either of these two steps: there are errors due to faulty dilution, and photometry errors.

The dilute solutions of cyanmethemoglobin in current use do not provide an adequate control. They are suitable for calibrating and checking photometers, but not for compensating for dilution errors depending on micropipettes or dilutors. These solutions are also costly, since each vial can be used as a rule only once. Consequently, the majority of the analysts check with the reference solutions now and again only, and this can be a source of error.

Another possibility is to use the samples of human blood that a few factories have recently put on the market. These samples, which were designed for checking hemoglobinometry as well as automatic multiple blood analyses, must be subjected to thorough agitation before use: otherwise the results may be seriously distorted. Furthermore, it is not easy, at least as yet, to evaluate their stability.

We have tried another approach. We have succeeded in preparing concentrated solutions of cyanmethemoglobin and of azide-methemoglobin, and we have found that they exhibit a good stability and permit to control simultaneously the dilution of the blood specimens as well as the photometer readings. Each vial or test tube can be used many times, since each control requires only 20 microliters solution; the cost of the daily control is therefore negligible.

Franzini has prepared a concentrated standard solution of azide-methemoglobin by dialysis of the red blood cells; his results were reported at the Round Table discussion on the Standardization of Hematological Methods held in Florence last year [1].

We have prepared concentrated reference solutions of azide-methemoglobin and cyanmethemoglobin more simply, by diluting washed red blood cells with the solutions A and B of table 1, respectively:

1) One volume of washed centrifugated erythrocytes is diluted with 0,6 volume of mixture A: thanks to the hemolytic action of Sterox SE a concentrated solution containing 18-19 g of azide-methemoglobin per 100 ml is obtained.

2) After diluting 1 to 251 with water, the exact hemoglobin concentration of this solution is determined by reading the absorbance in a Beckman DU spectrophotometer at 542 nm.

274

Table 1 – Composition of diluent solutions containing sterox SE

A) Conc. Solution of na Azide–K Ferricyanide:

THAM	1.0 g
Potassium Ferricyanide	1.5 g
Monohydrated Citric Acid	0.5 g
Sodium Azide	0.5 g
Sterox SE	2.0 ml

Make up to 100 ml

B) Conc. Solution of K Cyanide–K Ferricyanide:

Monobasic Potassium Phosphate	1.4 g
Potassium Ferrycyanide	1.5 g
Potassium Cyanide	0.5 g
Sterox SE	2.0 ml

Make up to 100 ml

---

3) On the basis of this reading the starting solution is diluted so as to obtain a concentration of exactly 16 g of hemoglobin per 100 ml, that is the concentration found in the blood of normal subjects.

The 16 g/100 ml azide-methemoglobin solution thus prepared can be stored in small plastic test tubes in the refrigerator [2], and used as reference for the azide-methemoglobin method [3]. A concentrated solution of cyanmethemoglobin can be prepared by a similar procedure by means of reagent B, and used as reference for the cyanmethemoglobin method [4, 5].

Since March 1967 we have been using the concentrated reference solution of azide-methemoglobin as daily control for hemoglobinometry. The results obtained have been reasonably good, although the stability was not entirely satisfactory (see fig. 1). If the test tubes containing the concentrated reference solution are kept at room temperature they often become contaminated; to improve the stability it was imperative to prepare sterile solutions.

We tried using the filtering membranes of Sartorius Membranfilter for this purpose, but we found that the filtration was hindered very soon, due to clogging of the pores by the stromata of the erythrocytes. We tried to remove the stromata by centrifugation, but with little success, probably because their specific weight is similar to that of the concentrated hemoglobin solution in which they are suspended. We tried hemolysis by freezing and thawing, but the results were not satisfactory. Finally we tried organic solvents like toluol and carbon tetrachloride as

Figure 1 - *Stability test of a non-sterilized concentrated reference solution of azide-methemoglobin: optical density at 542 nm.*

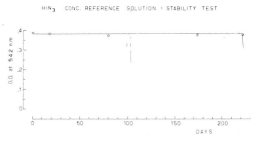

Figure 2 - *O.D. spectra of a 4 months old sterile solution of azide-methemoglobin (A) and of a freshly drawn blood specimen diluted with the azide-ferricyanide reagent (B). The reference solution was stored in an ampoule kept in the refrigerator.*

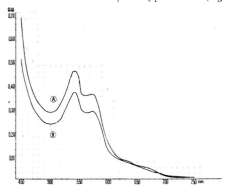

Figure 3 - *O.D. spectra of a 4 months old sterile reference solution of cyanmethemoglobin (A) and of a freshly drawn blood specimen diluted with the cyanide-ferricyanide reagent (B). The reference solution was kept at room temperature. The Hb concentrations are lower than those of the solutions of fig. 2.*

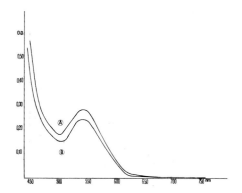

hemolytic agents, using solutions A and B of table 1 without Sterox SE [2].

After hemolysis with carbon tetrachloride it becomes possible to remove the stromata of the erythrocytes by centrifugation, probably because carbon tetrachloride imbibes the stromata thereby increasing their specific weight. After removal of the stromata membrane filtration becomes possible, and the resulting sterile concentrated solutions can be distributed in sterile vials.

Controls were performed by diluting the sterile concentrated solutions 1 to 251, reading the extinction at 542 nm and checking the absorption spectrum of several control specimens; fig. 2 and 3 illustrate the spectra of 4 months old sterile reference solutions and of freshly diluted blood specimens analyzed either by means of the azide-methemoglobin or by means of the cyanmethemoglobin method. The sterile concentrated solutions of cyanmethemoglobin and azide-methemoglobin have shown good stability not only when stored in the refrigerator, but also at room temperature.

These results are encouraging, but obviously extensive controls are required in order to establish the long term stability of these solutions.

And now a few words on the daily control of hemoglobinometry. Our control system comprises the following determinations:

1) Duplicate determination of the absorbance given by a concentrated reference solution of azide-methemoglobin (or cyanmethemoglobin, according to the method adopted). This solution is diluted along with the blood specimens using the same micropipettes (or dilutors). The daily average of the absorbance values of the standards is used for calculating the hemoglobin concentration of the unknown blood specimens. The absorbance values obtained in subsequent days are plotted on a control chart; if there is a trend in these values, the hemoglobin concentration of the reference solution must be rechecked with a high resolution spectrophotometer.

2) Duplicate determination of the hemoglobin concentration of a randomly selected blood specimen (« within-run » control).

3) Determination of the hemoglobin concentration of a randomly selected blood specimen (« carry-over » specimen) already analysed the day before and stored in a refrigerator (« between-run » control).

The data obtained are plotted every day on difference control charts. At the end of each month the control chart data are used for statistical analysis and for calculating the « within-run » variability (within-run controls) and the « between-run » variability (between-run controls).

In table 2 we report the confidence limits of hemoglobin determina-

Table 2 – Confidence Limits of Hemoglobin determination expressed as per cent

Months	Confidence Limits %	Months	Confidence Limits %
November/67	1.82	May	2.06
December	1.77	June	2.86
January/68	1.50	Jule	2.37
February	1.09	August	2.65
March	2.72	September	2.74
April	2.40	October	2.49

tion during the period November '67-October '68: the confidence limits are calculated percentagewise on the basis of the results supplied by the carry-over specimens.

Our control system can be applied not only to hemoglobinometry, but also to most routine biochemical analyses; a detailed description will be given elsewhere.

In conclusion further investigations are required to assess the long term stability of the concentrated reference solutions of azide-methemoglobin and cyanmethemoglobin, and will possibly lead to improved methods of preparation, but our results suggest that these concentrated solutions can contribute already now to a better control of the blood hemoglobin determinations.

References

[1] Franzini, C., *Il Lab. nella Diagn. Med.*, 1968.
[2] Vanzetti, G. and Franzini, C., *Clin. Chim. Acta, 24*, 417, 1969.
[3] Vanzetti, G., *J. Lab. Clin. Med., 67*, 116, 1966.
[4] Van Kampen, E. J. and Zijlstra, W. G., *Clin. Chim. Acta, 6*, 538, 1961.
[5] Van Kampen, E. J. and Zijlstra, W. G., *Bibl. haemat., 18*, 68, 1964.

5.5. The Estimation of the Maximum Red Cell Sedimentation Rate from a Single Reading at the 90th Minute

I. Brambilla and L. Cantoni, Ospedale Maggiore Ca' Granda di Milano, Italy

If the height of the plasma column during the red cell sedimentation (RCS) is recorded against time a triphasic curve with the shape of an italic S is obtained. The first and the third phases of the curve are nearly exponential, while the second phase, corresponding to the maximum sedimentation rate is linear (Fig. 1). This phenomenon, found

278

by Curtler in 1932 [1] was confirmed by Wintrobe [2, 3], Frimberger [4], Ordway [5] and Olmsted [6].

By this procedure the analyst can measure the maximum sedimentation rate in mm/h, instead of relying on empirical measurements such as the height of the plasma column read at the 60th minute from the start of the sedimentation, or as Katz's quotient [7]. The procedure is nevertheless too complex for routine use.

In order to obtain the maximum RCS rate in mm/h without computing it by means of the time-consuming procedure of Curtler, we have subjected to statistical analysis the three components of the RCS curve.

Method

4 ml of blood taken from an arm vein were diluted with 1 ml of 3.8% solution of sodium citrate, and placed in Westergren's tube [8]. The time required for a 1 mm increase of the plasma column along the tube was recorded, until the sedimentation rate decreased to 0.25 mm/h.

Cases without a clear separation between the plasma and the red cells, in which a correct reading of the height of the plasma column was difficult, were discarded. By means of this technique we carried out 76 experiments on 50 male subjects, either healthy or sick, in order to obtain and analyze their RCS curves.

Results and discussion

Fig. 1 shows the RCS curve of subject N. 26: the RCS rate increases gradually from the start to the 140th min (first phase): then a steady state with the maximum sedimentation rate of 12 mm/h is reached (second phase), followed at the 240th min by a third phase in which the RCS rate decreases gradually with time (third phase).

Fig. 2 shows another curve concerning subject N. 1: the RCS rate increases from the start to the 20th min (first phase); then a steady state with a constant rate of 120 mm/h is reached (second phase), followed after 50 mins by a third phase in which the rate gradually decreases with time.

The second phase, corresponding to the maximum sedimentation rate is the most important of the RCS curve; we have therefore studied the relation between the maximum RCS rate in mm/h and the height of the plasma column at 30, 60, 70, 75, 90, 120 and 180 mins after the start of the sedimentation.

Figure 1

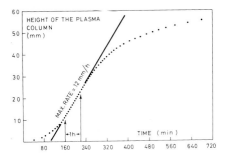

Figure 2

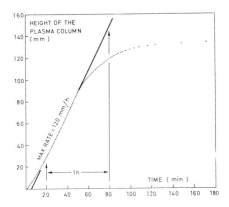

Figure 3

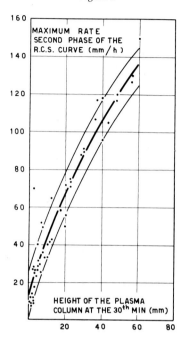

Figure 4

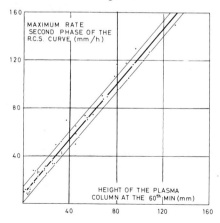

281

Figure 5

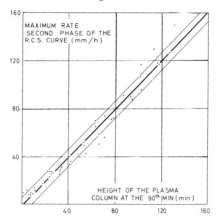

Figure 6

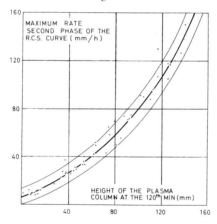

Figure 7

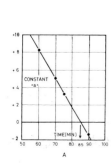

A

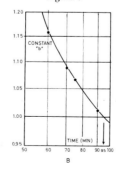

B

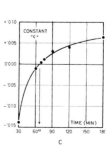

C

Table I

Time (t) after the start of the Red Cells Sedimentation (RCS) (min)	Regression equations $y = a + bx$ or $y = a + bx + cx^2$	Maximum rate of the RCS (second phase) against the height of the plasma column at the «t» times	t	P
30 mins	Rectilinear	$y = 18,383 + 2,185\ x \pm 11,485$	$-2,329$	$>0,02$
	Curvilinear*	$y = 13,992 + 2,918\ x - 0,014\ x^2 \pm 10,989$	$8,907$	$<0,001$
60 mins	Rectilinear*	$y = 8,218 + 1,157\ x \pm 6,474$	$13,982$	$<0,001$
	Curvilinear	$y = 5,902 + 1,308\ x - 0,001\ x^2 \pm 6,354$	$-1,683$	$>0,05$
70 mins	Rectilinear*	$y = 5,066 + 1,085\ x \pm 6,018$	$11,563$	$<0,001$
	Curvilinear	$y = 6,341 + 1,009\ x + 0,0006\ x^2 \pm 6,029$	$0,903$	$>0,3$
75 mins	Rectilinear*	$y = 3,180 + 1,062\ x \pm 6,109$	$10,484$	$<0,001$
	Curvilinear	$y = 6,043 + 0,901\ x + 0,001\ x^2 \pm 5,939$	$1,944$	$>0,05$
90 mins	Rectilinear*	$y = -1,533 + 1,009\ x \pm 7,243$	$7,128$	$<0,001$
	Curvilinear*	$y = 6,188 + 0,628\ x + 0,003\ x^2 \pm 6,128$	$4,477$	$<0,001$
120 mins	Rectilinear	$y = -8,827 + 0,960\ x \pm 9,339$	$3,443$	$>0,05$
	Curvilinear*	$y = 6,682 + 0,318\ x + 0,004\ x^2 \pm 7,228$	$7,159$	$<0,001$
180 mins	Rectilinear	$y = 19,047 + 0,958\ x \pm 12,714$	$-0,247$	$>0,8$
	Curvilinear*	$y = 9,305 + 0,032\ x + 0,006\ x^2 \pm 8,453$	$7,712$	$<0,001$

* Highly significant

In figs. 3 to 6 we have plotted the maximum RCS rate of each of our 50 subjects against the height of the plasma column (abscissa) at different times.

From the 60th to the 90th min a linear relation is obtained (Figs. 4 and 5): before 60 mins a curve with downward concavity (Fig. 3), while after more than 90 mins a curve with upward concavity is obtained (Fig. 6).

We calculated the regression equations of all these functions with the least squares method, assuming that the function was either $y = a + bx$ or $y = a + bx + cx^2$: the data found for the constants a, b and c are given in Table 1 and in Fig. 7.

The constant « a » has a zero value when the sedimentation is read after 85 mins. The constant « b » has a value of 1 when the sedimentation is read after 95 mins. The constant « c » has a zero value when the sedimentation is read after 68 mins, but its value is negligible between 50 and 90 min.

At the 90th min « a » and « c » are sufficiently small to be neglected (-1.533 and $+.003$ respectively) and « b » is very near the unity (1.009): therefore the function can then be assumed to be $y = x$.

The height in mm of the plasma column at the 90th minute is therefore nearly equal to the maximum sedimentation rate in mm/h.

In conclusion the maximum rate of the RCS in mm/h can be obtained with good approximation by means of a single reading of the height of the plasma column at the 90th min.

References

[1] Curtler, J. W., « The Practical Application of the Blood Sedimentation Test in General Medicine », *Am. J. Med. Sc.*, *183*, 643, 1932.
[2] Wintrobe, M. M. and Landsberg, J. W., « A Standardized Technique for the Blood Sedimentation Test », *Am. J. Med. Sc.*, *189*, 102, 1935.
[3] Wintrobe, M. M., « The Erythrocyte Sedimentation Test », *Internat. Clin. 46th serv.* 2, 34, 1936.
[4] Frimberger, F., « Untersuchungen über die reversible Ballung und Sedimentierung der roten Blutkörperchen », *Erg. Inn. Med. Kinderh.*, *61*, 680, 1942.
[5] Ordway, N. K. and Singer, R. B., « A Simplified Sedimentation Rate Technique with Combined Chart and Correction Nomogram », *J. Lab. Clin. Med.*, *33*, 511, 1948.
[6] Olmsted, F. and Hainline, A., « Automatic Photographic Recording of Sedimentation Rates », *Am. J. Clin. Path.*, *24*, 1030, 1954.
[7] Katz, G. und Leffkowitz, M., « Die Blutkörperchensenkung », *Erg. Inn. Med. Kinderh.*, *33*, 266, 1928.
[8] Westergren, A., « Die Senkungsreaktion », *Erg. Inn. Med. Kinderh.*, *26*, 577, 1924.

Acknowledgments

We are indebted to Dr. R. Margaria and to Dr. G. Vanzetti for suggestions and criticism during this work. We are also indebted to Dr. R. Saracci who performed the statistical calculation with the computer.

Chairmen: G. Astaldi, J. Jürgens, V. Zambotti

6.1. *The Kinetics of Iron*
S. Ventura, Department of General Clinical Medicine and Therapeutics, University of Perugia, Italy

The study of iron metabolism emerged from its empirical stage only in 1937, when Heilmeyer and Plötner initiated quantitative studies of the iron contained in blood serum. A further and valid contribution toward an understanding of iron kinetics in the human body came in 1947, when Laurell discovered transferrin, i.e. the beta$_1$-globulin that operates the transport of serum iron. However, it was not until 1951 that Huff and his associates identified all the stages and components of iron kinetics with the help of Fe^{59}, a radioactive iron isotope. In 1961 Pollycove and Mortimer elaborated their mathematical model of iron kinetics.

As the phrase clearly indicates, by « iron kinetics investigations » we mean studies affording analytical evaluation of all movements of iron in the body. These are now well known in their complexities, and may be outlined essentially as follows.

Iron moves in the human body under the control of the transferrin bond in the blood serum. Along this pathway, the iron originating from intestinal absorption, from storage, or from hemocatheretic tissues reaches the erythroblastic tissues or storage tissues. In physiological conditions, the rate of iron transport in the plasma is regulated by the activity of the erythropoietic bone marrow, i.e. by the rate of hemoglobin synthesis.

The iron that is liberated daily by catabolism of hemoglobin goes back in its entirety to the plasmatic pool, and hence is made available for further synthesis of hemoglobin.

All these movements can be monitored by administering radioactive iron intravenously: the tracer is subject to the same displacements as the iron already existing in the plasma, and thus reveals its itinerary through suitable detection of radioactivity.

Any attempt at standardization of the methods designed for monitoring the movements of iron must take into account two distinct groups of problems.

The first group of problems has to do with the technicalities of radioactive iron administration and of detection of radioactivity in the body. The amount of Fe^{59} being administered must be very small, so as not to modify the amount of circulating iron significantly; its radioactivity, on the other hand, must be enough to warrant detection by suitable instruments. Currently available preparation are quite satisfactory on both counts, since their specific activity is 2 μc per μg of iron.

Furthermore, the radioactive iron can follow the same metabolic path as the iron naturally present in the plasma only if it is likewise bound with transferrin. For many years the tracer dose of iron was linked to transferrin in vitro through utilization of fraction IV_7 of Cohn. But since transferrin can undergo denaturation during preparation, and therefore behave differently from natural transferrin in the body, it was proposed to use a 0.1 % solution of sodium citrate, which accelerates the linking of radioactive iron ions to transferrin. Today, however, the preferred procedure consists of incubating the radioactive iron in 10 ml of serum, homologous serum being acceptable for the purpose. When the iron-transferrin bond is obtained, the 10 ml dose is injected intravenously: this amount replaces the amounts collected at various times for determinations of radioactivity.

In effect, the problem of samples has a considerable importance. The study of iron kinetics is based on repeat determinations of radioactivity in the plasma and erythrocytes; this calls for several collections of blood over the first hours and days following administration of the iron tracer—and of course if too much blood is taken out of the subject, this alters both the total amount of radioactivity and the fractions of radioactivity in the circulating blood. In the past, when the well counter was used, this sort of thing could not be avoided. But now we have liquid phase scintillation counters with a sensitivity for iron from 10 to 15 times greater than that of the gamma ray well counter; this makes it possible to utilize remarkably small blood samples (0.1-0.4 ml).

Concerning measurements of surface radioactivity, obviously the application of the probe to the skin over the liver, spleen, and so on is an empiric method of limited usefulness. More accurate results can probably be obtained with new technics utilizing the positron scintillation chamber and Fe^{52}, which has a half-life of 8.4 hours and emits positrons. As of today, however, we can safely say that standardization of the technicalities of iron kinetics studies must rest on (a) the introduction of 5 µc of Fe^{59} previously bound to the transferrin contained in 10 ml of homologous plasma, (b) the collection of small blood samples (less than 1 ml), and (c) evaluation of blood radioactivity with a liquid-phase scintillation counter.

The second group of problems concerns standardization of methods and technics by which the movements of iron in the body are analyzed. The kinetics of iron in the human body can be broken down into three separate phases, each with a measure of autonomy and with characteristics of its own.

The first phase is represented by the movements of iron in the plasma, which regulate the whole process of iron metabolism. The equilibrium of iron in the blood plasma is highly dynamic, as can be seen by plotting the gradual reduction of plasma radioactivity on semilog paper: the decrement curve is represented by a segment with a well-defined exponential velocity. Its half-time, i.e. the time in which plasma radioactivity goes down to one-half its original value, expresses the slope of this curve and affords evaluation of plasma turnover by indicating the amount of iron that leaves the plasma in a certain period of time. From this value, the titer of iron per 100 ml of plasma and the total volume of plasma being known, one can calculate the amount of iron that leaves the plasma and goes back to it in 24 hours; this value may also be expressed relative to one kilo of body weight. This is the kind of information we obtain from analysis of the behavior of iron in the plasma during the first several hours after administration of the tracer. On the other hand, if we continue to monitor these phenomena over the next several days, we find that the radioactivity curve does not present a uniform slope but undergoes certain changes of the exponential velocity constant, with the appearance of a second and sometimes a third segment, expressing the return of certain fractions of iron to the plasma.

The second phase that can be subjected to analytical evaluation is the passage of iron into the tissues. Suitable scintillation probes applied to utilization sites (e.g. the sacrum) and to storage organs such as the liver and spleen show that as the tracer dose disappears from the plasma, erythroblastic tissues gradually accumulate more and more radioactivity until they account for the whole administered dose; the fraction that goes directly to storage tissues is negligible. The erythroblastic phase is obviously the most important of all: the capacity of erythroblasts for synthetizing hemoglobin, and their absolute need for iron, make these cells the only haven for the iron-transferrin molecule. The molecular complex becomes affixed to the cell membrane, liberates the iron, and then goes back to the blood stream to pick up more iron, while the iron delivered into the cytoplasm of erythroblasts reaches the cristae of the mitochondria, there to become bound to protoporphyrin in the form of heme. This stage of the process can be monitored by reading radioactivity over the sacrum. On the other hand, quantitative data can be obtained by determining the amount of iron used up daily in the synthesis of hemoglobin: this is done according to the mathematical model proposed by Pollycove, which gives the amount of iron that reaches the bone marrow daily, and the amount of hemoglobin that goes into erythrocytes daily. An index of these values is the hemoglobinization time of the erythron, i.e. the time lapse from iron uptake in the erythroblastic tissue to detection of radioactive hemoglobin in the peripheral blood. Concerning the passage of iron into storage tissues, this can be evaluated both by direct measurements of surface radioactivity and by calculation. At this point, however, I must mention a problem of considerable practical import. Is the Pollycove model correct and corresponding to reality as regards the magnitude of exchanges between the plasma and storage tissues? This American investigator says that the daily movements of plasmatic iron amount to as much as 35 mg, of which 32 mg leave the plasma and reach the erythropoietic bone marrow, where about 21 mg is utilized in the synthesis of hemoglobin; the fraction that reaches the liver and hence goes back to the plasma is less than 1 mg, i.e. negligible. Other authors, however, believe that as much as 10 mg of iron a day goes into storage (Finch et al.). This contrast of opinions cannot be solved momentarily, and certainly represents the first problem one meets on the way to standardization of iron kinetics methods.

The third (and last) phase is the analytical evaluation of the turnover of hemoglobin iron. If we monitor circulating erythrocytes after administering a radioactive iron tracer, we find that as radioactivity gradually decreases in the bone marrow, it increases in the erythrocytes, indicating the passage of radioactive hemoglobin into the peripheral blood. This curve reaches a peak and becomes stabilized at about 14 days of administration of the tracer, the value representing the percentage of administered iron that has been incorporated in the erythrocytes. This evaluation is not difficult to carry out and contributes information of practical value in the matter if iron kinetics. Likewise, a simple calculation will disclose the more complex index of the amount of erythrocyte iron that is renewed daily.

References

[1] Finch, C. A., Hosain, F., Morgan, E. H., Marsaglia, G., Giblett, E., Hillman, R. S., *Series Haematologica*, Copenhagen-Munksgaard, 6, 30, 1965.

[2] Garby, L., Schneider, W., Sundquist, O., Vuille, J. C., *Acta Physiologica Scandinavica*, 59 suppl., 216, 1963.

[3] Heilmeyer, L., Plötner, K., *Das Serumeisen und die Eisenmangelkrankheit*, Fischer, Jena, 1937.

[4] Huff, R. L., Elmlinger, P. J., Garcia, J. F., Oda, J. M., Cockerell, M. C., Lawrence, J. H., *J. Clin. Invest.*, 30, 1512, 1951.

[5] Larizza, P., Ventura, S., *Atti Accad. Med. Lomb.*, 20, 1953, 1965.

[6] Laurell, C. B., *Acta physiol. Scandinav.*, 14 suppl., 46, 1947.

[7] Pollycove, M., Mortimer, R., *J. Clin. Invest.*, 40, 753, 1961.

6.2. The Desferrioxamine and Differential DTPA-^{59}Fe Tests

E. Fiaschi, L. A. Scuro, G. Dobrilla, O. Bosello, G. Cartei, V. Lo Cascio, Department of Special Medical Pathology, and Clinical Methodology, University of Padua, Italy

Desferrioxamine has been used for several years in the diagnosis and treatment of hypersiderosis [1-12]. Desferrioxamine is a chelating agent with a high affinity for iron (stability constant 10^{31}); the substance is obtained from cultures of *Streptomyces pilosus*.

The test of induced sideruria with desferrioxamine consists of administering a suitable parenteral dose of the substance and then assaying the iron excreted with the urine. The test provides a rough estimate of iron deposits in the body. Its principal use is in the diagnosis of hypersiderosis; however, the same test is also useful in hyposiderosis, as it provides evidence of insufficient iron storage.

In December 1965 the Italian Committee for the Standardization of Methods in Hematology organized a panel discussion in Milan, in which the problem of standardizing the desferrioxamine test was discussed. On that occasion a scheme proposed by Scuro, summarized in Table I, was accepted.

The dose that we find most suitable for an adult is 1 gram given by intramuscular injection in the morning, as recommended by the majority of authors [10-14; 19, 20, 23, 31], since it has been observed that larger amounts of the substance do not lead to a significantly greater sideru-

Table I — Desferrioxamine Test

Dose	1 g
Administration	intramuscular
Urine collection	24 hours
Assay of urinary iron	method with 2,2 –dipyridyl–dithionite
Evaluation of results	sideruria < 2 mg/day: normosiderosis
	2-3 mg/day: baseline hypersiderosis
	> 3 mg/day: overt hypersiderosis

Table II — Dosage of desferrioxamine in various age groups

Age of Subjects	Desferrioxamine Dosage
Less than 3 years	250 mg
3 to 6 years	500 mg
6 to 12 years	750 mg
12 years and above	1 g

Table III — Optimal duration of desferrioxamine test according to several authors

Urine Collection	Authors
6 hours	Wöhler (3); Cimino (26); Rosen and Tullis (18)
12 hours	Masera and Leggio (31) (in pediatrics)
24 hours	Walsh et al. (10); Erlandson et al. (2); Dagg (7); Vannotti (41); Goldberg (9); Scuro and Dobrilla (15)
48 hours	Unseld (13)

ria. For children, Masera and Leggio [31] have recommended proportionally smaller doses of desferrioxamine (Table II).

Concerning the duration of the test, we feel that 24 hours is ideal, although some men have collected the urine for 6 to 12 hours [3, 5, 18, 25, 26, 28, 31] and some for 48 hours [9] after the administration of desferrioxamine (Table III).

Our own investigations confirm that most of the iron chelated by desferrioxamine is excreted during the first six hours; on the other hand, there are cases in which the excretion of iron is delayed, so that a 6-hour test may be negative, whereas the 24-hour test is positive (Fig. 1). For this reason we agree with numerous other authors [1, 10, 12, 14, 16, 20, 21, 23, 24, 26, 27, 29, 32] that the 24-hour test should be preferred, while longer test periods are unrewarding.

Coming now to the choice of methods for the assay of iron in the urine, if the test is to be adopted on a large scale, we must have a method that is reliable but also sufficiently expeditions and simple in actual performance. Thus we have abandoned the laborious method of humid incineration and we recommend the method utilizing dithionite-dipyridyl. Whereas the former method is certainly more accurate, the latter is still accurate enough for the results to be meaningful. The dithionite-dipyridyl method was advantageously modified by Dobrilla [33] so as to avoid the dismutation of dithionite to colloidal sulfur and the resulting opalescence interfering with spectrophotometry. The modification consists of using a buffer made of an equimolecular monobasic and dibasic sodium phosphate (10^{-1} M). In theory one might object that bivalent iron tends to make poorly soluble compounds with acid phosphates, whereas trivalent iron easily originates complex salts. In our case, however, both the trivalent and the bivalent iron in the test material are bound to desferrioxamine or to dipyridyl, and therefore the problem does not arise.

Our experience with this method has been highly satisfactory. The relatively low sensitivity may constitute a problem in cases with a very low sideruria (in the order of a few $\mu g \% ml$); but at such levels, differences between methods lose all practical significance.

Concerning the evaluation of results, we believe that the test should be pronounced positive when the iron mobilized by the chelating agent is more than 3 mg in 24 hours. Amounts between 2 and 3 mg should be regarded as borderline, possibly indicating initial hypersiderosis.

At this point we wish to give a brief report of our 478 observations (Table IV), the first 400 of which are shown graphically in Fig. 2. Our clinical material included 150 normal control subjects, 25 patients with

Table IV — Average values of siderinuria after DFOX in normal control subjects; comparison with averages observed in patient groups

Sideruria After Desferrioxamine

Group	No. observ.	Average ±	S.D.	Min. μg/24h	Max.	P
I Normal controls	150	956.45	37.09	100	2,000	—
II Iron-deficiency anemia	25	425.92	48.63	100	800	< 0.01
III Primitive siderochromatosis	27	17,301.92	2,286.94	1,593	48,600	< 0.001
IV Siderochromatosis sec.to Liver disease	40	6,504,32	715.45	3,000	21,000	< 0.01
V Cirrhosis of the liver	60	1,642.41	107.67	100	3,093	< 0.01
VI Alcoholism without liver disease	26	1,536.46	1,200.20	230	4,870	< 0.01
VII Acute viral hepatitis	93	2,668.33	164.52	650	7,575	< 0.01
VIII Pulmonary silicosis	18	1,824.61	267.61	240	4,060	< 0.01
IX Chronic renal insufficiency	11	515.70	75.34	100	860	< 0.01
X Mitral stenosis	15	907.80	92.94	156	1,420	< 0.90
XI Hemolytic anemia	13	6,858.84	5,766.01	1,610	17,799	< 0.01
Total	478					

Figure 1 - *Subjects affected with primitive (cases No. 6 and 22) and secondary hepato-pathic (case No. 14) hemochromatosis giving negative risulte after 6 hours DFOX test, but positive after 24 hours.*

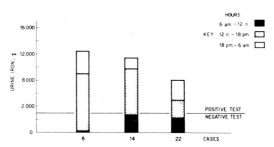

Figure 2 - *Desferrioxamine test in various pathological conditions (data up to 1967)* I - Normal control subjects (130 cases); II - Iron-deficiency anemia (22 cases); III - Primitive siderochromatosis (20 cases); IV - Siderochromatosis secondary to liver disease (25 cases); V - Cirrhosis of the liver (40 cases); - VI - Chronic alcoholism without liver disease (25 cases); VII - Acute viral hepatitis (84 cases); VIII - Pulmonary silicosis (18 cases); IX - Chronic renal insufficiency (11 cases); X - Mitral stenosis (15 cases); XI - Hemolytic anemia (11 cases).

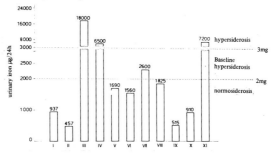

Figure 3 - *Distribution areas of per cent variations of iron plasma levels after administration of desferrioxamine in the group of patients with hypersideremia.*

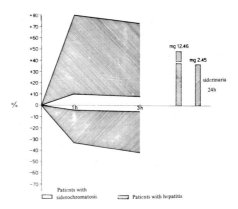

iron-deficiency anemia, 27 with primitive siderochromatosis, 40 with siderochromatosis secondary to liver disease, 60 with chronic cirrhogenous hepatitis, 26 chronic alcoholists without definite evidence of liver disease, 93 with acute hepatitis of probable viral origin, 18 with pulmonary silicosis, 11 with chronic renal disease and insufficiency, 15 with mitral valve pathology, and 13 with hemolytic anemia. The differences between the various groups were highly significant in statistical terms (Table IV).

From our results, as well as from available data in the literature, it is apparent that the desferrioxamine test represents a very useful tool for the recognition of hypersiderosis. The main advantages of the method are its applicability to ambulant patients, remarkable ease in performance, good reproducibility of results, low cost, and freedom from adverse side actions.

On the other hand we must admit that the test has certain limitations: one may get false negative results (eg in chronic renal insufficiency) and false positive results (in acute hepatitis). We found that in patients with renal insufficiency the sideruria after administration of the chelating agent was significantly less than in normal controls, and very close to the values observed in patients with iron-deficiency anemia. As other authors have pointed out, this probably reflects a low clearance of the iron-desferrioxamine complex, whereby patients with hypersiderosis and associated renal insufficiency may give false negative results with this test. The same may happen if the iron mobilized by the chelating agent is immediately utilized for the synthesis of hemoglobin, as might be the case in situations of abnormally active hematopoiesis.

A high sideruria following administration of desferrioxamine is often observed in cases of acute hepatitis of probable viral origin. This does not indicate abnormally large iron deposits, which are easily ruled out by the patient's history and by the findings of liver biopsy. The high sideruria observed in such cases indicates the presence in the blood stream of ferritin iron originating from the lysis of liver cells, and perhaps of hemoglobin degradation products.

We find it interesting to point out that acute viral hepatitis and hypersiderosis, both conditions being associated with hypersideremia and hypersiderinuria, can be told apart by looking at the behavior of iron plasma levels in the hours immediately after administration of desferrioxamine (Fig. 3, 4). Whereas in the presence of increased iron deposits there is an evident rise of plasmatic iron, in acute viral hepatitis the iron plasma level drops appreciably (Table V) [34, 35].

Table V – Statistical significance of variations of iron plasma levels at 1 hour and 3 hours of desferrioxamine administration (1 g I.M.)

	Basal values (Average ± S.D.)	% Variation at 1 h (Average ± S.D.)	% Variation at 3 h (Average ± S.D.)
Normal subjects	133.77 ± 13.25	– 3.86 ± 1.45	– 6.08 ± 2.10
Siderochromatosis	275.13 ± 14.22 P < 0.001	+ 18.78 ± 4.66 P < 0.001	+ 16.16 ± 4.23 P < 0.001
Hepatitis	197.62 ± 10.8 P < 0.005 > 0.001	– 15.98 ± 1.06 P < 0.001	– 17.74 ± 1.85 P < 0.005 > 0.001

Figure 4 - *Average per cent variations of iron plasma levels after administration of DFOX (1 g I.M.).*

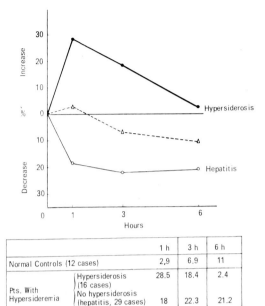

	1 h	3 h	6 h
Normal Controls (12 cases)	2,9	6.9	11
Pts. With Hypersideremia — Hypersiderosis (16 cases)	28.5	18.4	2.4
Pts. With Hypersideremia — No hypersiderosis (hepatitis, 29 cases)	18	22.3	21.2

Figure 5 - *Schematic representation of FIELDING's differential test* (from Williams, 42).

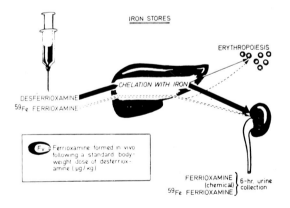

296

Thus, with these few limitations in mind, we can accept the desferrioxamine test as a fully legitimate diagnostic tool for states of hypersiderosis. Of course, if we want more precise information concerning the total amount of iron captured by the chelating agent in the tissues, and concerning the mode of chelation, we may have recourse to one of the following two tests:

a) the differential test of Fielding [36], in which the patient receives intravenous desferrioxamine and ^{59}Fe-ferrioxamine simultaneously (Fig. 5 and Table VI);

Table VI – Differential ferrioxamine test

^{59}Ferrioxamine (excreted) (Fex)	:	^{59}Ferrioxamine (injected) (F)	=	Ferrioxamine excreted (Fd)	:	Ferrioxamine formed after injection of DFOX (Fv)

$$Fv = \frac{Fd \cdot F}{Fex}$$

b) the diethylenetriaminopentaacetic acid (DTPA) differential test, in which the patient receives intravenous DTPA instead of desferrioxamine, and ^{59}Fe-DTPA instead of ^{59}Fe-ferrioxamine [37, 41].

The purpose of these two tests is to inject simultaneously a free chelating agent and a chelating agent saturated with ^{59}Fe, in order to explore the dynamics of iron mobilization from the tissues and obtain more reliable information on the ratio of iron actually captured by the chelating agent to iron excreted with the urine. It appears that the test utilizing DTPA offers certain definite advantages over the Fielding test. DTPA has the property of diffusing rapidly into the extracellular space, so that it is practically eliminated with the urine within six hours of administration, along with the chelated iron. Further, this chelating agent is not metabolized in the body and not eliminated into the intestinal lumen appreciably [38].

The simultaneous administration of DTPA and ^{59}Fe-DTPA makes it possible to assess the total amount of iron chelated in vivo through measurements of urinary radioactivity. The advantages over the Fielding test are as follows:

a) the range of normal values is much narrower [37, 38, 40] (Fig. 6, 7);
b) one does not get the false positive results observed with the Fielding

Figure 6 - *Desferrioxamine-chelatable iron in liver disease.*

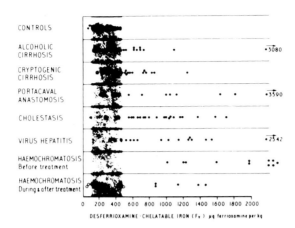

Figure 7 - *DTPA-chelatable iron in liver disease.*

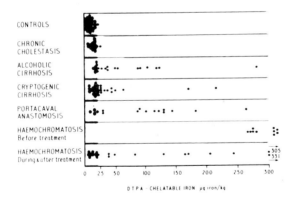

298

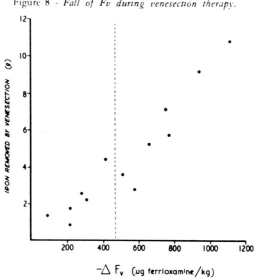

Figure 8 - *Fall of Fv during venesection therapy.*

$-\triangle\ F_v$ (µg ferrioxamine/kg)

Figure 9 - *Fall in DTPA-chelatable iron during venesection therapy.*

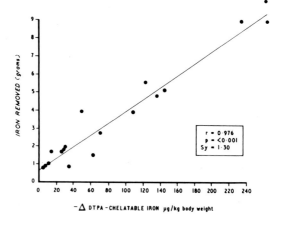

r = 0.976
p = <0.001
Sy = 1.30

$-\triangle$ DTPA-CHELATABLE IRON µg/kg body weight

test in cases of chronic cholestasis, and sometimes also in chronic liver diseases with moderate liver insufficiency [21];　·

c) all the chelating agent is excreted with the urine, whereas in the case of desferrioxamine a small portion is excreted into the bile [40];

d) one can calculate total body storage iron with better approximation [37, 40];

e) testing with ^{59}Fe-DTPA offers a better guidance in the matter of planning venesection treatment for patients with hypersiderosis [37, 40].

In this last connection (Fig. 8, 9) the values of total chelatable iron in a given subject, as obtained with the ^{59}Fe-DTPA test, closely reflect the actual iron overload, whereas with the Fielding test one may get apparently normal results in subjects deprived of as much as 4 g of iron by venesection. The reason of the superiority of the ^{59}Fe-DTPA test in this respect is that its range of normal values for chelatable iron is much more restricted.

In conclusion: for the ready discrimination of hypersiderosis the desferrioxamine test is quite adequate, and we recommend the standardized method currently used in our Department at Padua University. On the other hand, in cases calling for more precise information on the amount of iron removable or actually removed by the chelating agent, and on the metabolic fate of the chelated metal, one may carry out a Fielding test in addition, or even better, a ^{59}Fe-DTPA test.

References

[1] Bannerman, R. M., Callender, S. T., Williams, D. L., « Effect of Desferrioxamine and DTPA in Iron Overload », Brit. Med. J., 5319, 1573, 1962.

[2] Erlandson, M. E., Gobulow, J., Wehman, J., Smith, C. A., « Removal of Iron from Patients in Secondary Hemochromatosis », Blood, 22, 815, 1963.

[3] Wöhler, F., « Diagnosis of Iron Storage Diseases with Desferrioxamine (Desferal Test) », Acta Haemat. (Basel), 32, 324, 1964.

[4] Wöhler, F., « The Treatment of Haemochromatosis with Desferrioxamine », Iron Metabolism, Springer Verlag, Berlin, pag. 551, 1964.

[5] Moeschlin, S., Schineder, V., « Treatment of Primary and Secondary Haemochromatosis and Acute Iron Poisoning with a New Potent Iron Eliminating Agent (Desferrioxamine B) », Iron Metabolism, Springer Verlag, Berlin, pag. 525, 1964.

[6] Scuro, L. A., Broccia, G., Dobrilla, G., Tagliamonte, A., « Una nuova prova per l'accertamento degli stati di siderosi: il test della desferrioxamina », Policlinico, Sez. Prat., 71, 1101, 1964.

[7] Dagg, J. H., « The Excretion of Iron in Normal Sideropaenic and Iron Deficient Subjects after Giving Desferrioxamine », A Symposium on Desferrioxamine in the Diagnosis and Treatment of Abnormalities of Iron Metabolism, Ciba Foundation, London, pag. 21, 1964.

[8] Schnack, H., Wewalka, F., « Ergebnisse eines Tests zum Nachweis vermehrter Eisen Speicherung im Organismus bei Leberkrankheiten », Verh. Dtsch. Ges. Inn. Med., 70° Kongr., pag. 411, 1964.

300

[9] Goldberg ,A., *A Symposium on « Desferrioxamine » in the diagnosis and treatment of abnormalities of iron metabolism*, Ciba Found., London 1964.

[10] Walsh, R., Mass, R. E., Smith, F. W., Lange, V. E., « Iron chelation with desferrioxamine », *Ann. Int. Med., 60*, 728, 1964.

[11] Ventura, S., Coli, L., « Ricerche sulla desferrioxamina B. Nota III. L'impiego clinico della desferrioxamina B », *Haemat., 49, 3*, 1964.

[12] Hwang, Y. F., Brown, E. B., « Evaluation of Deferoxamine in Iron Overload », *Arch. Int. Med., 114*, 741, 1964.

[13] Unseld, D. W., « Ein neuer Test ('' Desferal test '') zum Nachweis von pathologischen Eisenablagerungen im Organismus », *Med. Welt, 11*, 569, 1964.

[14] Tura, S., Ricci-Bitti, M. L., Lodi, L., Pascucci, E., « Utilità e limiti del test al '' desferal '' nella diagnosi della ipersiderosi », *G. Clin. Med., 46*, 1167, 1965.

[15] Scuro, L. A., Dobrilla, G., « Il test della desferrioxamina nella diagnostica delle siderosi », *Policlinico, sez. prat., 72*, 155, 1965.

[16] Lenoir, P., Allanic H., Chauvel, A., Danon, G., Bourel, M., « Epreuve d'hypersidérurie provoquée à la desferrioxamine B dans les hémochromatoses », *Sem. Hôp.*, Paris, *47*, 2715, 1965.

[17] Walsh, J. R., Mass, R. E., Frederic, W. S., Mange, V., « Iron Chelation with Deferoxamine in Hepatic Disease ». *Gastroenterology, 49*, 134, 1965.

[18] Rosen, B. J., Tullis, J. L., « Simplified Deferoxamine Test in Normal, Diabetic, and Iron-overload Patients », *JAMA, 195*, 21, 1966.

[19] Ploem, J. E., De Wael, J., Verloop, C., Punt, K., « Sideruria Following a Single Dose of Desferrioxamine B as a Diagnostic Test in Iron Overload », *Brit. J. Haemat., 12*, 396, 1966.

[20] Aron, E., Weill, J. D., Galand, A., Mlle Domenech, « Variation respective de la sidérémie et de la sidérurie chez les cirrhotiques et les alcooliques après épreuve à la desferrioxamine », *Arch. Franç. Mal. App. Dig., 55*, 1159, 1966.

[21] Harker, L. A., Funk, D. D., Finch, C. A., « Evaluation of Storage Iron by Chelates », *Am. J. Med., 45*, 105, 1968.

[22] Scuro, L. A., « Su la standardizzazione del test della desferrioxamina », *Acta Med. Lomb., 20*, 2269, 1965.

[23] Eridani, S., Pozza, G., « Aspetti genetici e clinici dell'emocromatosi idiopatica », *Acta Med. Lombarda, 20*, 1993, 1965.

[24] Broccia, G., Massacci, E., Luxi, G., « Studi sulla eliminazione urinaria di ferro indotta dalla desferrioxamina B in soggetti normali, sideropenici e siderotici », *Rass. Med. Sarda, 68*, 243, 1965.

[25] Polosa, P., « Risultati clinico-ematologici dopo impiego di desferrioxamina B in un gruppo di talassemici e talassodrepanocitici », *Acta Med. Lombarda, 20*, 2175, 1965.

[26] Cimino, R., « Esperienze sul test al Desferal », *Acta Med. Lombarda, 20*, 2231, 1965.

[27] Gallinelli, R., « Contributo alla standardizzazione del Desferal test nella diagnostica delle emocromatosi primitive e secondarie », *Acta Med. Lombarda, 20*, 2251, 1965.

[28] Dal Co, C., « Esperienze con il test della desferrioxamina », *Acta Med. Lombarda, 20*, 2283, 1965.

[29] Taglioretti, D., Ponti, G. B., Petrella, A., « Il test della sideruria provocata da desferrioxamina nei soggetti emocromatosici », *Acta Med. Lombarda, 20*, 2285, 1965.

[30] Priolisi, A., intervento in discussione, *Accad. Med. Lombarda, 20*, 2295, 1965.

[31] Masera, G., Leggio, M. L., « Il test al Desferal nell'infanzia ».

[32] Pannacciulli, I., intervento in discussione, *Acta Med. Lombarda. 20*, 2293, 1965.

[33] Dobrilla, G., Lechi, A., Innecco, A., Cartei, G., Cavallini, G., « Osservazioni sulle tecniche impiegate per la determinazione del ferro urinario nel corso del test della desferrioxamina », *Quad. Sclavo Diagn., 2*, 343, 1966.

[34] Scuro, L. A., Dobrilla, G., Lechi, A., Innecco, A., Lo Cascio, V., Ponte, E., «La curva sideremica dopo desferrioxamina », *Riforma Med., 11*, 286, 1967.

[35] Scuro, L. A., Dobrilla, G., « Siderosis, Haemolysis or Hepatonecrosis in Increasing

Post-desferrioxamine Sideruria in Acute Viral Hepatitis? », *Postgrad. Med. J.*, 43, 708, 1967.

[36] Fielding, J., « Differential Ferrioxamine Test for Measuring Chelatable Body Iron », *J. Clin. Path.*, 18, 88, 1965.

[37] Barry, M., Cartei, G., Sherlock, S., « Accurate Determination of Body Storage Iron », *Submitted to Clin. Sci.*

[38] Smith, P. M., Studley, F., Williams, R., « Assessment of Body-iron Stores in Cirrhosis and Haemochromatosis with the Differential Ferrioxamine Test », *Lancet I*, 133, 1967.

[39] Stevens, E., Rosoff, B., Weiner, M., Spencer, H., « Metabolism of the Chelating Agent Diethylentetramine-pentaacetic Acid », *Proc. Soc. Exp. Biol. Med.* III, 235, 1962.

[40] Barry, M., Cartei, G., « Chelatable Iron in Liver Diseases », *Symposium Internazionale su « Siderosi e siderocromatosi »*, Padova, 1968.

[41] Vannotti, A., *Introduction in « Les Hémochromatoses »*, Masson Ed., Paris, 1963.

[42] Williams, R., « Iron in Chronic Liver Diseases », *Conv. Farmitalia*, Milano 1966.

6.3. *Vitamin B$_{12}$ and Folic Acid Determinations*
G. Izak, M. D., Department of Hematology, Hebrew University-Hadassah Medical School, and Hadassah University Hospital, Jerusalem, Israel

Among the biologically active and important compounds the two groups of vitamins, namely, B$_{12}$ and Folates have raised considerable interest during the last 3 decades, which — considering their vital role in cell metabolism — is not surprising. It is my task today to summarize briefly the procedures available to estimate quantitatively these compounds in blood, serum, tissues, tissue fluids and foodstuffs. If it is expected of me, that by the end of 15 minutes at my disposal, you should get up from your chairs and go away with the knowledge that by following well standardized procedures — clearly defined by me — you would end up with reasonably accurate, reproducible results, let me disappoint you at the very outset, as no such procedures are at present available.

Before we get into the discussion of some aspects of the efforts concerned with standardization procedures, allow me to devote a few moments to the brief summary of the field, to which these procedures have to be applied. I should also like to deal with the requirements one has to fulfil in establishing standard laboratory procedures for the estimation of these hematinics.

Nutritional anemia is extremely widespread, and although it varies a great deal in severity and frequency, it has been found to occur in all areas of human habitation, wherever the problem has been studied. Lack — or depletion of vitamin B$_{12}$ and of folates in humans have been

found to go hand in hand with under, — or malnutrition and one of
the most important clinical manifestation of these deficiencies is macrocytic anemia with all its consequences. As malnutrition is the ground
upon which B_{12} and folate depletion prosper, it is the under-privileged
and under-developed population groups, still so enormously large —
which are most affected. You all know, that B_{12} and folates have each
their specific metabolic functions, hence, they cannot replace each other.
Consequently, whenever we are faced with a population group or for
that matter, with an individual patient with macrocytic anemia, we
have to have means at our disposal to establish which of these two
hematinics is missing. It follows from the above, that one expects from
a standardized procedure to give a reliable answer to this question. This,
however, is not all; one also demands a method which is simple, does
not require sophisticated equipment for its performance and be as little
dependent on outside conditions — like temperature, humidity, bacterial
contamination, etc., as possible.

Let us see now, how do the available laboratory procedures stand
up to these requirements.

The structure of the cobalamins is well known, and once these vitamins have been isolated from the blood, tissues, or tissue fluids, there
are perfectly good spectroscopic and colorimetric methods to establish
their concentration. The problem is, that to get B_{12} to this form repeated
chromatographic procedures are required to free them from other inactive cobolamins and impurities, which render this path completely impractical for the purposes we have outlined. A somewhat simpler method
is based on initial acid hydrolysis of the vitamins, yielding through a
number of additional steps dimethylphenylenediamine, which, when
cleared from a good number of impurities can be estimated colorimetri-
cally. These methods, however, besides being extremely laborious, do
not estimate errors arising from impurities or inactive analogues.

It is for these reasons, that increasing attention has been paid to
microbiological assays, the principles of which need not be described
here in detail. A large number of B_{12}-dependent bacterial strains have
been identified, the growth rate of which is proportional to the B_{12}
concentration present in the medium; simple turbidimetry or bacterial
cell counts will then give us the required results. *E. Coli, Euglena
Gracilis, Ochromonas Malhamensis* are some of the micro-organisms
employed most frequently. Here too, the B_{12} has to be liberated from
its organic bonds, which can be achieved by heating the specimen, but
no further purification steps are required, as the discrimination is done
by the micro-organism. While this procedure is much simpler than the

ones mentioned before, it is still a far cry from the requirements we set down earlier. Hence, the attempt to estimate vitamin B_{12} by an isotope dilution technique described by Herbert was a welcome addition. The method consists essentially of adding a measured amount of Co^{57}-vitamin B_{12} to the unknown cobolamin liberated from the tissues. Part of the « B_{12}-mixture » is then bound to a purified, potent intrinsic factor preparation, while the unbound cobolamin is absorbed to albumin-coated charcoal. The B_{12} concentration of the unknown sample can be easily calculated from the degree of the dilution of the labelled B_{12} by its unlabelled congener in the supernatant.

These two procedures are the most widely employed ones, and it was the initial task of the expert panel of the International Committee for Standardization in Hematology (I.C.S.H.) set up to produce an international standard, to find out how reproducible and accurate these procedures were. The first important requirement in establishing standard procedures, namely, the simplicity of the test had to be abandoned. As a trial, six participating laboratories, from almost as many countries have estimated the B_{12} content in solutions mailed to them on 10 occasions. Each of these laboratories are well known in the literature for their contributions to the knowledge of B_{12} metabolism. Each laboratory used the method they usually employ. The mean values of three determinations have been collected by the secretary of the panel and the results were not very encouraging. True, very low values tended to give low readings in every laboratory, just as very high ones were similar everywhere. However, when you consider that with any one batch of samples differences amounted up to 100%, the conclusion seems to be inevitable, that the procedures as performed in the participating laboratories are far from the required standard we discussed before. At present, the efforts of the panel are aimed at working out a uniform procedure to be followed by all participants. It is hoped, that suitable modifications will be worked out to correct the inaccuracies uncovered by this cooperative effort.

The situation with the folate group is — if possible — more complicated. The substance referred to as folic acid is, as you know, pteroylglutamic acid, — which in this form is biologically inactive and it has to be reduced through a series of steps in the body to endow it with its vital function of one carbon transfer. It should be mentioned that a variety of folates are involved in a large number of metabolic reactions. The problem is further complicated by the fact, that a substantial proportion of folates in the body is present in conjugated forms as bi,-tri-hepta-glutamates, which in turn may be reduced or not. The reduced forms of folates are rather labile and special care has to be taken to preserve them in their reduced forms, during the process of their liberation from tissues. Once in solution as free compounds, concentrated and purified, their quantitative estimation can be achieved with perfect ease. However, as with the B_{12}, — here too the procedures required to achieve this, render these procedures entirely impractical for the purposes outlined above. Indirect methods were and are still employed to estimate the availability of folates in the body the best known of which is the determination of formiminoglutamic acid in the urine after histidine load. This method, besides it being indirect, has been found to be inadequate in a number of conditions (i.e. pregnancy). To our luck, the microbiological assay came to the rescue here too. Micro-organisms have been isolated, each of which was found to be dependent on a varying, though specific range of folates present in the medium. Thus, *L. casei* would respond to PGA, reduced or nonreduced, conjugated or deconjugated folates, hence, one could estimate with this bacterium the overall folate content of a given solution. A strain of *P. cerevisiae* was found to be sensitive to all reduced folates except N-5-methyl THFA; while *S. foecalis* would measure all this and in addition PGA too. With the use of these organisms a fair map of folate content could be obtained in a given sample.

The expert panel of I.C.S.H. on folate set out to test the accuracy and reproducibility of these procedures. The participating laboratories are here too, experts in the field. Samples mailed to them were estimated with *L. casei* and the results of 10 such samples were summarized. The same wide range was obtained here as was the case in the preliminary trial with vitamin B_{12}. The present efforts of this panel are also aimed at working out a uniform procedure to be used by each participating laboratory. A new approach has been introduced recently by Ricker and associates, based on the work of Sela, when it was shown that antibodies can be prepared against p-aminobenzoyl-L-glutamate as a heptene — when this compound was covalently linked to a large synthetic polypeptide or bovine serum albumin. The antiserum would then precipitate the folic acid from the solution. Not enough is known about this procedure yet, but it may be the beginning of an immuno-assay, which may be the answer to our problem.

In summary, the available procedures for the quantitative estimation of B_{12} and folates in blood, serum, tissue and foodstuffs are elaborate, difficult to perform and at present are not sufficiently standardized to give accurate and reproducible results. They are of considerable clinical use, but much has to be done to make out of it the tool needed in a large areas of the world. I hope that a few years hence, I shall be in a position to report the successful solution of these problems, mainly as a result of the cooperative effort of the members of the I.C.S.H. expert panels.

References

[1] Grossowicz, N., Aronovitch, J. and Rachmilewitz, M., *Proc. Soc. Exp. Biol. Med.*, *87*, 513. 1954.
[2] Grossowicz, N., Mandelbaum-Shavit, F., Davidoff, R. and Aronovitch, J., *Blood*, *20*, 609, 1962.
[3] Ungar-Waron, H., Sela, M., *Biochim. Biophys. Acta*, *124*, 149, 1966.
[4] Ricker, R., Stollar, B. D., *Biochemistry*, *6*, 2001, 1967.
[5] Gottlieb, Ch., Lau, K. S., Wasserman, L. R. and Herbert, V., *Blood*, *25*, 875, 1965.

7.1. The Standardization of the Common Blood Coagulation Procedures
J. Jürgens, II Med. Univ.-Klinik, Frankfurt am Main, Germany

Among the problems encountered in haematological research, the standardization of techniques for assaying the blood coagulation system presents inordinate difficulties. The reason is, that no practicable methods have yet been devised for isolating the individual coagulation factors in pure form, so that their plasma concentration can be expressed as a gravimetrical unit. An indirect manner of determining the various coagulation factors has therefore to be resorted to. This consists of determining a specific coagulation activity of each particular factor, which can only be expressed as a time measurement relating to the course of a coagulation process or system under stipulated conditions.

The one exception is the assay of fibrinogen (Factor I). This can be done gravimetrically and the plasma concentration expressed in milligrams percent. With some of the coagulation factors whose specific activity can be determined, the activity can be expressed as a percentage of normal, whereby the normal value is regarded as 100 percent of norm, as in Sahli's assay for haemoglobin. In other methods, where either the complete process or one particular phase of coagulation is determined, it is however not possible to convert the results into percentage of norm. The only thing to do in such cases is to strictly define all the conditions of these particular methods and to express the result as coagulation time in minutes or seconds. To date, this is a necessity for the following methods:

1. Whole blood coagulation time;
2. Recalcification time (Calcium Clotting Time);
3. Heparin tolerance test;
4. PTT (partial Thromboplastin Time);
5. Thrombin - time.

These methods especially need standardisation for the following considerations:

a) If the tests are carried out conscientiously and with technical accuracy they are relatively efficient. At least the middle-grade forms and certainly the serious forms of haemophilia, as well as a variety of coagulation dysfunctions, in particular those due to fibrinogen deficiency and overdosage of anticoagulants during therapeutical treatment, can be recognised or inferred. This also applies to the determination of hypercoagulability which possibly could provide an indication of whether or not to proceed with anticoagulant therapy.
b) Technically the tests are fairly simple and because of this they are universally used.
c) Unfortunately all the methods for analysing the mechanism of coagulation and fibrinolysis are fundamentally affected by various and dissimilar laboratory conditions, and this lack of consistency can of itself lead to severe mistakes.

The most important factors, which generally exert a substantial influence on the result of coagulation investigations, are presented in the following synopsis:

I. *Collection of blood*

a) Cannula — size, bore polished or ordinary.
b) Syringe — of glass, plastic, inside surface paraffin-coated or untreated.
c) Anticoagulant citrate, oxalate blood-volume-part.
d) Duration of compression for venipuncture.
e) Blood extraction in laboratory? — or transported blood?

II. *Age of blood sample — duration of transport?*

III. *Shaking*

IV. *Duration of centrifugation*
V. *Types of tubes used for the coagulation mixture*
a) Glass tubes — effect of cleaning and drying.
b) Glass tubes — siliconised.
c) Plastic tubes.

VI. *Factors dependant on coagulation mixture*

a) Dilution of plasma.
b) Temperature.
c) pH.
d) Jonic strength.
e) Type of specific reagent.
f) Ca^{++} — optimal concentration.

VII. *Technic for ascertaining onset of coagulation*

a) Loop method.
b) Tilting in test tube.
c) Thread-pulling in watchglass.
d) Turbidimetric measurement.
e) Measurement of electrical resistance.
f) Thrombelastography — other mechanical procedures.

VIII. *Method of calculation*

a) In minutes/seconds.
b) In percent of norm.
c) In units.
d) In milligrampercent.

Use of thin cannulas when extracting a blood sample leads, on account of facilitated disintegration of the thrombocytes, to shorter coagulation times than the use of wide-calibre needles or cannulas with shiny bores. Glass syringes with their relatively rough inside surfaces lead, for the same reason, to shorter coagulation times than do plastic syringes. Longer coagulation times are obtained by applying a paraffin coat (paraffinum liquidum) to the chambers of glass syringes. Furthermore it is not a matter of indifference if sodium citrate or sodium oxalate are used as anticoagulants. The ratio of anticoagulant to blood is also a decisive factor. For most coagulation tests, citrate in the blood in the ratio of 1 : 10 (1 to 10) is to be recommended. However, even at the present time there are methods in use where this ratio is 1 : 5. Since, when recalcifying, the object is not just to neutralise the citrate portion but also to achieve an excess of calcium ions, a deviation from the prescribed ratio can lead to uncommon results and even cause incoagulability of the test (Figure 1).

Overlong stricture of the vein when taking a blood sample should be strictly avoided. It can lead, through activation of the coagulation system (process) and of concurrent platelet metabolism to considerably changed coagulation times (Fig. 2). Venipuncture should be performed

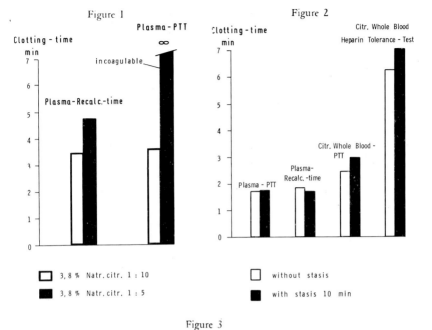

Figure 1

Clotting - time
min

Plasma-Recalc.-time

Plasma - PTT

incoagulable

∞

☐ 3,8 % Natr.citr. 1 : 10
■ 3,8 % Natr.citr. 1 : 5

Figure 2

Clotting - time
min

Citr. Whole Blood
Heparin Tolerance - Test

Citr. Whole Blood -
PTT

Plasma-
Recalc. -time

Plasma - PTT

☐ without stasis
■ with stasis 10 min

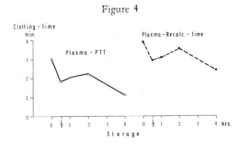

Figure 3

Changes of PTT and Plasma - Recalc. - time by Shaking
the Blood sample.

min

Clotting - time

Plasma-Recalc.-time

PTT

0 1   5 10 20   0 1   5 10 20 min

Shaking - time

Figure 4

Clotting - time
min

Plasma - PTT

Plasma - Recalc. - time

0 ½ 1   2   3   4   0 ½ 1   2   3   4 hrs.

Storage

without hitches. Unsuccessful puncture with lesion of the vessel wall, or even paravenous puncture, brings about a mixture of the blood sample with tissue thromboplastin, and as a result the coagulation time is shortened.

Blood withdrawing is best performed in the haematological laboratory. Blood which has been obtained at a distance from the research building or clinic is no longer suitable for tests 1 - 5 due to unavoidable shaking during transport. This causes disintegration of the thrombocytes with ensuing activation of all the coagulation processes. Transport within the same clinic, for example from a ward to the laboratory, is however permissible provided the assay is carried out within minutes after extraction, with every possible care being taken to avoid shaking (Fig. 3, 4).

The type of centrifugation, too, affects substantially all those assay methods where substances other than thromboplastin are used as reagents — for example recalcification time and PTT. Centrifuged plasma should be as nearly as possible platelet-free for these tests (Fig. 5).

Another factor that can affect markedly the result of assays is the consistency of the inside surfaces of test tubes used in the water bath for establishing the course of coagulation. Ordinary, non-siliconised centrifuge tubes exert a further influence, depending on the type of cleaning and pre-treatment to which they have been submitted. Prolonged pre-immersion in *chromic sulphuric acid* induces, in consequence of an alteration to the glass surface, shorter coagulation times than is the case with thickly siliconised or plastic tubes.

As for the coagulation mixture itself, a whole row of factors are involved. Here the plasma final dilution and hence the final volume of the coagulation mixture play a leading role. Temperature should be maintained at a constant 37° centigrade. In those methods where strong plasma dilutions are used, the pH should be adjusted by addition of buffer to 7.6. A careful maintenance of ionic strength should be observed, as even fairly trivial changes of concentration affect the determination of all the coagulation factors.

It is obvious that when different reagents are used for determining one and the same factor, differing coagulation times are obtained. Thus when setting out to standardize assay methods, a single reagent should be stipulated as a standard, and when tests are undertaken with other reagents these should be named. Unfortunately all reagents have a limited and varying durability. Supervision of the stability of certain reagents should be taken over by an international commission.

Figure 5

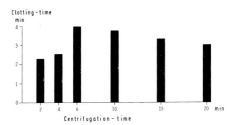

Figure 6

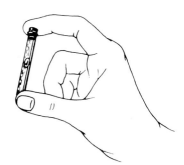

Figure 7

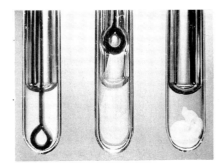

Figure 8

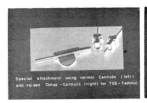
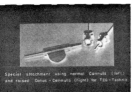
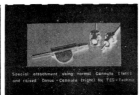

Figure 9

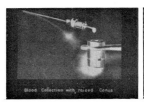
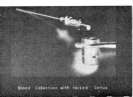
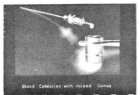

Finally, the methods used for observing the coagulation process can also considerably affect the result of tests. When applying the loop method, for example, it is of significance whether the formation of a fibrin thread on the metal loop occurs in a narrow micro test-tube in a water bath, or in a thin watchglass or in an ordinary test tube (Fig. 6, 7). Still other results are obtained when the instant of coagulation is noted while lightly shaking or tilting the blood-probe mixture in a narrow test tube. In all these mechanical procedures the speed with which one tilts, stirs or pulls is of great consequence.

If the centrifugal charge is mixed too quickly, an initial defibrination of the blood-probe occurs which is not visible and this gives rise to substantially longer coagulation times. Most reliable are the photometric or electrical methods, or thrombelastrography, for which however a standardisation of the various assay tests — worked out to the last details — is imperative.

Finally, for standardizing methods of determining blood-coagulation factors and activities, the modes of calculation should also be uniform. Here considerable difficulties stand in the way, because the means of carrying out individual tests vary so widely from one laboratory to another.

Methods of conducting assays

1. *Whole-blood coagulation time* (clotting time)
Method of Lee and White [6]
Withdrawing of Blood:
Briefest possible compression of the upper arm and puncture of the vena cubitalis.
Cannula: No. 1.
Syringe: Plastic 5 ml.
Test tubes: Plastic - 2.1/2 × 3/8 in.
Thermostat: Water bath 37 °C.
Technic:
5 ml spontaneous blood is collected and transferred to 4 plastic test tubes in amounts of 1 ml. The test tubes are then placed in the water bath and tilted every 30 seconds so as to ascertain onset of coagulation. Shaking should be avoided. With the aid of a stopwatch the clotting time of the whole-blood sample is registered.
Normal value 18-25 min.

1a. *Modifications of the whole-blood clotting time* [1]
As an alternative to the plastic tubes, siliconised test tubes can be used, but if the silicone coating is in any way defective, errors arise.
It is also possible to use non-siliconised test tubes that have been pre-

treated in chromic sulphuric acid and washed with special care, but this method is not so accurate and the clotting time is shorter (5-10 min.).

2. *Recalcification time (calcium clotting time)* [2]
   Withdrawal of blood
   Puncture of the vena cubitalis as in 1.
   Cannula: No. 1.
   Syringe: Plastic.
   Anticoagulant: Sodium citrate 3.8 %.
   Preparation for test: 1 part citrate to 9 parts blood.
   Withdrawal of blood should be performed fairly quickly so that the mixing with the anticoagulant ensues speedily. As soon as the blood has been sucked into the syringe a little air should be drawn in too and by means of tilting well mixed with the blood, so as to prevent partial coagulation in the syringe.

   Centrifugation:
   To obtain fairly platelet-poor plasma, the citrated blood is transferred from normal glass tubes to centrifuge glass tubes and centrifuged for at least 10 min. at 3,000 r.p.m.
   Thermostat: Water bath at 37 °C.
   Test tubes: normal glass 2.1/2 × 3/8 in.
   Visualisation of instant of clotting: (loop) method.

   Technic:
   Into pre-warmed test tubes the following reactive mixture is pipetted:
   0.1 ml platelet-free plasma
   0.1 ml NaCl solution 0.85 % (physiol, saline)
   0.1 ml M/40 CaCl$_2$.
   By slowly dipping and withdrawing a platinum loop, the moment of coagulation is determined - visually ascertainable by the withdrawal of a coagulum.
   Normal clotting time: 90-250 sec.

3. *Partial-Thromboplastin-Time (PTT)* - Quick [13]
   Reagents:
   a) Tachostyptan - obtainable from Hormon-Chemie AG, Munich/Germany. The reagent is supplied solubilised in ampoules and must be diluted 1 : 50 with Michaelis buffer pH 7.6;
   b) PTT-reagent supplied by The Ortho-Research-Foundation, Raritan, New Jersey, U.S.A. The reagent is in the form of dry ampoules - 1 ampoule to be dissolved in 1 ml distilled water.
   Technic:
   As in 2. - recalcification time - but the reactive mixture is made up of the following:
   0.1 ml plasma
   0.1 ml reagent

0.1 ml $CaCl_2$ solution.

Normal value: 1 min. 0.5 sec. to 1 min. 20 sec.

Controls:

To counter-check the normal value a control determination can be made using commercial normal dry plasma. For this, the following preparations can be recommended:

a) Reagent hp 65 - human plasma - normal coagulation - test control supplied by The Ortho-Research-Foundation, Raritan, New Jersey, U.S.A.
1 ampoule to be dissolved in 1 ml distilled water.

b) Diagnostic Plasma obtainable from the firm of Warner-Chilcott, NI, U.S.A.
1 ampoule to be dissolved in 0.5 ml distilled water.

4. *Heparin tolerance test* - Marbet and Winterstein [8]
Reagent:
Complete reagent for the heparin tolerance test is obtainable from the Hoffmann-La Roche Co., Basel/Switzerland - Code No. Ro 1-2232/760.
1 dry ampoule is dissolved in 5 ml H_2O = 10 I.U./ml heparin.
From this heparin solution, 0.2 ml is diluted with 9.8 ml M/40 $CaCl_2$ solution.

Withdrawing of Blood
As in 2. - recalcification time - except that the non-centrifuged, citrated whole blood is used.

Test tubes: Siliconised glass tubes 2.1/2 × 3/8 in.

Technic:
The reagent is first warmed in the water bath. Into the silicon tubes prepared as above, 0.5 ml citrated whole blood is pip likewise pre-warmed in the water bath. Subsequently 0.5 n Heparin-$CaCl_2$ reagent mixture is added with a pipette.
Determination of the instant of clotting:
The probe is withdrawn every 10 seconds from the water bath and the moment of coagulum formation established by careful rotatory shaking.
Normal values: 2 min. 30 sec. ± 15 sec.

5. *Rapid method for determination of isolated prothrombin in* one stage principle following Koller, Loeliger, Duckert [4]
With commercial reagents.
Reagents:
1. Reagent for assay of prothrombin supplied by Hoffmann-La Roche Co., Basel/Switzerland. Code No. Ro 1-8977
1 dry ampoule is dissolved in 1 ml distilled water.
2. Michaelis buffer pH 7.6.
Technic:
Procedure as in 2. - recalcification time. But the reactive mixture is as follows:

0.1 ml test plasma, already diluted 1 : 10 with Michaelis buffer pH 7.6
0.1 ml Prothrombin reagent
0.1 ml thromboplastin
0.1 ml M/40 CaCl$_2$ solution
Moment of clotting is ascertained with the eyelet method.

Calculation:
The clotting time of normal plasma is determined by means of the above method - whereby the buffer dilution 1 : 10 counts as 100 % prothrombin.
Through further thinning of the original plasma-dilution to 50 %, 25 % and 10 %, clotting times are obtained that correspond to the respective prothrombin values in percent. The recording of these values in a double-logarithmic coordinate system gives a straight line which can then be used as a standard curve for converting the coagulation times into prothrombin-percent (percentage of prothrombin).
If commercial reagents are not available the technic can be modified using self-prepared reagents [10].
In this case the reactive mixture is the following:
0.1 ml test plasma diluted 1 : 10
0.1 ml Al (OH)$_3$ - adsorbed normal plasma
0.1 ml stored human serum
0.1 ml thromboplastin
0.1 ml M/40 CaCl$_2$-solution.

Preparation of Al (OH)$_3$ - absorbed normal human citrate-plasma:
to 1.0 ml citrate-plasma 0.1 ml Al (OH)$_3$-suspension (1 %) is added.
The mixture is shaken three minutes, centrifuged and the supernatant stored in the refrigerator.

Preparation of stored human serum:
To 1.0 ml cellfree centrifuged fresh human serum 0.1 ml thromboplastin is added and the mixture incubated for one hour in the water-bath of 37 °C.
Storing of this serum in the refrigerator.

6. *Rapid method for determining Factor V*
Owren [12]

With commercial reagents [9]:
Procedure as in 5. - except that a specific reagent for Factor V supplied by the Hoffmann-La Roche Co. - No. Ro 1-8498/1 - is used.
The dry ampoule is dissolved in 1 ml distilled water.
If commercial reagents are not available the Factor-V-reagent can be prepared as follows:
Cellfree centrifuged normal human oxalated plasma (1 part 1,34 % Sodium oxalate + 9 parts blood) are kept for 24 hours at 37 °C in the incubator.

316

Keep this factor-V-free plasma until use in the refrigerator.

7. *Determination of Factor VII using the one stage principle* of Koller, Loeliger and Duckert [4, 5, 7]

With commercial reagents:

Procedure as in 5. - except that the specific reagent suplied by the Hoffmann-La Roche Co. - No. Ro 1-8497/1 - is used.
The dry ampoule is dissolved in 1 ml distilled water.
If the commercial reagent ist not available Factor-VII-reagent can be self prepared following the original method of Koller et al. [11]:
Cellfree centrifuged oxalated ox-plasma (1 part 1,34 % Sodium oxalate + 9 parts blood) are filtered using Seitz-Asbestos-Filter containing 30 % asbestos.
A second filtration follows using a filter containing 40 % asbestos. Storing of the factor-V-free plasma in the refrigerator.
With the following method the complex consisting from Factor-VII- and Factor-X is estimated.
If between the activity of this both factors should be differenciated other methods using Russels's Viper venom together with Cephalin must be performed. Because these methods are relatively complicated and therefore less common there is no possibility to describe them here.

8. *Thrombin time*

Reagent: Topostasin Roche.
1 flask contains 3,000 I.U.
Preparation and standardisation of the thrombin solution: 1 oese of thrombin dry substance is dissolved in 5 ml Michaelis buffer pH 7.6. By adding more buffer the activity is adjusted to a coagulation time of 10 seconds.

Reactive mixture:

0.1 ml platelet-poor plasma (obtained according to 2.)
0.1 ml Michaelis buffer pH 7.6
0.1 ml thrombin solution (solubilised thrombin)
The results are registered in sec./thrombin-time.

9. *Fibrinogen*

Photometric Principle of Ebbecke and Knüchel [3] (own modification)
Principle: Photometric measurement of scattered light before and after the coagulation of a platelet-free centrifuged plasma.

Reagents:

1. Optimal platelet-poor centrifuged citrated plasma - obtained as in 2.
2. Physiol. saline 0.85 %
3. Thromboplastin solution - all the commercial preparations of this can be used.

   a) Thromboplastin Hoffman-La Roche

b) Thromboplastin supplied by The Ortho-Research Foundation, NI, U.S.A. - reagent No. ORF 4276 G.

Technic:

Apparatus: Light scattering attachment fitted to suitable photometer - e.g. the Eppendorf Photometer supplied by the firm of Netheler & Hintz.

Adjustment of apparatus: With aid of standard gauge No. 1155, optical density should first be adjusted to 0.350 E.

Reactive mixture: Made up in a cuvette of 20 mm as follows:

0.1 ml phatelet-poor centrifuged plasma, obtained as in 2.

3.0 ml physiol. saline 0.85 %

0.1 ml solubilised thromboplastin

1.0 ml M/40 $CaCl_2$ solution

After brief mixing by careful, tilting (3-4 times), the scattered Light of the recalcified plasma is read and noted as E_1. Due to the slow onset, of coagulation after an incubation period, the scattered Light gradually increases. The optimum is noted as E_2.

Calculation:

According to the formula: $0.7 \times (E_1 - E_2)$ = fibrinogen in milligrams-percent.

For fibrinogen determination with concomitant fibrinolytic activity, a 0.85 % physiological saline containing pro ml 0.1 mg AMCHA or 1 mg epsilon-aminocaprone acid is used in the above reactive mixture.

10. *Thrombelastogram*:

Blood Collection: Cuvettes are filled with spontaneous blood.

Cannulas: special types with raised conus or special attachment (Fig. 8, 9) for preventing adherence of droplets.

Cuvettes: of plastic - obtainable from the firm of W. Fischer, Frankfurt-on-Main (Kiesstrasse 36).

Normal values: the r-value when using plastic cuvettes is 2.5 - 4.5 minutes longer than when using steel cuvettes.

The above-described procedures for assaying coagulation-potential or individual clotting factors represent only a small selection of the most important of a much greater number of physiological methods which, on account of their technical simplicity, can be performed in clinical laboratories not equipped with highly specialised apparatus. Having regard to the still more numerous, widely scattered modifications and complementary tests, it is plain that standardisation in this field can only be tackled by the setting up of an international committee, for whose task the suggestions made here are merely intended as a basis for discussion.

318

References

[1] Biggs, R. and MacFarlane, R. G., *Human Blood Coagulation and its Disorders*, Blackwell Scientific Publications Oxford, 3. Edition, 1962, p. 381.
[2] *Idem*, p. 384.
[3] Ebbecke, V. and Knüchel. *Pflügers - Arch.*, 243, 54, 1939.
[4] Koller, F., Loeliger, A. and Duckert F., *Acta haematol.*, 6, 1, 1951.
[5] Koller, F., Loeliger A. and Duckert, F., *Rev. hématol.*, 7, 156, 1952.
[6] Lee, R. I. and White, P. D., *American J. med. Sci.*, 145, 495, 1913.
[7] Loeliger. A., *Wien. Zschr. inn. Med.*, 33, 169, 1952.
[8] Marbet, R. and Winterstein, A., *Aerztl. Forsch.*, IX, 10, 1/460, 1955.
[9] Marbet, R. and Winterstein, A., « Faktor V », *Hoffmann-La Roche - Information* from 21-4-1954.
[10] Jürgens, J. and Beller, F. K., *Klinische Methoden der Blutgerinnungsanalyse.* Thieme, Stuttgart, p. 197, 1955.
[11] Jürgens, J. and Beller, F. K., *Klinische Methoden der Blutgerinnungsanalyse.* Thieme, Stuttgart, 1955, p. 211.
[12] Owren, P. A., *Lancet*, 254, 466, 1947; *Bull. Schweiz. Akad. med. Wiss.*, 3, 163, 1947; *Biochem. J.*, 43, 136, 1948.
[13] Quick, A. J., *Thromb. et Diathesis Haem.*, 1, 9-15, 1957.

7.2. Standardization of Measurements of prothrombin time

P. De Nicola, Chair of Gerontology and Geriatrics,
University of Pavia, Italy

Standardization of methods for the measurement of prothrombin time, or prothrombin activity, is concerned with the technicalities and suitable criteria toward a greater uniformity and reliability of results. We shall consider first the general technicalities, such as are applicable also to other tests of coagulation, and then those more closely related to the prothrombin time, such as the choice of thromboplastin, the calculation of percentages, and the limits of normal values.

General technicalities have to do with the separation of plasma and with its preservation up to the time of use for testing. In the case of prothrombin time these technical details are of limited importance—far less, at any rate, than the mode of separation and preservation of the plasma influences the determination of recalcification time or the thrombo-elastogram, or than the mode of preservation of the plasma modifies the activity of factor V. Concerning anticoagulants, the times obtained with citrate are usually a little shorter than with oxalate: hence the need

(*) The text of this presentation is derived from that of a similar lecture by the same author in cooperation with P. Boccaccio, S. Coccheri, G. Crolle, A. G. Dettori, F. Gobbi, and M. Marcacci, read on behalf of C.I.S.M.E.'s Panel for the Study and Standardization of Methods Pertaining to Coagulation and Fibrinolysis, at the Florence Meeting of 4 November 1967 (Proc. Nat. Symp. on Standardization in Hematology: *Haematologica Latina* II, 7, 1968).

for adopting one or the other substance as standard, not only for one-stage prothrombin testing but also for other tests of coagulation. The substitution of citrate for oxalate is recommended on the ground that citrate is being increasingly used in testing for thromboplastin generation and for work on blood platelets.

In the matter of temperatures, there is a general preference for using a water bath adjusted at 37 to 37.5 °C, though it is recognized that the temperature inside the test tubes may be somewhat lower if the reagents are not left for some time in the water bath preparatory to testing.

The pre-incubation of reagents among themselves is again a general technical problem that applies also to prothrombin time independently of pre-heating of each reagent separately. It has been observed that a prolonged pre-incubation of calcium and thromboplastin, like that of thromboplastin and plasma, may lead to shortening of coagulation time values. Still, a short incubation of calcium and thromboplastin may be advisable.

The last aspect of general technicalities is evaluation of the endpoint in coagulation. Any of the various available criteria is defendable, as long as the operator has enough experience with coagulation tests. It would be desirable to have automatic, or at least semi-automatic, methods also for measuring the endpoint of coagulation, as has been increasingly the case with other laboratory tests. Unfortunately, complete data on the reliability of automatic recorders are still wanting—though some of these instruments lend themselves admirably for serial work.

The central problem in the study of prothrombin activity in terms of prothrombin time is the choice of thromboplastin and the use of suitable curves for the calculation of percentages, the latter defining the limits of normal values in seconds and in per cent prothrombin activity. This applies equally to the classical Quick method and to other methods derived therefrom. In addition to thromboplastin itself, we must take into consideration the calcium chloride, the sodium oxalate, and the veronal buffer used for the preparation of dilution curves. Both in view of standardization and for the sake of simplification it may be a good idea to use thromboplastin preparations that contain calcium, aside from other preferences. Though thromboplastins made in the laboratory (eg from rabbit brain according to Quick, or from human brain) may be excellent, commercially available thromboplastins are obviously preferable from the point of view of standardization. Today there are several commercial brands of thromboplastin whose standard of purity is quite good.

The evaluation of various thromboplastins can be done through a study of plasma dilution curves, which become straight lines when reported on double-log scale. In many cases the course of these straight lines is approximately parallel even if the starting points are taken at different time values. But even with the same thromboplastin there is a considerable variability of these straight lines in normal and pathological conditions.

According to Quick's original definition, the prothrombin time is the coagulation time that, in the presence of optimal amounts of calcium and of excess thromboplastin, is influenced by variations of prothrombin concentration—or in more up-to-date terms, of factors II, V, VII and X, plus a few others that are generally not taken into consideration (fibrinogen, anticoagulants in the blood stream, and the like). The shortest prothrombin times obtained with thromboplastins in current use are in the region of 11 or 12 seconds; however, there are thromboplastins that give longer times. The problem is to decide how far we can go beyond 12 seconds. It has been said that with short times one cannot demonstrate small differences in the range from 50 % to 100 %, or more, prothrombin activity. With longer times, one would obtain a better differentiation of individual results; but this would be at the cost of the principle that calls for the addition of thromboplastin in excess. If the thromboplastin preparation is not very active, one may find inordinately long times, and not easily reproduced, when the prothrombin activity is low. As the time results increase, so does the standard deviation of repeat assays with the same plasma, to the point where the results become unreliable or poorly reproducible.

By using diluted plasma, as is currently done for the determination of numerous factors by methods derived from prothrombin time, one can obtain a greater differentiation of values even if one uses a very active thromboplastin preparation. Between using a low-activity thromboplastin and diluting the plasma for better differentiation of results, the latter device appears preferable.

It is generally thought that no thromboplastin should give readings in excess of 15 or 16 seconds in normal conditions; and many authors are in favor of more active thromboplastins.

In our own experimental investigations we have often found that the time readings are slightly longer than shown in the instructions, even though the latter are followed scrupulously. The same is true of lyophilized control plasma preparations, of which we have used a large number to evaluate the possibility of using them instead of normal plasma obtained from incidental donors, or instead of pooled normal plasma.

The experience gathered in the course of these trials has fortified our conviction that each laboratory should first of all verify time readings and curves and make sure that these data are valid in their own experimental conditions. This is probably the crucial point in the matter of standardization of the measurement of prothrombin time, even though in our experimental work we found a fairly good degree of correlation between the data obtained in various laboratories with different thromboplastins. Our results are currently undergoing statistical analysis.

Once the measurement of prothrombin time is standardized satisfactorily, several other methods derived from it will easily be standardized accordingly.

Synopsis of points to be considered in standardization of prothrombin time and allied methods

1. Technic of sample collection:
   (a) with plain or silicone-treated syringe;
   (b) with citrate or oxalate.
2. Plasma separation:
   (a) by centrifugation;
   (b) by natural sedimentation.
3. Preservation of sample (and its duration):
   (a) at room temperature;
   (b) at $+4$ °C in the refrigerator.
4. Optimal temperature (for testing).
5. Pre-heating of reagents.
6. Pre-incubation of reagents.
7. Evaluation of coagulation endpoint:
   (a) by the eye;
   (b) with a platinum loop;
   (c) with bits of paper;
   (d) with glass beads;
   (e) with automatic recording instruments.
8. Characteristics of thromboplastin:
   (a) commercial;
   (b) prepared in the laboratory;
   (c) optimal time readings.
9. Preparation of curve for calculation of percentages:
   (a) plasma dilution:
       i - with physiological salt solution;
       ii - with adsorbed plasma;
       iii - with buffer;
   (b) characteristics of the curve.
10. Choice of normal plasma:
    (a) pooled normal human plasma;
    (b) standard lyophilized plasma:
        i - commercial;
        ii - prepared in the laboratory.
11. Limits of normal values:
    (a) prothrombin time;
    (b) prothrombin activity.

7.3. *Erythrocyte Enzyme Determinations*

Paul E. Carson, Section of Genetics and International Health, Department of Medicine University of Chicago, Chicago, Illinois, USA *

Erythrocyte enzyme determinations have proven to be of great value in several medical and biological fields and their use has, therefore, become common and widespread throughout the world. They are used in the diagnosis and study of primary and secondary hematological disorders, in metabolic and biochemical investigations, and in genetic studies both of families and of populations.

The modern phase of the use of these determinations probably began with the studies on blood preservation initiated just before and during the second World War, but perhaps the greatest impetus to increased use of these procedures has occurred because of the discovery of specific genetically determined erythrocytic enzyme deficiencies associated with increased hemolytic susceptibility. These are, for the most part, enzymes of carbohydrate metabolism. They can, furthermore, be divided into two groups, clinically as well as biochemically, namely, the enzymes of the pentose phosphate pathway (PPP) and those of the glycolytic pathway of glucose catabolism. The principal distinction between the two pathways appears to be that deficiencies of the PPP render the affected individual susceptible to oxidative hemolysis induced by ingestion of exogenous agents such as fava beans, primaquine and various other drugs whereas deficiencies of the glycolytic pathway present as chronic nonspherocytic hemolytic anemia (CNSHA) without susceptibility to drug induced hemolysis. (This is not an absolute rule as cases of CNSHA can also occur with deficiencies of the PPP; even then, however, the manifestations are worsened by oxidative stresses.) (Carson and Frischer, 1966; Carson, 1968).

The extension of the use of erythrocyte enzyme determinations to metabolic studies is a natural step. For example, alteration of glucose-6-phosphate dehydrogenase (G-6-PD) activity has been reported in thyroid disease and changes in basal metabolic rate in subjects with G-6-PD deficiency have been observed (Powell et al., 1966). Changes in glutathione reductase activity in association with altered carbohydrate metabolism have been found in G-6-PD deficiency, diabetes, during the

---

* On leave at The Galton Laboratory, Department of Human Genetics and Biometry, University College London.

administration of nicotinic acid, and in certain malnourished populations (Carson, 1968).

In genetics there is increased use of red cell enzyme surveys not only to characterize populations for anthropological purposes (Bowman, 1966) but also for ascertaining molecular variants in the search for various polymorphisms (Harris, 1968). Thus, the list of red cell enzymes which are commonly determined is already large and still increasing. The developments which have brought us to this stage have not, however, occurred systematically, having arisen in many different laboratories at various times and there are no generally agreed upon procedures. Therefore, it is often difficult if not impossible to compare erythrocyte enzyme determination from one laboratory to another. From this background a need for standardization of these procedures seems almost self evident and the possibilities as well as the necessary criteria will be examined.

A program for international standardization of erythrocyte enzyme determinations would require the exchange of both normal and abnormal blood samples among several laboratories in all parts of the world. The advent of jet transportation, inexpensive lightweight styrofoam containers, and solutions for the preservation of blood has now made such exchange possible. A preliminary meeting of cooperating investigators would be needed to establish agreement on the protocols and procedures to be used. Where agreement was not reached, experiments could be arranged to resolve the differences. As a basis for such a meeting some help is already available from two previous international agreements. One is the acceptance of the cyanmethemoglobin method for measuring hemoglobin and the other is the definition of the enzyme unit stated by the International Commission on Enzymes.

«One unit (U) of any enzyme is defined as that amount which will catalyze the transformation of 1 micromole of substrate per minute, or, where more than one bond of each substrate molecule is attacked, 1 microequivalent of the group concerned per minute, under defined conditions. The temperature should be stated and it is suggested that where practicable it should be 25 °C. The other conditions including pH and substrate concentration, should, where practicable, be optimal» (1961).

With this basis, let us now be more specific and consider some of the properties of erythrocytes and details of the procedures as they pertain to possible standardization.

Although the normal circulating red cell has no nucleus, it is not simply an inert bag of hemoglobin but an actively metabolizing cell

324

with a finite life span. For practical purposes its enzymes may be divided into two groups — those associated with the membrane and those associated with the cytoplasm, the soluble enzymes (Carson and Tarlov, 1962). The latter vary in activity not only among themselves but also as a function of the age of the red cells. Many of the soluble enzymes are more active in young cells than in old cells. This statement, nevertheless, cannot be made as a generalization. In one series studied in our laboratory, for example, the magnitude of the mean differences in enzyme activity between young and old red cells prepared by differential centrifugation, was pyruvate kinase > G-6-PD > phosphofructokinase > glutathione reductase (Eppes, et al., 1966). Glutathione reductase, in fact, scarcely changes, or may even increase, during normal red cell aging. During reticulocytosis the activities of many of these enzymes may increase several fold, often sufficiently to obscure the diagnosis of an enzyme deficiency.

In addition to the variations associated with cell age the comparative activities of many of the enzymes within a given cell are probably quite different. In hemolysates of normal erythrocytes, for example, the activity of G-6-PD or of pyruvate kinase is many times less than that of glyceraldehyde-3-phosphate dehydrogenase (GA-3-PD) and several hundred times less than that of triose isomerase.

From this discussion, it is evident that even for normal blood, many difficulties lie in the path of achieving standardization of red cell enzyme determinations. These difficulties will, of course, be multiplied for abnormal conditions where significant differences in cell number, age, size, shape and hemoglobin content will have to be taken into account.

Despite these difficulties let us, nevertheless, consider the procedures themselves; the considerations may be divided into three parts, I. the collection and preparation of blood for enzyme assay, II. the conditions of assay, and III. the standards of reference for expression of enzyme activities.

I. *Collection and Preparation of Blood for Enzyme Assay*

A. *Medical Status*

The individuals from whom blood is to be drawn should have complete blood counts including a blood smear and reticulocyte count. A brief statement of medical status even for the healthy normal individuals should be included.

B. *Choice of anticoagulant*

To enable separation of red cells from the plasma and other formed elements of blood an anticoagulant must be used. This should be one which is in universal use, is relatively inexpensive and in which the enzyme activities do not change for at least several days. For this purpose the acid-citrate-dextrose (ACD) solutions used for storage of blood for transfusions are quite adequate. We have found the commercially prepared vacutainer tubes containing ACD especially useful both for collecting and transporting large numbers of blood samples. Prompt and continued refrigeration (but *not* freezing) is necessary until performance of the enzyme determinations. For transportation of the samples we have placed the tubes with ice into lightweight styrofoam containers. When these are properly sealed (with tape) the ice does not melt for 48-72 hours; we have successfully received samples handled in this way from Europe, Asia, and Africa at the University of Chicago.

C. *Separation of red cells*

Centrifugation of blood, removal of the « buffy » coat by aspiration, and subsequent « washing » of the red cells with an isotonic solution and repeated centrifugation is already universal practice. Choice of the washing solution and the number of times of washing will require prior agreement. For routine enzyme assays use of buffered balanced salt solutions with added glucose has not offered any advantages in our hands over inexpensive isotonic NaCl solutions. It is our practice to use a refrigerated centrifuge and cold solutions throughout the preparation for assay. This may not be necessary in all cases but seems advisable especially for standardization by comparison in several laboratories.

D. *Preparation of hemolysate*

The activities of most of the enzymes of present interest are determined in hemolysates. The cells can be hemolyzed after washing by freezing and thawing, by addition of hypotonic solutions (usually water), or by addition of an agent such as saponin. There are relative advantages and disadvantages to each of these and prior agreement on which method of hemolysis to use will be required. Presumably, for universal use, addition of water would be the simplest and most economical method.

E. *Removal of stromata*

After hemolysis the red cell membranes i.e. stromata or « ghosts » remain in the hemolysate. Enzymes e.g. NAD-ase and NAD(P)ase which remain attached to the stromata can under certain conditions alter the activities of at least three cytoplasmic enzymes, G-6-PD, 6-phosphogluconic dehydrogenase and glutathione reductase (Carson et al., 1963; Ajmar et al., 1968). These stromal effects do not interfere with routine assays if refrigeration is maintained during the preparation of hemolysate and if undue time (i.e. several hours) does not elapse before performance of the assay. Interference by turibidity due to stromata depends on the dilution of hemolysate in the final reaction mixture; in fairly concentrated hemolysates turbidity due to stromata can be significant. Removal of stromata requires an additional centrifugation at forces from 9,000 - 20,000 g and, hopefully, could be avoided for routine assays.

II. Conditions of assay

Space does not permit discussion of the specific assay for each enzyme which might be a candidate for inclusion in a program for international standardization. Most of the assays of current interest are spectrophotometric and utilize the change in absorbancy at 340 nm occurring with formation of NADH from NAD or NADPH from NADP, or vice versa. This is because most of the commonly determined enzymes either require or can be coupled to a reaction requiring one or the other of these coenzymes. For these and indeed for most of the enzymes of the red cell the following considerations will apply as indicated by the recommendations of the International Commission on Enzymes.

A. pH

Although a case might be made for using « physiological » pH i.e. 7.3 - 7.5, for all red cell enzymes thus making standardization easier the use of optimum pH does seem to be advisable. Whether or not intracellular pH is 7.3 - 7.5 has not been proven and one is far removed from this criterion at the time of assay. In addition most available data have been obtained using optimum pH's rather than « physiological » pH. Since most pH optima curves for these enzymes are relatively flat, use of optimum pH also allows for some error in buffering. This is especially significant for those enzymes for which the physiological pH range is also the slope of their pH optimum curve. For most of these enzymes, use of pH optima will mean in practice the use of a pH range of approximately 6-9.

B. *Choice of buffers*

Many different buffers have been used by many investigators for assays of many red cell enzymes, i.e. no systematic comparison of buffer effects on red cell enzyme activities has been accomplished. In this instance establishing prior agreement on choice of buffers for a standardization program may require prior experimental comparison of buffer effects in different laboratories. The most spectabular buffer effect of which I am aware is the inhibition of triose isomerase by tris buffer. This buffer, triethanolamine, glycylglycine and phosphate buffers give essentially equivalent results for most of the enzymes of glucose catabolism in the red cell. Triose isomerase, however, which in hemolysates is several hundred times more active than G-6-PD or pyruvate kinase is so markedly inhibited by Tris buffer that to detect its activity in this buffer, it is necessary to use hemolysate concentrations like those used for G-6-PD and pyruvate kinase (Carson, P. E. and Blau, N. unpublished observations).

C. *Temperature*

For any standardization program, the regulation of temperature will be critical. Maintenance within 0.5 °C limits of the 25 °C recommended by the International Commission will require thermostatted devices e.g. circulating water around the cuvette compartments of the spectrophotometer. In many parts of the world, room temperatures may never reach 25 °C; in others it will be above this level is some seasons and below in others. In many areas the variation even during the day is significant. Because some device to regulate the temperature of the assays, will, therefore, be necessary, attention should be called to the advantages of using 37 °C: (1) the increased rate of reaction decreases the time necessary to follow the reaction, (2) to maintain 25 °C requires both a heating and a cooling system whereas since ambient temperatures above 37 °C are rare only a heating system would be necessary, and (3) although similar criticisms as described above (II A) would apply, use of 37 °C would be « physiological » insofar as we know that the cell reactions, take place at or near this temperature *in vivo*. Whatever the eventual choice of temperature for a standardization program, it is likely that the temperature coefficients for each enzyme assay will need to be determined — at least between 20° - 40°C.

D. *Substrates and Coenzymes*

Every investigator in this field has probably had the experience of having previously established normal ranges of enzyme activities sud-

328

denly change with use of a different batch of even the best grade of a chromatographically pure reagent whether obtained commercially from the same or different manufacturers. At present the only way to handle this situation is to be certain to run several assays with both new and old reagents and record the factor of change. For a standardization program it will be necessary initially to obtain enough of given batches of reagents for use in all cooperating laboratories until agreement of data is confirmed; subsequent monitoring of reagents among cooperating laboratories will be required on a regular basis.

The recommendation of the International Commission that optimum substrate concentrations be used is clearly advisable especially for a standardization program. Note should be made, however, that once again this is non-physiological. The actual concentrations of substrates and coenzymes within the red blood cell may be such as to alter the Michaelis-Menten relationships significantly compared to those found with optimal levels of the cofactors (Kirkman, 1968).

III. *Units of activity and standards of reference*

For reporting the units of activity, the recommendation of the International Commission should be followed. The standards of reference, however, continue to present problems. « Haemoglobin has been used as a standard of reference because in the non-nucleated erythrocyte it is present in large amounts, is metabolically inert, and can be accurately determined. However, the enzymatic activities are a function of the cell rather than the hemoglobin and in those instances where there is change in size or shape of the cell, e.g. microcytosis in iron deficiency, or macrocytosis in pernicious anemia, reference to this standard will not give accurate results » (Carson, 1960). Use of the volume of packed cells as a standard of reference is also subject to error. Even if calculation of « trapped » plasma (which varies with the force and time of centrifugation) is neglected the volume will also vary with altered size and shape of the cells. The development of instruments which can be used to count cells accurately and give a quantitative spectrum of the cell sizes offers a rational approach to these problems.

At the stage of preparation of red cells for enzyme assay just prior to hemolysis (i.e. after washing the cells) hemoglobin, cell counts, cell volume and cell size are determined. After hemolysis subsequent dilutions and enzyme assay, the hemoglobin of the final reaction mixture is determined. The enzyme activity can then not only be referred to hemoglobin but also to the cell count (and size). These results could in turn be correlated with the blood indices obtained at the time of drawing the blood. A normal series obtained in this way would then give a rational basis for the study of abnormal hematological conditions. (Determination of hemoglobin in the final reaction mixture has other advantages in that hemolysate dilution errors are eliminated and calibrated pipettes except for the final hemoglobin determination are not required.)

Summary and Conclusions

Erythrocyte enzyme determinations have proven to be of great value in several medical and biological fields and their use has, therefore, become common and widespread throughout the world. The developments which have brought this result did not, however, occur systematically and the methods and procedures presently used vary widely even though it is now apparent that international standardization of these determinations would be of significant value to clinicians and to investigators in several areas of study. Although many difficulties lie in the path of successful international standardization they do not appear to be insurmountable. The recommendation is made, therefore, that an international program for standardization of erythrocyte enzyme determinations should be undertaken.

References

Ajmar, F., Scharrer, B., Hashimoto, F. and Carson, P. E., *Proc. Nat. Acad. Sci.*, *59*, 538, 1968.
Bowman, J. E., International Pathology, *7*, 92, 1966.
Carson, P. E., *Federation Proc.*, *19*, 995, 1960; *Ann. N. Y. Acad. Sci.*, *151*, 2, 765, 1968.
Carson, P. E. and Frischer, H., *Am. J. Med.*, *41*, 744, 1966.
Carson, P. E., Okita, G. T., Frischer, H., Hirasa, J., Long, W. K. and Brewer G. J., *Proc. 9th Congr. Europ. Soc. Haemat.*, Lisbon, Basel - New York S. Karger, p. 655, 1963.
Carson, P. E. and Tarlov, A. R., *Ann. Rev. Med.*, *13*, 105, 1962.
Eppes, R. B., McNamara, J. V., Powell, R. D. and Carson, P. E., *J. Clin. Invest.*, *45*, 1005, 1966.
Harris, H., *Brit. Med. J.*, 2, 135, 1968.
Kirkman, H. N., *Ann. N. Y. Acad. Sci.*, *151*, 2, 753, 1968.
Powell, R. D., Brewer, G. J., De Gowin, R. L. and Carson, P. E., *Mil. Med.*, *9*, Supplement, 131, 1039, 1966.
Report of the Commission on Enzymes of the Int. Union of Biochem., Oxford, Pergamon Press, 1961.

Contribution number 528 from the U. S. Army Malaria Research Program. This work was supported by U. S. Public Health Service Grant HE-06078 and by U. S. Army contracts DA-49-193-MD-2413 and DA-49-007-968. Paul E. Carson is a Research and Career Development Awardee of the United States Public Health Service.

8th Session

Chairmen: P. De Nicola, S. M. Lewis, A. Giordano

8.1. *The Methemoglobin Reduction Test: A Valuable Screening Method for the Detection of G-6-PD Deficiency in the Red Cells Supported by U.S. Army Through its European Research Office*
E. Salvidio and I. Pannacciulli, Istituto Scientifico di Medicina Interna (Cattedra di Clinica Medica e Cattedra di Ematologia) Università di Genova, Italy

In order to evaluate the occurrence of G-6-PD deficiency, clinical criteria are not sufficient and some morphologic and chemical methods may be relatively insensitive. G-6-PD deficiency of the red cells may remain hidden for life if hemolytic drugs or vegetals are never administered to the sensitive subjects.

Several screening methods have been developed, but some of them have become obsolete either for lack of sensitivity in the detection of heterozygotes (GSH stability, Brilliant Cresyl Blue test) or for difficulties in standardization (Heinz body formation) [1, 2, 3].

The direct quantitation of G-6-PD activity in the red cells requires specialized equipment not available in all hematological laboratories, and expensive reagents. This procedure, according to some investigators [4, 2, 5], is not always suitable for the detection of female heterozygotes.

Some 8 years ago Brewer and associates [6] worked out the methemoglobin reduction test which has in general proved to be simple, sensitive, reliable, and easy to standardize.

The original methemoglobin reduction test introduced by Brewer et al. can be summarized as follows: to 2 ml of blood, freshly collected in ACD, 0.1 ml of a 0.18 M sodium nitrite solution and 0.1 ml of a 0.0004 M methylene blue solution are separately added. After 12 gentle inversions, the test tubes are incubated at 37 °C in a water-bath. At 60 and 120 minutes the blood is mixed by blowing one breath of air gently through a 0.1 ml pipette. At 180 minutes 0.1 ml of the red cells are hemolyzed in 10 ml of 0.02 M phosphate buffer (pH 6.6) and photometric readings of the remaining methemoglobin before and after the addition of a drop of 0.4 M sodium cyanide are taken at 640 nm.

The total Hb in the same sample is determined by transferring 2 ml of the hemolysate to 8 ml of 0.05 M phosphate buffer (pH 6.6): one drop of 0.6 M potassium ferricyanide and one drop of 0.4 M sodium cyanide are added to this second solution and the readings are taken at 540 nm.

The large-scale use of the methemoglobin reduction test has brought out some disavantages [7, 3] which can be listed as follows:

1. preparation of too many solutions;
2. instability of the sodium nitrite solution;
3. short storage period of the methylene blue solution;
4. the separate pipetting of the sodium nitrite and methylene blue solutions, which is time-consuming if a large number of samples has to be tested.

In order to overcome these disadvantages, we introduced some minor modifications to Brewer's test [8], which do not impair the high sensitivity of the original method.

(1) Sodium nitrite in distilled water and methylene blue in a sodium chloride solution are pipetted into dark-glass vials of 5 ml capacity, lyophilized, filled with nitrogen, and sealed. At the end of the lyophilizing procedure each vial contains 0.374 mg of methylene blue, 33 mg of sodium nitrite, and 20.25 mg of sodium chloride. The vials, kept in the dark, can be stored for several years without alterations in the activity of the reagents. Immediately before use the content of each vial is dissolved into exactly 5 ml of distilled water, and 0.1 ml of this solution is pipetted into the test tube containing 1 ml of blood.

(2) The amount of both buffer solutions necessary for the methemoglobin and hemoglobin readings is reduced respectively to 5 ml and 4 ml; 0.1 ml of blood is transferred from the test tube to the first buffer solution and 1.0 ml of the hemolysate is transferred to the second buffer solution.

Table I shows that the sensitivity and reliability of Brewer's methemoglobin reduction test are not altered by our modifications.

Table 1

	Number of case	MetHb as percent of total Hb mean values		^{2} for paired samples
		Brewer's method	modified vial method	
Normal subjects	57	3.72	3.63	0.0004 (n.s.)
Mutant subjects	58	62.40	63.58	0.41 (n.s.)

With these minor modifications the test is time-saving particularly in screening of a large number of samples. With an appropriate schedule of several batches we can perform the « clinical test » in more than 100 cases in a single working day.

5412 Italians were screened by means of the methemoglobin reduction test. Mean normal value of remaining methemoglobin % in 5019 samples was 4.10 % (ranging from 0 to 7 %). 393 samples showed a positive methemoglobin reduction test. Among males, no subject with a positive methemoglobin reduction test had G-6-PD activity values higher than 3 U/g/Hb/'; a few had values ranging from 1 to 3 U; the greatest number showed values below 1 U/g/Hb/'.

In these cases the remaining methemoglobin ranged from 60 to 99 %.

In females with a positive methemoglobin reduction, the values of remaining methemoglobin ranged from 20 to 90 %.

The mean G-6-PD activity was 55 % of the norm, with a wide range. Some cases showed an overlapping with the normal values of G-6-PD.

The erythrocytes of these subjects had a normal G-6-PD activity and a positive MetHb test; but when they were tagged with Cr^{51} and tested in vivo with primaquin, they were destroyed [9].

This discrepancy between a positive methemoglobin test and a normal G-6-PD activity can be explained if the theory of mosaicism is accepted. In fact it is thought that erythrocytes of female heterozygotes may be a mixture of normal red cells and G-6-PD-deficient ones. Therefore if one measures the G-6-PD activity in the hemolysate of a heterozygote, the enzyme level assayed reflects the level of the red cell population as a whole, and may give normal values. Also if the mixture is composed of a relatively high percentage of abnormal cells and a smaller percentage of cells with high G-6-PD activity, the end results of the G-6-PD determination may be in the normal range. The methemoglobin reduction test, instead, is based on the reduction of methemoglobin to hemoglobin by individual red cells. If a fraction of a population is G-6-PD-

deficient, the remaining methemoglobin will be higher than normal [2].
From all the above it follows that the methemoglobin reduction test
allows to detect the highest percentage of female heterozygotes [2].
Finally, this test is extremely reliable in detecting hemizygous males.
For a proper standardization the following recommendations should
be borne in mind:

1. Inosine should be added to the ACD solution if the methemoglobin
   reduction test is to be delayed for more than a few days;
2. Blood of anemic patients should be readjusted to normal values
   of hematocrit in order to avoid false positive results;
3. Lyophylized reagents should be used in order to insure stability of
   the solutions of sodium nitrite and methylene blue.

References

[1] Motulsky, A. G., « Theoretical and Clinical Problem of Glucose-6-Phosphate Dehy-
    drogenase Deficiency », *Abnormal Haemoglobins in Africa: A Symposium F. A.
    Davis Co.*, Philadelphia P. A., 1965.
[2] Stanatoyannopoulos, G., Papayannopoulou, Th., Bakopoulos, Chr. and Motulsky,
    A. G., « Detection of G-6-PD Deficient Heterozygotes », *Blood, 29*, 87, 1967.
[3] Salvidio, E., Pannacciulli, I. and Tizianello A., « Evaluation expérimentale de
    quelques méthodes biochimiques permettant de déceler la succeptibilité à l'émolyse
    due aux médicaments », *Nouv. Rev. franç. Hémat., 3*, 233, 1963.
[4] Alving, A. S., Kellermeyer, R. W., Tarlov, A., Schrier, S. and Carson, P. E.,
    « Biochemical and Genetic Aspects of Primaquine-sensitive Hemolytic Anemia »,
    Ann. int. Med., 49, 240, 1958.
[5] Salvidio, E., Pannacciulli, I. and Tizianello, A., « Studium über die Medikamenten-
    sensibilitaet der italiener Mittels dem Test der Methaemoglobinreduktion nach Brewer
    und Mitarbestern », *Proc. of VIII Congress of Europëan Soc. Hemat. Wien, 1961,*
    2 vol., Karger édit. Bâle, vol. II, 319, 1962.
[6] Brewer, G. J., Tarlov, A. K. and Alving, A. S., « Methemoglobin Reduction Test:
    A New Simple in Vitro Test for Identifying Primaquine Sensitivity », *Bull. World
    Health Ass., 22*, 633, 1960.
[7] Fairbanks, V. F. and Beutler, E., « A Simple Method for Detection of Erythrocyte
    Glucose-6-Phosphate Dehydrogenase Deficiency (G-6-PD Spot Test) », *Blood, 20*,
    591, 1962.
[8] Tizianello, A., Pannacciulli, I. and Salvidio, E., « A Simplified Procedure for
    Brewer's Methemoglobin Reduction Test », *Acta haemat., 35*, 176, 1966.

8.2. *Diagnostic Tests for Thalassemias*

G. Sansone, Pediatric Hospital « S. Filippo » of the
« Ospedali Galliera », Genova, Italy

The problem of standardizing laboratory methods for the diagnosis
of thalassemia has been raised by several investigators at various meetings
and congresses. The need for such standardization cannot be overstated,

334

since according to recent calculations there are about two million carriers of this defect in Italy alone.

But the whole problem has become quite involved from the moment it was shown that thalassemia is in reality a heterogenous rather than unitary disease entity. We must make a distinction today between alpha and beta thalassemia; and in beta thalassemia we must distinguish between typical and atypical forms (beta-delta thalassemia, with normal hemoglobin A_2 and with increased or normal hemoglobin F).

Obviously the problem, as seen from our point of view, is urgent with regard to heterozygous beta thalassemia and not urgent for the homozygous form (*thalassemia major* or Cooley's disease), with the exception of the rare atypical cases of *thalassemia intermedia* and those with double heterozygosis.

There are essentially two common occurrences in which the diagnosis of heterozygous thalassemia is concerned: one is the screening of populations, and the other is the study of individual patients or separate family groups. The methodology involved differs radically in the two situations.

Methods for Population Screening

For obvious practical reasons, methods employed for the screening of whole populations must be simplified as much as possible. It is difficult to secure sufficient amounts of blood taken from the veins: so we must make do with small specimens obtained from a stab wound in the finger. Two tests are essential in mass screening, namely (a) the test of maximal osmotic resistance, with a single pipette and 0.40% Simmel solution, and (b) testing for alterations of erythrocyte morphology as evinced by conventional blood smears. To these two tests we might add the test of acid denaturation on smears according to Kleihauer, which in our experience offers some additonal information of a certain value.

Needless to say, these simplified tests require the utmost care and experience from the responsible operator, precisely because they are simplified.

Now, according to the policy above we have screened several hundred thousand subjects in Italy, in a program of mass investigation that may be regarded as unique. But no matter how careful and accurate we try to be in this work, obviously some of the carriers remain undetected—though probably not many. Now, failure of detecting carriers is not nearly so important in mass screening as it is in individual cases: suffice it to mention the ethical implications, for instance, in marriage counsel.

Methods for Individual Investigation

The minimal program for individual assessment comprises (a) the study of osmotic resistances; (b) complete hemochromometry including hemoglobin assay, RBC count, erythrocyte morphology, a search for RBCs with a basophilic stippling, and the hematocrit value. An *in vitro* search for intra-erythrocytary inclusions with brilliant cresyl blue is also recommended; and (c) biochemical tests such as assay of hemoglobin A_2, hemoglobin F, and blood iron.

Some Comments on the Various Tests

Osmotic Resistances. It is surprising to see how the results of this test still vary from one laboratory to another. In Italy we have used in the past the method of Viola, which gives acceptable results if correctly performed. In many cases, however, one fails to specify whether the maximal resistance is determined macroscopically or microscopically. Dacie's method has gained increased acceptance in hematological laboratories; the results are satisfactory also in our own experience. Hopefully the use of the « fragilograph » will simplify this important basic test.

Hemochromometry. An important parameter for the diagnosis of heterozygous thalassemia is the determination of mean corpuscular hemoglobin. To obtain reliable results it is indispensable to assay hemoglobin by the method of cyanmethemoglobin, and to count red blood cells with an electronic counter.

Another important parameter is true microcytosis (microvolumnia), which implies the standardization of hematocrit technics. With regard to the evaluation of morphological alterations in the erythrocytes, experience is a major requisite. Smears with slight but significant alterations are often wrongly tagged « normal ». A rather obvious but surely needed remark is that one should first of all learn to make perfect blood smears—a virtue far less common than one would believe.

Biochemical Tests. The assay of hemoglobin A_2 is fundamental. There are various methods available, roughly divided into chromatographic and electrophoretic methods. Concerning the latter, it would be desirable to reach a general agreement on the choice between paper electrophoresis and electrophoresis on starch, starch gel, cellulose acetate, polyacrylamide, and so on. It would be desirable to give preference to a relatively simple method that would at the same time give a precise quantitative assay of this lesser hemoglobin fraction. For quantitation, we are still relying on starch block electrophoresis.

The study of hemoglobin F is also important, particularly in the rare cases in which the levels of hemoglobin A_2 are normal. For many years the one-minute Singer method has been in general use, but the results are not very accurate because hemoglobin F occurs in small concentrations. Accordingly, Jonxis and Visser have proposed a modification of this method. Excellent separation of hemoglobin F can be obtained by agar gel electrophoresis.

The assay of iron in the blood plasma may contribute valuable diagnostic information: hypersideremia is an element in favor of a positive diagnosis of thalassemia; conversely, hyposideremia may account for cases of pseudothalassemia (nonspecific alterations of erythrocyte morphology and increased osmotic resistances); this is particularly true in the case of small children.

Early (Neonatal) Diagnosis of Thalassemia

A separate problem is that of recognizing thalassemia in the newborn baby; for several reasons, this is far more important with regard to *thalassemia major*. In two cases we have been able to make a very early diagnosis by starting our work with blood from the umbilical cord. The methods are the classical ones repeated serially over the first several weeks of life; to these, one may add examinations of the bone marrow (testing for PAS-positivity and for Fessa's inclusion bodies). Recently, interesting results were reported from studies of the synthesis of beta chains with labeled aminoacids.

No consistent data are yet available on the diagnosis of heterozygous thalassemia at birth. We believe that much is to be gained by the study of fractional erythrocyte populations.

Diagnosis of Thalassemia Major in Multitransfused Patients

Multiple transfusions given to children before making a definite diagnosis sometimes interferes with diagnosis itself. If the patient was over-transfused, and there is a secondary aplasia of the bone marrow, diagnosis will be quite impossible and must be postponed. In the absence of erythroblastic aplasia of the bone marrow, bone marrow studies are of great assistance.

This study may be carried out both with current staining methods, which afford accurate examination of erythroblast morphology, and with special staining methods, such as Hotchkiss's method for the detection of PAS-positivity in the erythroblasts, and methyl violet staining for the detection of Fessas's inclusions.

From what I have just said it is apparent that standardization is badly needed, particularly in methods that are indispensable for diagnosis. Recognition of carriers should always be possible, even though some cases may be difficult to handle and additional investigations may be in order. In doubtful cases, one should never confine oneself to examining the given subject: the investigation should include as many of the subject's kin as feasible.

In conclusion, and with due allowance for shadings and special problems, the same need for refinement and standardization of laboratory methods exists in regard to thalassemia as it obtains in the case of all other diseases of the erythrocytes.

8.3. Blood Group Determination Procedures
K.L.G. Goldsmith, W.H.O. International Blood Group Reference Laboratory, London, England

An error occurring in a Blood Transfusion Laboratory can easily result in the death of the recipient of a transfusion. It is essential, therefore, that all tests are meticulously performed, that the results are correctly interpreted and that the findings are correctly recorded. It is important to remember that more deaths due to mismatched blood transfusion are the result of clerical error than due to mistakes in practical serology.

In this paper the determination of ABO and Rh blood groups of patients and of blood donors will be considered beginning with regulations for the preparation of grouping sera. Specifications for the latter will be based on those laid down in the European Agreement on the Exchanges of Blood-Grouping Reagents [1].

Anti-A of human origin must be tested for potency and for specificity. It should be titrated separately against suspensions of A_1, A_2 and $A_2 B$ corpuscles in parallel with the reconstituted but undiluted International Standard Preparation of Anti-A blood-grouping serum [2] or an equivalent reference preparation. The potency of the serum shall in each case be not less than 64 International Units per ml. The avidity of the anti-A serum is determined by mixing it on a slide with an equal volume of a 5% to 10% suspension of A_1, A_2 and $A_2 B$ corpuscles, when agglutination of each suspension should first appear in not more than twice the time taken when the reference anti-A preparation is used with the same cell suspension.

Tests for specificity of the anti-A grouping serum are also essential.

In the British Blood Group Reference Laboratory all batches of the reagent are tested to exclude the presence of anti-B, —M, —N, —S, —s, —Mi^a, —V^w, —P, —P$_1$, —C, —c, —C^w, —D, —E, —e, —Lu^a, —Lu^b, —K, —k, —Fy^a, —Fy^b, —Jk^a, —Jk^b, —Xg^a and —Wr^a. In addition the reagents are shown to be free of antibodies to Gm antigens.

Anti-B must be similarly tested with appropriate red cells, in parallel with the International Standard Preparation of anti-B blood grouping serum [2] or a similar reference preparation for potency, avidity and specificity.

Anti-A$_1$ and *Anti-A + Anti-B (Group 0 Serum)* must be equally exhaustively tested though international reference preparations do not exist for these preparations. The anti-A + anti-B should be chosen so that it will agglutinate A$_x$ cells.

Rh Grouping Sera, whatever their specificity may be either « complete » or « incomplete ». « Complete » anti-D should have a titre of not less than 32 against CcDee red cells in saline suspension. « Incomplete » anti-D in tested against CcDee corpuscles in albumin suspension in parallel with the International Standard Preparation of « Incomplete » anti-D (anti-Rh$_o$) [3] or equivalent reference preparation, and shall have a potency of not less than 32 International Units. Anti-D sera to be used for slide tests must also be examined for avidity just as are anti-A and anti-B. As with anti-A and anti-B, no unwanted antibodies may be present.

All grouping reagents must be free of haemolytic properties, bacterial products, pseudo-agglutinins and prozone phenomena. All reagents must be issued with precise instructions for their use and these must always be followed.

International Standards for anti-A, anti-B and for « incomplete » anti-D blood typing sera, prepared at the request of the World Health Organization, are held by the Department of Biological Standards, State Serum Institute, Copenhagen. Only limited quantities are available but they may be obtained for the standardization of National Standard Preparations for these three antibodies.

Performance of grouping tests

ABO grouping should be performed by checking the presence of antigens on the red cells and of the agglutinins in the serum of the specimens. Adequate controls must be used throughout. Whatever technique is used, be it tube or slide, it must be so performed so that apparent negative results can be checked by microscopical examination. Different people have different ideas on the techniques to be used, but it is intended here to lay down minimum criteria and the techniques which are to be described are put forward as examples of these basic requirements. The layout of a block for ABO agglutinogen tests is shown in Figure 1.

In addition, this figure shows the distribution of positive and negative results that may be seen. Note particularly the layout of control cells, the strong A_1 antigen excluding the presence of anti-A in the anti-B grouping serum while A_2 cells are used to check that anti-A and anti-A + anti-B are potent. The latter serum is particularly useful in detecting cells carrying weak forms of A antigen. Anti-A_1 has not been used to determine the $A_1 A_2$ status of A and A B cells but this may be done if desired. The unknown samples appear to be O, A, B and AB, these findings being confirmed when the next block is examined for the presence of agglutinins in the serum samples. Details are shown in Figure 2.

Note the use of not only Group A_1 and Group B cells to check for the presence of anti-A and anti-B but also of Group O cells which are used as a negative control to check that another antibody, pseudo-agglutinin or rouleaux maker in the serum samples is not the cause of the agglutination of the Group A_1 and B cells.

Rh grouping. Potential recipients of blood transfusion should be grouped with anti-D serum. Two such anti-D sera should preferably be used in parallel and the tests with each antiserum may be set up as in Figure 3.

Again notice the presence of positive and negative controls. All cells which react as apparently Rh-negative in this test must be further tested for the presence of the D^u antigen.

Rh grouping of all blood donors must be performed with at least anti-C, -D and anti-E and each serum must be adequately controlled with appropriate cells for positive and negative controls. In the case of positive controls, every effort should be made to use cells that are heterozygous for the antigen in question. The presence of the D^u antigen must be sought in all who are apparently D-negative.

In other cases, including the determination of the probable Rh-genotype, anti-C and anti-E may well have to be used, but the principles are the same, and the use of adequate controls is essential.

The problems involved have been considered only in outline and the suggestions made are minimum requirements. Many will already be doing all that has been suggested, but there is room for improvement in some of the world's laboratories. Only by education of those who fall behind and bringing to their notice these basic rules can the standard of blood group serology be raised.

Figure 1 - *ABO agglutinogen block.*

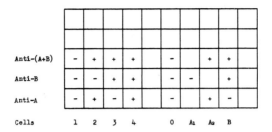

Anti-(A+B)	-	+	+	+		-		+	+
Anti-B	-	-	+	+		-	-		+
Anti-A	-	+	-	+		-		+	-
Cells	1	2	3	4		0	A₁	A₂	B

Figure 2

ABO AGGLUTININ BLOCK

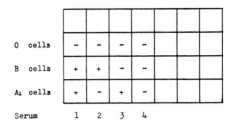

0 cells	-	-	-	-
B cells	+	+	-	-
A₁ cells	+	-	+	-
Serum	1	2	3	4

Figure 3

Rh(D) TYPING BLOCK

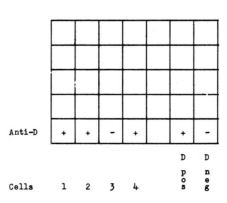

Anti-D	+	+	-	+		+	-
Cells	1	2	3	4		D pos	D neg

341

In conclusion, it should be remembered that problems concerning blood group serology, including the obtaining of an independent opinion on blood grouping reagents, should be first referred to one's own National Blood Group Reference Laboratory. This laboratory may in turn refer problems to the W.H.O. International Blood Group Reference Laboratory in London, England.

References

[1] Council of Europe, *European Treaty Series No. 39*, 1968.
[2] Miles, A. A., *Bull. World Health Org.*, 3, 301, 1950.
[3] Goldsmith, K. L. G., Mourant, A. E. and Bangham, D. R., *Bull. Wld. Hlth. Org.*, 36, 435, 1967.

8.4. The Routine Detection of Erythrocyte and Leucocyte Isoantibodies

G. Sirchia, F. Mercuriali and S. Ferrone, Institute of Medical Pathology, University of Milan, Italy

The hospital blood transfusion service is faced with an increasing demand for tests for the detection of abnormal red blood cell isoantibodies. This investigation is now strongly recommended as a routine procedure for every pregnant woman (Giblett, 1964; Hanson and Rutkowski, 1964; Pirofsky, 1965; Allen et al., 1967; Smith et al., 1967; Bowman, 1968), for the recipients of blood transfusion (Grove-Rasmussen, 1964; Kissmeyer-Nielsen, 1965; Iammarino, 1966) and for blood donors (Zettner and Bove, 1963; Myhre et al., 1965; Iammarino, 1966; Franciosi et al., 1967). Moreover, the major cross-match, that is the indispensable preliminary to every blood transfusion, is also an antibody detection procedure, in which the recipient's serum is allowed to react with the donor's red cells. Therefore the laboratory must carry out each day a large number of investigations. Moreover, every search for antibody must include at least 2 or 3 tests, since it is known that no single technique is sufficient to detect all the clinically significant antibodies (Griffitts and Schmidt, 1962; Kissmeyer-Nielsen, 1965; A.A.B.B., 1966; Tovey and Jenkins, 1967). The practical importance of the choice of the type and number of tests, as well as the continuous effort to find safe, simple and rapid tests is therefore easily understood. Different procedures have been developed, but still no single one can be considered fully satisfactory from a clinical standpoint (see Rosenfield, 1966).

342

In our laboratory a five-tube procedure has been in use for a number of years (Fig. 1).

In the first tube are placed 2 drops of the fresh serum to be tested, together with 2 drops of 22% bovine albumin; the same mixture, in half volume, is employed in the second tube. One drop of serum is put in the 3rd and 4th tubes and one drop of serum plus one drop of bromelin in tube No. 5. To each tube is then added a 5% saline suspension of red cells, equal in volume to that of the serum being tested. Tubes Nos. 4 and 5 are left for 1 hour at room temperature (approximately 20 °C), while the first 3 tubes are incubated for 30 to 60 minutes in a waterbath at 37 °C. At the end of the incubation period all the tubes, except the first, are examined for haemolysis (naked eye) and/or for agglutination (microscope-100x). If no agglutination is found in tubes Nos. 2 and/or 3, the antiglobulin test with immediate centrifugation is carried out with tube No. 1, using a broad-spectrum reagent.

If needed, the time required for this procedure may be shortened by carrying out the immediate centrifugation of tubes Nos. 4 and 5 and the centrifugation of tubes Nos. 2 and 3 after only a 15 minute incubation, that is sufficient also for the antiglobulin test.

The type of red cells used in the test will obviously vary according to the purpose of the test itself: red cells of the potential blood donor in the case of the cross-match, red cells carrying all the clinically significant antigens in the other cases. In the case of pregnant women, the husband's red cells may be used if ABO-compatible.

The described procedure is in fact a combination of 5 different tests: saline test at 20 °C and 37 °C, haemolysin detection test, albumin test, enzyme test and antiglobulin test « sensitized » with albumin (Griffitts et al., 1964; Stroup and Mac Ilroy, 1965; Clayton et al., 1965). Moreover, it allows microscopic reading of the agglutination, that, in our opinion, is definitely helpful.

The above procedure does not claim to be fully satisfactory. In fact, it is not one of the simplest. Furthermore, it makes use of bromelin instead of other proteolytic enzymes such as papain, preferred by some Authors (Kissmeyer-Nielsen, 1965). However, regarding this latter point it must be remembered that enzyme tests are usually considered as auxiliary tests (Croucher, 1966; A.A.B.B., 1966) because of their limitations. In fact enzyme tests are very sensitive to the presence of cold antibodies of little or no clinical significance (Mollison, 1967; Tovey and Jenkins, 1967), and, on the other hand, enzymes may not detect antibodies of the Duffy, MNSs and Kell systems (see Morton, 1962; Sacchi

Figure 1 - *Five-tube procedure for erythrocyte isoantibody detection.*

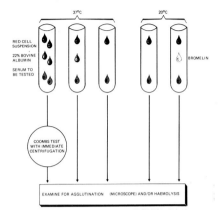

Figure 2 - *Procedure for leucocyte cytotoxic isoantibody detection.*

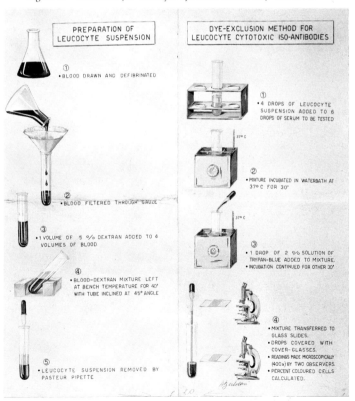

344

et al., 1967). Bearing this in mind, the easy-to-do one-stage bromelin test has been preferred in our laboratory to other more complicated enzyme tests.

Another point that may be discussed is the albumin test. In discussing this test, one must consider concentration of bovine albumin (Jones, 1964; Pollack, 1964; Hossaini, 1966), the technique used to perform the test [the layering technique might be preferable (Dodge, 1952)] and the possible advantage of using instead a mixture of albumin-inert AB serum (Stratton and Diamond, 1955).

The five-tube procedure described above can be considered as a combination of 3 fundamental tests (Coombs test, saline test at 20 °C and 37 °C and detection of haemolysins) and 2 auxiliary tests (albumin test and enzyme test). While it is not a perfect technique, in our opinion it balances perfection and practicability.

In addition to the routine detection of red cell isoantibodies, it may be expected that the routine detection of leucocyte isoantibodies will in a short time become another task of the blood transfusion service. In fact, leucocyte isoantibodies are known to occur frequently after pregnancy (see Jensen, 1966; Ferrone et al., 1968) and blood transfusion (see Engelfriet, 1966; Cabibbo and Brunetti, 1968) and to be the cause of non-haemolytic transfusion reaction (see Engelfriet, 1966; Perkins et al., 1966; Cabibbo and Brunetti, 1968). Different serologic types of these antibodies have been found, and different techniques developed for their detection (see Lalezari, 1966; Curtoni and Mattiuz, 1967; Ferrone et al., 1968). No single technique is sufficient to detect all types of antibodies (Engelfriet, 1966; Bodmer et al., 1966; Payne et al., 1967).

According to the literature (Engelfriet, 1966), and in our own experience, cytotoxic tests appear to be the most suitable from the clinical standpoint. Several variations of cytotoxic tests are now extensively used for leucocyte typing (see Curtoni and Mattiuz, 1967; Ferrone et al., 1968). Among these, the dye-exclusion (trypan-blue) technique described by Engelfriet et al. (Engelfriet and Eijsvoogel, 1965; Engelfriet and Britten, 1966) appears to meet the routine requirements of the blood transfusion service.

The test is based on the property of damaged leucocytes to assume the dye becoming coloured, while living cells do not. The procedure is carried out as follows (Fig. 2):

Leucocyte suspensions are prepared from defibrinated blood by the dextran sedimentation method immediately before use. Six drops of fresh serum to be tested are incubated with 4 drops of leucocyte suspension for 30 minutes in a waterbath at 37 °C. After a 30 minute incubat-

ion, 1 drop of 2% solution of trypan-blue in distilled water is added
to the leucocyte-serum mixture and the incubation is prolonged for a
further 30 minutes. At the end of the incubation period, the leucocytes
are gently resuspended and the percentage of coloured cells is determined microscopically. Each sample of serum to be tested must be
challenged with the leucocytes from at least 5 different normal donors,
possibly carrying most of the known leucocyte antigens.
Proper positive and negative controls must be performed simultaneously. Moreover, since it has been demonstrated that a prozone
phenomenon can occur in cytotoxic reactions (Terasaki and McClelland, 1963; Walford et al., 1965; Ferrone et al., 1967), in our laboratory
we screen the sera for cytotoxic antibodies using the serum to be tested
both undiluted and diluted 1/4 in fresh normal serum.
The test shows good reproducibility, in our hands 88%. Other
investigators, using pure lymphocyte suspensions and selected antisera,
have reported even higher figures (Dausset et al., 1966; Peacocke et
al., 1966).
From the practical point of view, it is important that the serum to
be tested be fresh or properly stored, in order, not only to ensure the
presence of complement, but particularly to avoid the development of
anticomplementary activity. Ferrone et al. (1967) have in fact shown that
anticomplementary factors can hamper cytotoxic reactions and be the
cause of false negative results.
The dye-exclusion technique can be recommended because of its
sensitivity, reproducibility, simplicity and rapidity. According to Engelfriet (1967) and ourselves, its use, in addition to a test for the detection
of leucoagglutinins, should prove satisfactory for clinical purposes. The
choice of the second test, however, is open to discussion, since it is not
as yet clear to what extent different tests detect different types of
antibodies (see van Rood and Eernisse, 1968).
In summary, simple and reliable techniques for erythrocyte and
leucocyte isoantibody detection are available at present. There is much
to be said for making them part of the routine work of every blood
transfusion laboratory.

References

American Association of Blood Banks (A.A.B.B.), *Technical Methods and Procedures,* 4th edn., 1966.
Allen, S. T., Dubner, M. S. and Mockler, N. D., *Am. J. Obst. Gynec.,* 99, 274, 1967.
Bodmer, J., Bodmer, W. F., Payne, R., Terasaki, P. I. and Vredevoe, D., *Nature, 210,* 28, 1966.
Bowman, H. S., *Am. J. Obst. Gynec., 101,* 614, 1968.
Cabibbo, S. and Brunetti, M., *Rec. Progr. Med., 44,* 435, 1968.

346

Clayton, E. M., Brown, R. B. and Bove, J. R., *Transfusion*, 5, 344, 1965.
Croucher, B. E. E., *Canad. J. med. Technol.*, 28, 133, 1966.
Curtoni, E. S. and Mattiuz, P. L., *La trasfusione del sangue*, 12, 205, 1967.
Dausset, J., Ivanyi, P. and Feingold, N., *Ann. N.Y. Acad. Sci.*, 129, 386, 1966.
Dodge, O. G., *J. clin. Path.*, 5, 102, 1952.
Engelfriet, C. P., *Cytotoxic isoantibodies against leucocytes*, Thesis, Amsterdam, 1966; personal communication, 1967.
Engelfriet, C. P. and Britten, A., *Vox Sang.*, 11, 334, 1966.
Engelfriet, C. P. and Eijsvoogel V. P., *Vox Sang.*, 10, 228, 1965.
Ferrone, S., Sirchia, G., Farina, C. and Dambrosio, F., *Ricerca Clin. Lab.*, in press.
Ferrone, S., Sirchia, G., Farina, C. and Dambrosio, F., *Ricerca Clin. Lab.*, 7, 56, 1968. Copenhagen, 1967, p. 357.
Franciosi, R. A., Awer, E. and Santana, M., *Transfusion*, 7, 297, 1967.
Giblett, E. R., *Clin. Obst. & Gynec.*, 7, 1044, 1964.
Griffitts, J. J. and Schmidt, R. P., *Transfusion*, 2, 385, 1962.
Griffitts, J. J., Frank, S. and Schmidt, R. P., *Transfusion*, 4, 461, 1964.
Grove-Rasmussen, M., *Transfusion*, 4, 200, 1964.
Hanson, D. J. and Rutkowski, I., *Presented as an exhibit*, A.A.B.B. Annual Convention, Washington, D. C., 1964.
Hossaini, A. A., *Am. J. clin. Path.*, 45, 348, 1966.
Iammarino, R. M., *Am. J. clin. Path.*, 46, 573, 1966.
Jensen, K. G., *Leucocyte Antibodies and Pregnancy. A Survey*, Munksgaard, Copenhagen, 1966.
Jones, A. R., *Transfusion*, 4, 481, 1964.
Kissmeyer-Nielsen, F., *Scand. J. Haemat.*, 2, 331, 1965.
Lalezari, P., *Seminars Hemat.*, 3, 87, 1966.
Melief, C. J. M., van der Hart, M., Engelfriet, C. P. and van Loghem, J. J., *Vox Sang.*, 12, 374, 1967.
Mollison, P. L., *Blood Transfusion in Clinical Medicine*, 4th edn., Blackwell Scientific Publications, Oxford and Edinburgh, 1967, p. 417.
Morton, J. A., *Brit. J. Haemat.*, 8, 134, 1962.
Myhre, B. A., Greenwalt, T. J. and Gajewski, M., *Transfusion*, 5, 350, 1965.
Payne, R., Bodmer, W. F., Troup, G. M. and Walford, R. L., *Transplantation*, 5, 597, 1967.
Peacocke, I., Amons, B. and Laszlo, J., *Blood*, 28, 665, 1966.
Perkins, H. A., Payne, R., Ferguson, J. and Wood, M., *Vox Sang.*, 11, 578, 1966.
Pirofsky, B., *Am. J. Obst. Gynec.*, 92, 720, 1965.
Pollack, W., *Transfusion*, 4, 481, 1964.
Rood van, J. J. and Eernisse, J. G., *Seminars Hemat.*, 5, 187, 1968.
Rosenfield, R. E., *Med. Clin. N. Amer.*, 50, 1643, 1966.
Sacchi, R., Reali, G. and Sermasi, G., *La trasfusione del sangue*, 12, 1, 1967.
Smith, B. D., Haber, J. M. and Queenan, J. T., *Obst. & Gynec.*, 29, 118, 1967.
Stratton, G. and Diamond, E. R., *J. clin. Path.*, 8, 218, 1955.
Stroup, M. and Mac Ilroy, M., *Transfusion*, 5, 184, 1965.
Terasaki, P. I. and McClelland, J. D., *J. exp. Med.*, 117, 675, 1963.
Tovey, G. H. and Jenkins, W. J., *Association of Clinical Pathologists*, Broadsheet 57, 1967.
Walford, R. L., Gallagher, R. and Troup, G. M., *Transplantation*, 3, 387, 1965.
Zettner, A. and Bove, J., *Transfusion*, 3, 48, 1963.

8.5. *Closing Remarks*
S. M. Lewis, Secretary of ICSH

As Chairman of this session my next duty is the sad one of ending the symposium. It is customary for the Chairman to review the proceedings of such a meeting, but we have had such an intensive meeting with so wide a range of different subjects that it would require a further two days to do this adequately. But the proceedings will give us all an opportunity to remember the papers and the discussions which were stimulated by them. There have been many new ideas and facts offered to us and we go home with this stimulus for further research and study.

ICSH is proud to have been associated with a symposium of the high standard we have had. We hope that there will be an opportunity for another symposium of a similar type, with the same collaboration we have here enjoyed, in order that we may see how the ideas formulated in this meeting will have developed and to review the advances in standardization which will surely follow. Even more important, another symposium will give us the happy opportunity of meeting again with our Italian friends to whom we owe thanks for a warm hospitality and a most memorable visit to Milan.

On behalf of ICSH I would like to endorse the opening remarks by our President-elect, Dr. J. Spaander, and to thank, again, the organizing committee of CISMEL, and the Centro di Biochimica Analitica of Milan. We thank, also, all the participants and especially we thank Professor Sirtori and the Carlo Erba Foundation for making the symposium possible.

Stampa Franco Angeli Editore — Milano